PSYCHOLOGY LIBRARY EDITIONS: SPEECH AND LANGUAGE DISORDERS

Volume 6

I0131340

SPEECH AND VOICE

SPEECH AND VOICE
Their Evolution, Pathology and Therapy

LEOPOLD STEIN

Routledge
Taylor & Francis Group

LONDON AND NEW YORK

First published in 1942 by Methuen & Co. Ltd

This edition first published in 2019
by Routledge
2 Park Square, Milton Park, Abingdon, Oxon OX14 4RN

and by Routledge
52 Vanderbilt Avenue, New York, NY 10017

Routledge is an imprint of the Taylor & Francis Group, an informa business

British Library Cataloguing in Publication Data
A catalogue record for this book is available from the British Library

ISBN: 978-1-138-34553-9 (Set)
ISBN: 978-0-429-39880-3 (Set) (ebk)
ISBN: 978-1-138-35883-6 (Volume 6) (hbk)
ISBN: 978-1-138-35889-8 (Volume 6) (pbk)
ISBN: 978-0-429-43406-8 (Volume 6) (ebk)

Publisher's Note
The publisher has gone to great lengths to ensure the quality of this reprint but points out that some imperfections in the original copies may be apparent.

Disclaimer
The publisher has made every effort to trace copyright holders and would welcome correspondence from those they have been unable to trace.

SPEECH AND VOICE

THEIR EVOLUTION, PATHOLOGY
AND THERAPY

by

LEOPOLD STEIN

M.D. (VIND.)

*Formerly Director of the Speech Department of the Policlinic, Vienna
Hon. Speech Therapist to the Tavistock Clinic (The
Institute of Medical Psychology), London*

WITH A FOREWORD BY

J. R. REES, M.D.

*Medical Director of the Tavistock Clinic, London
Consulting Psychiatrist to the Army*

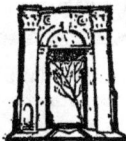

METHUEN & CO. LTD. LONDON
36 Essex Street, Strand, W.C.2

First published in 1942

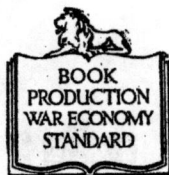

PRINTED IN GREAT BRITAIN

FOREWORD

BY J. R. REES, M.D.

It is indeed a privilege to be associated with this book, which will certainly be recognised as setting new standards in the scientific approach to speech problems.

Like every other psychiatrist who is called on to deal with neurotic and allied difficulties in children and adults, whether in peace or in war, I am frequently puzzled by the speech problems which present themselves. Much of the speech therapy of the past has been unsatisfactory because of its emphasis upon the purely mechanical aspects of the condition, while at the same time the purely psychological approach has not been sufficient to lead to satisfactory and radical treatment.

Throughout this book Dr. Stein gives us evidence of his wisdom in combining the two approaches, and by setting out the basic pathology of the various conditions he throws a flood of new light upon them.

It is fortunate, I think, that this book should appear now, during the war, when so much of our technique and methods is in the melting-pot. This work will lead to advances in this particular field of medical and educational work.

J. R. R.

May 1942.

PREFACE

"A man should never be ashamed to own he has been in the
wrong, which is but saying, in other words, that he is wiser
to-day than he was yesterday."

DEAN SWIFT
Thoughts on Various Subjects

This book has a curious history. For more than twenty years I had
been treating disorders of speech and voice and had become convinced
that the Viennese School of Speech Therapy was right in reading
the *Book of Speech*—to use George Meredith's words [1]—"by the
watchmaker's eye in luminous rings eruptive of the infinitesimal."
When I came to this country I found many excellently trained speech
therapists practising our young science with much ardour, sympathy
and—not least—intuition. The English and American textbooks
supply a considerable volume of facts, "raising in bright relief minutest
grains of evidence;" and though among them I found many that I
had previously overlooked or neglected, it seemed to me that the
collection of facts had gone ahead of the comprehending of them
within a suitable coherent unit and of their elucidation.

While still pondering how to remedy this condition, I was greatly
encouraged to set to work by Dr. Boome, Miss Baines and Mrs. Harries,
who in their book *Abnormal Speech* express the view that "the centre
of Speech Therapy is now here." I felt, however, that it would be
better not to contribute to the efforts already made by speech therapists
in this country by grafting on to existing ideas those that I had brought
with me. Convinced that theoretical knowledge in itself is of no
account unless methods of practical application can be deduced from
it, I had to find a basis on which our diagnostic and therapeutic
endeavours could be consolidated.

The right outlook can, to my mind, be attained only by realising
that the data provided by the evolution and development of Speech
and Voice are those from which we may best hope that our efforts
to understand and to help will achieve success.

This book is far from being a translation of my former articles
and books. The broad outlook of this country and its liberal but
cautious methods have shown me a better approach. My concepts
have undergone a further integration which, as will be seen in such
chapters as those on the Evolution of Speech, Dyslalia, and Stammering,
justifies, I think, this attempt to write anew on these matters. Other
chapters, as for instance, those on voice disorders, and on Rhinophonia,
are based on my former papers and books as no considerable advances
have been made recently.

I have maintained an eclectic point of view in so complex a matter
as speech and its changes, but I have not included many valuable
findings that do not seem to contribute to a solution of the *problems*

[1] *The Egoist*, Prelude.

vi

with which we are faced. To my mind eclecticism should be applied in such a way as to show that "between the most opposite beliefs there is usually something in common—something taken for granted by each ; and that this something, if not to be set down as an unquestionable verity, may yet be considered to have the highest degree of probability." [1]

This book is not and cannot be regarded as an Encyclopedia of Speech Pathology. To give it the character of a handbook would, in view of the multitude of contributions, exceed one man's powers. Nor can it supply the special knowledge that must be presupposed in order to understand one of the most complex responses of mankind. In the *Book of Human Speech* there is "a constant tendency to accumulate excess of substance, and such repleteness, obscuring the glass it holds to mankind, renders us inexact in the recognition of our individual countenances." [2]   And—to avail myself once again of Meredith's words—this is what I have learnt from the great thinkers of this country, that the *Book of Speech* needs a "powerful compression" to give us "those interminable mile-post piles of matter . . . in essence, in chosen samples, digestibility." [3]

Every effort has been made to point out the basic mechanisms of those organ systems which carry out speech-patterns. This aim, however, created a difficulty in that the concepts of speech and its deviations must naturally be based on ideas elaborated by branches of knowledge serving us as auxiliary sciences. I have tried to overcome this, and hope I have kept the golden mean in giving the essential data. If desirable details appear missing to some it is for this reason.

Some subjects have been given preference on account of their import in treatment, e.g. Stammering and Dyslalia. If some seemingly equally important items are comparatively short, it is either because we know nothing more about them or because what is known lacks, to my mind, probability, the correlation of the facts not having been cogently established. Other chapters, such as that on the evolution of language, may appear perhaps rather aphoristic or arbitrary, not because there is not enough knowledge but because to explain the data provided by sciences such as Comparative Philology would lead us too far afield. The relevant examples given are designed to induce further study with which the writer himself is profitably occupied. Books which the reader might find useful as an introduction to the specialities concerned are mentioned in the Bibliography.

I have endeavoured to do justice to the demands made of the candidates in this country for qualification in Speech Therapy. This has necessitated the frequent use of simple examples, pictures and similes. I have taken care to keep the happy medium between common parlance and scientific modes of expression. This ' Socratic method ' has been adopted because both the layman and the scientist must try to discover "which of our terms are undefined or partially defined

---

[1] Spencer, H. (1880). *First Principles*, H. M. Caldwell, New York–Boston, p. 7.

[2] Meredith, G., l.c.   [3] Ibid.

or draggled with fringes of connotation "[1] so as to reach a *common* basis of understanding.

This book may also serve as a guide for all who are concerned with child welfare and education. It is a book for the nurse, teacher, psychologist and singing master. Doctors may also find subjects in the book which should be of use in their daily practice.

This is a personal confession. Reference is therefore made only to those workers whose findings seem to support my views. Thus the Bibliography is necessarily somewhat arbitrary, for I have tried to avoid controversies which would not be compatible with our pragmatic line of thought. Therefore, eminent writers are not quoted who "tell quite a different story;" . . . "it is mine, not theirs, I am trying to tell in such wise as to render it, if I can, at least comprehensible."[2]

I am conscious that at the present stage of our knowledge my explanations can be only tentative. But having learnt from experience that my improved method of approach has enabled me to help my suffering fellow-men, I feel no hesitation in setting out my principles and practice for the consideration of all workers in this field. If they gain from my mistakes, my aim is achieved. And finally, "there is no book so bad but something good may be found in it."[3]

I should not have been able to undertake this work without the previous knowledge gained in years of collaboration with my teacher, Prof. Fröschels. If in many respects I follow my own way and directions taken from workers such as W. Meyer-Lübke, Hughlings Jackson, Alfred Adler, M. Seeman, and others, he will now understand that it is the natural and inevitable course of spiritual integration.

Substantial progress in knowledge I owe to the manifold help I have received in this country. I owe an especially great debt of gratitude to the Directors of the Institute of Medical Psychology (Tavistock Clinic), London, for having offered me the opportunity to work and to verify my ideas. Discussions with the members of the staff have contributed much to my work.

I have received much encouragement, too, from my work at the Central School of Speech Training and Dramatic Art, from Miss E. Fogerty's friendly support in my teaching and searching and her never-flagging interest, and from the friendly spirit of the Association of Teachers of Speech and Drama. Not least I feel I must express my profound thankfulness to John S. L. Gilmour. Our many discussions on questions of genetics, classification, phylogeny and epistemology have not only been a source of intellectual stimulation, but have also helped me to master the subtleties of the English language. Others, especially Mrs. T. L. Gilmour, Miss Baines, Dr. D. Murray, Mr. McNae, and Miss Bennett have helped me greatly over questions of English diction. The latter and Dr. H. Fleischhacker bestowed many pains

[1] Bloomfield, L. (1939). *Linguistic Aspects of Science*, The University of Chicago Press, Chicago, p. 46.

[2] Lloyd Morgan, C. (1929). *Mind at the Crossways*, Williams & Norgate, London, p. 94.

[3] *John O'London* (no date). *Treasure Trove*, George Newnes Ltd., London, p. 28.

upon discussing the whole subject with me.   I wish to thank Mr. C. Joliffe for the diagram on p. 181.

I should like also to pay tribute to Messrs. Methuen & Co. for publishing the book in these troublous days.

Many friends who have supported and helped me in this work prefer not to be acknowledged publicly.   One who has been working for many years in this sense is my faithful wife, who in good and evil days, in joy and sorrow, has sacrificed all her personal interests unmurmuringly on my behalf.   To her I owe my greatest debt.

L. STEIN

KEW, *July* 1942

CONTENTS

CHAPTER I

GENERAL PRINCIPLES

For many thousands of years men have been living together in communities. A community, by its very nature, implies the existence within itself of certain links which connect the individual members with one another. One of the most outstanding of these links is communication by means of sounds, known as 'language' or 'speech.'

The terms 'language' and 'speech' are so familiar that the ordinary man may think it unnecessary to give them any deeper consideration. He may assume that they are part of the make-up of every normal person, here for him to use, just as he does any other tool; and he attributes to them certain qualities such as goodness, badness, beauty, and so forth.

However, when he finds his tool proving inefficient, he is faced with the necessity of seeking some means by which he can improve it. During this process he may awaken to the fact that language *is* a tool, a tool which needs handling, and that this necessitates some knowledge of its structure. Take, for example, the man who tries to make himself understood in a foreign land. He may, because of this experience, ask himself, "What is language? What is speech? What is articulation?" These questions do not then seem to him so superfluous as they did before he encountered this difficulty in his own life.

He may then begin to observe aspects of language which until then he had taken for granted. He learns to distinguish sounds, letters, intonation, and so forth. Having separated them and named them he assumes at last that he has grasped the nature of his tool. But to his astonishment he finds still that he cannot handle it as he would or use it to accomplish his ends.

This experience may lead him to the conclusion that knowledge based only upon outward observation does not gain for him an understanding of the real nature of the thing itself. To take an example: he who merely sees the various parts of a locomotive—the wheels, axles, etc.—cannot be said to have a knowledge of the locomotive itself until he recognises some relation between all its different parts. Put into scientific language : "The ordering of the mass of experience into a special kind of structure or system is at once the principal aim of thought and the measure of its advance." [1]

Desiring in this work to avoid any pitfalls in clipping together the given sense data, let us not take anything for granted but begin on the very simplest level of thought and try to learn as many facts as possible, and to arrange them in an orderly manner. How can this be done ?

In our endeavour to find a simple basis from which to start, we must look for that which lies *behind* the vague and hazy idea which is

[1] Blanshard, B. (1939). *The Nature of Thought*, Allen & Unwin, London, i, p. 67.

I

presented to our thought by the word ' speech.' Having done this,
what do we find ? Beings like ourselves who act and behave in certain
ways and in so doing exhibit certain phenomena which can be perceived
by the senses of sight and hearing.

What then could be simpler than to examine the conditions under
which these phenomena arise ? Since we are convinced that the
phenomena in question have some sort of significance and we have
started to find a method by which they can be handled, we shall be
forced to submit the interpretation which we give to them to some
test as to its usefulness or practicability. " A true scientific theory
merely means a successful working hypothesis. It is highly probable
that all scientific theories are wrong. Those that we accept are variable
within our present limits of observation. Truth then, in science, is a
pragmatic affair. - A good scientific theory accounts for known facts
and enables us to predict new ones, which are then verified by observation. . . ." [1]

" This atmosphere of provisional hypothesis and practically veri-
fiable statements constitutes what has been called the ' homely air '
of science, and is one of its great charms. Science has adopted the
pragmatic criterion of truth, namely, success, and as a result science
has been successful." [2]

Here we must make clear what it is that characterises a tool as
useful or successful.

The history of the development of mankind shows us that at each
stage man has been faced with the necessity of mastering the circumstances in which he has found himself, in other words, of adapting
himself to his environment. Step by step, sometimes partly by what
seemed to be mere chance, he has discovered means for accomplishing
this task, and has rendered these means more effective by detecting
new and better methods. ·

The familiar things of everyday life, such as pens, motor-cars, or
spoons, are what they are because of a gradual process of development.
We are justified then in regarding tools and machines as mere extensions
or developments of the handling organs of those who have made them.
Can we not also infer that their mode of working is similar ? This is
the more likely as, when closely examined, new phenomena usually
prove not to be complete innovations but a further evolution of something already existing.

When we examine these familiar objects carefully, we discover a
complex mass of impressions (phenomena) with which our minds are
quite unable to deal. We instinctively wish to examine something
simple enough to be comprehensible. For example, some one interested in motor-cars naturally wants to understand its engine.
His teacher, therefore, will introduce him first to a less complicated
type of engine ; thus the process of simplification has been accomplished.

How can we apply this method in attempting to establish a theory
of speech and its variations ?

The answer is that we must look to nature. We must see how

[1] Sullivan, J. W. N. (1938). *Limitations of Science*, Pelican Books, p. 206.
[2] Ibid., pp. 212–13.

nature has built up the process of speech, and this will necessitate investigation in a new direction. Our investigations are therefore given a new orientation. " The aim of a scientific theory is to present a system of propositions logically connected, which system must be an expression and a classification of natural laws." [1]

We should remember, however, that a ' natural law ' is not something in itself, but only the *symbol* or outward expression of the nature of reality, the actual structure of things.

" We are no longer required to believe that our response to beauty, or the mystic's sense of communion with God, have no objective counterpart. It is perfectly possible that they are, what they have so often been taken to be, clues to the nature of reality. Thus our various experiences are put on a more equal footing, as it were. Our religious aspirations, our perceptions of beauty, may not be the essentially illusory phenomena they were supposed to be. In this new scientific universe even mystics have a right to exist." [2] All sciences dealing with speech are legitimately concerned, therefore, with such things as beauty, ease of expression, and so forth, and even mystical abstractions such as the feeling of ' grace ' may play their part.

[1] Lauwerys, J. A. (1938). " Scientific Instruments," *Proceedings of the Aristotelian Society*, 38, p. 236.
[2] Sullivan (1939), pp. 186–7.

CHAPTER II

DEVELOPMENT AND EVOLUTION

Fortunately the procedure employed by the scientists who have been elucidating the general principles of development provides us with what we need when confining our investigations to language and speech. This is a great help, since speech and voice pathology is still at a comparatively early stage of development. Material from which the framework of this science may be constructed has still to be collected.

Since language and speech are so essential a part of human behaviour let us try to understand how this has come about. The view is no longer held that the world has become what it is by an instantaneous act of creation, but that it has grown to its present state through aeons of time.

Mankind has always been puzzled by the phenomenon of growth —the gradual changing of a seed into a plant, of a child into a man. The original belief was that the completed flower existed from the beginning within the seed from which it unfolded, impelled by some mysterious power. From this belief were developed by analogy the expressions ' development ' and ' evolution.' These terms, now commonly in use, are Latin equivalents of our words unroll, unfurl, unfold.

This primary meaning of the words was held until the eighteenth century. Only then did the epigeneticists replace this by the assumption that primary tissues in the egg gradually adopted the form and structure seen later in the individual. This doctrine was then given the scientific name ' evolution.'

Lamarck asked himself how it was that these tissues changed into the particular forms and structures observable in any given individual. His answer was that it was due to a gradual transformation forced upon the individual, who during the course of his life was compelled to adapt his functions to differing surroundings. The following quotation shows to what extent biologists have been able to observe this process : " Under the microscope the set of genes—the chromosomes of the egg—are seen to go promptly to work. They suck up a quantity of material from the surrounding cytoplasm, becoming balloon-like. They transform this chemically, then give it off again into the cell body, visibly changed into something new. Diverse new substances thus formed move into different regions of the egg. By cell division some of the newly manufactured substances are passed into one cell, others into another. Thus the cells become diverse ; the different structures of the body are being made. This is repeated in each cell generation, the chromosomes by interaction with the cytoplasm changing the substance of the cells, until finally nerve, muscle, bone, gland and other tissues result." [1]

[1] Jennings, H. S. (no date). *Prometheus*, Kegan Paul, London, pp. 37–8.

4

In the course of time the modified habits and the effector organs were handed on to the offspring, that is, they were 'inherited.' This theory has been further developed by Wallace, Darwin, Lyell, Goethe, Haeckel, and others, and has led to the conception that the structures and functions have in some degree been handed down to successions of living beings. We are then able to detect a common fundamental pattern of structure, function, habit, and so on, which has been modified, specialised, and differentiated in various directions.

The fundamental laws governing this process have been put in general terms by Herbert Spencer. According to him the pattern of function in living beings can be accounted for by the principles observed in the inter-relation of the ultimate constituents of the world.

Haeckel has combined observations on the origin of the individual and inferences as to the origin of the race in his famous statement, that " the series of forms through which the individual organism passes during its progress from the egg-cell to its fully developed state is a brief compressed reproduction of the long series of forms through which the animal ancestors of that organism (or the ancestral form of its species) have passed from the earliest periods of so-called organic creation down to the present time." In brief terms, the development of the individual is a recapitulation of that of the race.

This bipartition of the process of descent into (1) the growth of the individual (ontogeny),[1] and (2) the origin of the ancestry (phylogeny),[2] enforced the use of the term ' development ' for the former and ' evolution ' for the latter.

We cannot, however, fail to realise that the aggregates of particles representing ' things ' manifest qualities which are not found in the individual particles. The knowledge has given rise to the theory of ' *emergent* evolution,' which states that " at various stages of material complexity, radically new properties emerge. According to this theory both Life and Mind are emergent properties of certain material aggregates. A complete knowledge of the constituents of these aggregates would not enable us to predict that, in combination, they would manifest the properties of life or mind." [3]

Our method of approach to our subject will now be based on the conception that " Body and Mind, man, is the outcome of his ancestry, and it is along that line that investigation appears to hold out the greatest promise of ultimate success," [4] and that " the selves mount upon the grand staircase of history " (Lord Acton).

In making the theory of evolution the basis of our investigations concerning speech and its variations, we are well aware that many links in the chain of development of human speech are missing. There is still much work to be done by biologists, psychologists, speech therapists and philologists, but the writer hopes to show in this work *which* links are missing and to suggest possible ways of supplying them.

The need of deriving the observable variations of speech from its

[1] *On* ' the being.'   [2] = *phylon*, ' race, tribe, kind.'
[3] Sullivan, l.c., p. 136.
[4] Douglas, A. C. (1932). *The Physical Mechanism of the Human Mind*, E. & S. Livingstone, Edinburgh, pp. 11-12.

development has apparently been felt by most of the writers on the subject since they preface their observations on disorders of speech and voice by a survey of normal speech development. We do not, however, feel that the connection between this development and the pathological facts has been made sufficiently clear.

In the following chapters we shall therefore attempt to use the evolutionary principles which we have thus briefly outlined, in explaining the structure of language in its variations.

NERVOUS FUNCTIONS

The nerve cell.—Having shown in the previous chapter that it is necessary to begin our investigations by always dealing with the simplest aspect of any phenomena, let us here take the cell as our ultimate structural unit. We shall not go into details concerning its principles, constituents, or properties, all of which are explained at length in the textbooks on anatomy and physiology. (See Bibliography.)

The cell manifests a simple but efficient form of reaction, the process by which an organism adapts itself to the changes in its environment.

When the organism, through propagation of its cells, grows more complex, it proves useful to subordinate the activities of its individual cells to the maintenance of the whole organism. As part of this process some cells are evolved for special purposes and acquire the function of regulating the relationship between individual parts and in bringing about their co-operation in the service of the whole organism.

Muscles were evolved before either nerves or sense organs. When muscles are stimulated to contraction through the influence of the nerves connected with them, they move the bones which with their connecting joints constitute the framework of the body.

The central organisation is provided by the nervous system, which co-ordinates the functions of the various systems of the body. Its work can be compared to that of the central office in a big establishment composed of many different departments all of which, working harmoniously together, are essential to the successful functioning of the whole.

The nervous system, to carry out its task efficiently, developed through differentiation three distinct types of nerves: (1) those possessing the power of receiving incoming messages; (2) those able to transmit what is received; and (3) those capable of carrying out the instructions which have been transmitted. They are called afferent, connector, and efferent neurons respectively.

This differentiation takes place as soon as in the metazoa certain cells have specialised in taking over certain activities of the unicellular organism, such as movement or secretion. All of these specialised cells, such as muscular cells, glandular cells, etc., possess a definite structure which enables them to carry out their particular task efficiently.

The nervous system is the fundamental unit with which we have to deal in our investigations into language and speech, as it is this system which governs the actions of the whole body. In describing the phenomena which it exhibits, we shall follow the theory of evolution, regarding it not as something already existing, but as something in the process of becoming.

A nerve unit consists of a cell with various branches. The nerve cells are grey and are usually gathered together in masses called ganglia. The grey matter of the nervous system consists of such aggregated cells. Bundles of nerves (axons) form the white matter. The nerve branches take on a different appearance as soon as they leave the body of the cell. One of these branches, the axon, is a fine thread of, at times, considerable length. It can be compared to a wire which, to prevent the electric current from escaping, has been surrounded by a sheath. The axon divides into many branches which terminate in various organs. Other ramifications resembling trees are called dendrites; these do not separate from the grey matter of the central nervous system, but connect the nerve cells with each other. The unit which consists of the body of the cell, the axon, and the dendrites, is named the neuron.

Two neurons can come into contact within the grey matter of the nervous system. The axon belonging to each neuron splits up and its branches touch the dendrites of the other neuron or its cell. This connection through contact is called synapse.

Reflex arc.—Afferent nerves, connector nerves, and efferent nerves are arranged in such a way as to bring about a response to incoming stimuli independently of voluntary control. The organic basis of this *reflex action* is the *reflex arc*. To illustrate what we mean by ' reflex action ' let us take the following simple example : a frog whose brain (' seat of consciousness ') has been separated from the spinal cord scratches himself if some sulphuric acid is spilt on him ; or if you put a fly in his mouth he will eat it, but should you only show him the fly, he will make no attempt to reach it.

These examples, simple as they appear, deserve further consideration. Though carried out by an elementary mechanism, these actions are not of a simple nature, for they show well-designed ' patterns,' viz. those of effectively removing a stimulus which causes pain or of swallowing something desirable.

Following along the path indicated by the theory of evolution, we must assume that the previous experience of the ancestors of the frog has impressed upon this fundamental unit of nerve function the particular action we have seen. This shows us a process which is going on in evolutionary time, as well as developmental time.

" The passage of a reaction along a nerve-path has the effect of sensitising that nerve-path (i.e. of endowing it with increased conductivity) to that particular reaction." This " sensitisation, or ' canalisation,' of a nerve-path by any specific stimulus—representing, as it does, a molecular modification—is in reality an incipient *structural* change." [1] Thus the outstanding feature of the nervous system is its response to changes of environment and its power of adapting the whole organism to them. The reactions of the nervous system show

[1] Douglas, l.c., pp. 27 and 37.

us a definite pattern, growing more and more complex as the individual reaches higher and higher levels of development.

Such structural and functional patterns are to a great extent inherited. The structure of any action, therefore, should always be regarded in the light of the many patterns of adaptation which have been impressed on its nervous mechanism at previous levels of evolution and development. Every action constitutes a hierarchy of patterns.

The spinal cord.—The nerves receiving messages from the outside world (afferent nerves), the nerves transmitting those stimuli (connector nerves), and those stimulating the effector organs (efferent nerves), are in higher animals bundled together in what is called the spinal cord.

The spinal bulb (Medulla oblongata).—The Medulla oblongata is, as its name indicates, the upper extension of the spinal cord. Here arise those nerves especially concerned with swallowing, breathing, the secretion of saliva, the movements of the heart, and dilatation and contraction of the blood vessels. In addition the bulb contains the pathways through which external stimuli can reach higher cerebral parts, and through which the impulses from those parts are conveyed to the efferent nerves and the effector organs.

Mind.—Man, when subjected to sensory stimulation, such as in tickling, shuddering, sneezing, coughing, laughing, and sucking in infancy, exhibits reflexes similar to those which occur in the frog. All these movements appear *almost* involuntary and beyond his control. If a fly settles on the nose of a sleeper, he brushes it away with a well-aimed movement of the hand. This is an example of automatic control, the sleeper being, it is assumed, unaware of the occurrence.

During consciousness such movements can be performed deliberately and with some awareness of them, or be left unperformed. A mystical being, the 'mind' or 'soul' has been assumed to be the controlling factor in such phenomena.

For centuries questions as to the genesis and the substantiality of mind have exercised the thoughts of men. But in accordance with our fundamental concept nothing need be said in answer to them. The same process may present itself in two aspects according to our point of vantage. This and the terminology used in an attempt to describe the sets of life-patterns in their gradations make them appear then as psychological or physiological patterns. In order to preserve the unity of the underlying acting whole we may at times find it helpful to use the behaviouristic method of approach.

The doctrine of Behaviourism, as expounded especially by Watson,[1] refuses to have any dealings with "introspectively observable facts." . . . "It refrains from describing or explaining emotions, desires, fantasy, thoughts, memory, etc. The psychologist must rely upon data of one kind only, the data or facts obtained by observing the movements and various bodily changes exhibited by human and other organisms."[2]

[1] Watson, J. B. and McDougall, W. (1928). *The Battle of Behaviourism*, Kegan Paul, London.
[2] McDougall, ibid., p. 52.

" Sane Behaviourists " combine those data with all the conclusions arrived at by means of introspection, thus directing attention from facts of consciousness to facts of *conduct.*

Instinct.—With a view to pursuing the hierarchy of action-patterns we will now modify our last example. Suppose we are talking to a friend who suddenly flicks away a wasp from his nose. We observe he uses the same kind of action as was exhibited by the sleeping man. Now, however, we can ask him why he acted in this way, and he naturally answers : " I felt something stinging me, and I instinctively put my hand up to remove it. I did not think about what I was doing."

We would doubtless agree, and we may therefore conclude that (1) man is able to act in response to external stimuli ; (2) no concentration on the particular action is necessary; (3) he is introspectively aware of a certain feeling ; (4) this precedes cognition.

How are these data to be accounted for ? The action itself possesses a striking similarity to that of the frog and of the sleeper. From this we infer that it is based on that evolutionary pattern. Such reflex actions, as far as they are " inherited habits, characterised by a high degree of sensitisation in their nerve-circuits, as evidenced by the promptitude and invariability of the response," are termed instincts.[1]

Sympathetic nervous system.—Our description of the symptoms was not quite exact. We might have noticed that (5) the man became pale, that his pupils had dilated, and that his pulse had quickened ; (6) on being questioned he would declare that he had heart palpitation and other vague bodily feelings of uneasiness, even that he was on the point of fainting.

But his report seems to indicate that there is more in this than meets the eye. ' Life ' itself was in danger. To maintain the life of a more specialised and differentiated organism organs have been developed—such as the intestines, heart, blood vessels, lungs, and glands —designed to effect metabolism. Their functions are controlled from a nerve-system constituting the oldest nerve-paths, viz. the *sympathetic* or *autonomic nervous system.* The autonomic nerves interact with the spinal nerves on the reflex principle already mentioned. In our example we saw how they unite in action to re-establish equilibrium. The processes going on in the sympathetic nervous system are highly canalised, and therefore hardly under our conscious control. This absence of conscious control is characteristic of reflex actions, instincts, and emotions.

Endocrine system.—In recalling instances of blushing, feeble pulse, sweating, etc., which have occurred in other subjects under observation, we may assume that these primitive reflex processes are governed by some as yet undiscovered influences. In fact they encroach upon the primary factors of life, viz. the activities of the *endocrine glands.*

The endocrine system consists of several glands producing substances (hormones) which get into the blood, and affect the metabolism of the body in every respect.

Emotion.—Let us revert to the man who was stung by the wasp.

[1] Douglas, l.c., p. 128.

He said he ' felt ' something ; that is the vital point. His experience was certainly a vivid one, but on the other hand, he found it difficult to give it a satisfactory description. We can discriminate between two types of feeling—pleasure and displeasure. Both types appear as an ' attack ' on those experiencing them, and not as an action which they themselves have taken.

The idea that we are in some way dominated by agencies which at the time we cannot discern, is expressed in common parlance by the verb ' to affect,' derived from the Latin *facere*, ' to do,' and *ad*, ' to.' The fact that some potentialities of movement are aroused is implied in the word ' emotion.' Its meaning originates from the Latin *movere*, ' to move,' and *e*, ' out of.'

Pleasure " may range from lukewarm appreciation to voluptuous delight ; desire or will may range from comparative indifference to intense longing, or to blind and impulsive action." Displeasure is felt as anger or frustration which " may pass from mild resentment to uncontrollable rage."

" Those stimuli which evoke the more active reactions upon which these sensations depend show a tendency to set in motion not only the voluntary muscular mechanism, but to overflow, as it were, into the muscular glandular department of organic response presided over by the sympathetic. We have seen stimulation of the lachrymal glands associated with frustration ; stimulation of the sweat glands may be associated with fear ; and stimulation of the suprarenal glands (resulting in rise of blood-pressure) is characteristic of anger, and so on."[1] Thus certain primitive behavioural patterns, such as reflexes, instincts, and emotions are not of a differing kind, but in reality one and the same action described in terms of physiology, biology, and/or psychology.

Interbrain.—The requirements of life give rise to further growth of the cell mass in the primitive nervous system and to definite structures capable of better adjustment. The next anatomical structures to emerge are the *thalamus* and the *hypothalamus*. The former acts as a higher reflex centre receiving incoming stimuli from all the sense organs.

This stage of development extends back as far as the evolutionary level of the fish. The long period throughout which the reflexes have worked explains why, according to Cannon, " emotional expression is a complex highly organised reflex act which differs from cortical activity in being far more uniform and stereotyped in character."

There is much evidence to show that " the sympathetic nervous system is under the control of the hypothalamus (diencephalon)."[2] This accounts for the visceral (vegetative) components in emotional reactions. Injuries to the interbrain often produce uncontrollable laughing or weeping.[3]

The mid brain (*mesencephalon*).—Pursuing the example of our friend who was stung, we reached the stage where he had removed the wasp. The time has come to investigate this activity in greater detail. We

---

[1] Douglas, l.c., p. 93.
[2] Wright, S. (1934). *Applied Physiology*, Oxford University Press, p. 86.
[3] Woodworth, R. S. (1935). *Psychology*, Methuen, London, p. 348.

can detect that it is executed with a certain tension in the muscles of the arm, while the whole body assumes a definite posture. What is it that influences the motor components of this process ? The counterpart of the thalamic sensory centre is played by a phylogenetically old aggregate of motor cells, the *strio-pallidar system*. It consists of various nuclei a description of which would lead us too far afield.

These grey nuclei are connected by white pathways conducting the afferent impulses from the thalamus exclusively. The motor impulses are sent out by the globus pallidus. They reach first the nuclei underneath the thalamus, thence they descend to the spinal cord and finally reach the efferent nerves and the effector organs.[1]

This system is known as the ' extrapyramidal tracts ' in contradistinction to other motor pathways which take their course through two swellings of the spinal bulb, the ' pyramids,' and which are therefore called the ' pyramidal tracts.'

Though the anatomical and physiological views on this system are still a.matter of much controversy, it seems highly probable that the function of the corpus striatum is to supply " a steady and appropriate basis for the final communal path, which controls the tonus and regulates the neuro-muscular rhythm." [2] " Foerster regards the globus pallidus as a centre for movements of reaction and expression, and as playing an important rôle in conducting cortical impulses concerned in voluntary movement, evoking and strengthening synergic movements and co-operating in movements of succession. In addition, it inhibits the reflex activity of lower centres, particularly certain postural reflexes mediated by the cerebellum, and a hypothetical hypothalamic centre concerned in plastic tonus." [3] The latter will be dealt with presently.

Tonus.—There is no living organism possessing a nervous and muscular system which does not exhibit under all circumstances a certain tension of the muscles.

At first any stimulus passing through the reflex system of the spinal cord causes a contraction of the muscles. The influences from the midbrain delineated above are superimposed on this mechanism. " An algebraic summation of all these conflicting influences takes place ; the anterior horn cell responds accordingly controlling in that way the degree of activity of its related muscle fibres, and consequently the posture of the part. . . . Posture is the basis of movement ; all movements start and end in a posture." [4] " The observations of the tonus of skeletal muscle in the mammal, therefore, go to show that the phenomenon is in skeletal muscle nothing more nor less than postural contraction." [5] Brain and Strauss add : " The tonus present in any muscle at any time forms part of a complete postural pattern of the whole body. Apart from volition, the body adopts by means of highly complicated systems of chained reflexes the posture most suited to its

[1] Wright, l.c., pp. 91–2.
[2] Kinnier Wilson (1924). *Arch. f. Neurol. and Psychiat.*, xi, p. 385.
[3] Brain, W. R. and Strauss, E. B. *Recent Advances in Neurology*, Churchill, London, pp. 198–9.
[4] Wright, l.c., p. 71.　　　　[5] Sherrington, C. S. (1915). *Brain*, **38**, p. 191.

actual needs. If this is true, characteristic postures have their bio-logical meanings ; . . . tonus is a beautifully graded service of pro-prioceptive reflexes, continuously and unconsciously playing its part in our every motor act. By its remarkable specificity it moulds our individual muscles ; by its universality it controls our postures." [1] Thus tension shows an evolutionary stratification corresponding to the layers already described.

The cerebrum.—Let us now further modify our example. Suppose our friend has seen the wasp approaching. By combining introspection with observation he develops awareness of the fact (which in the previous example he did not possess at the moment of action). He may in that case either (1) frighten the wasp away, or (2) ignore it. Posture and form of action are changed in tone (tension) and aim (judgment). Emotional expression is present but has weakened and changed in some way.

What at first strikes us is that activity and emotion linked together have receded into the background, whereas ' thought ' has emerged.

Numerous experiments and pathological facts, as well as develop-mental and evolutionary data, have made it clear that this is due to the " latest addition to the complexities of the nervous system," [2] viz. the cerebrum.

" Previous to the development of the cerebrum, the muscular reactions of the organism were dictated by the inherited experience of the species. The paucity of nerve-paths in the simpler organisms is responsible for unvarying reaction, and this gives place, with the march of neural evolution, to behaviour which becomes more and more variable. But even in the thalamic animal reflex-paths are com-paratively few and well worn, and its reactions, as compared with the cerebral animal, are relatively stereotyped and calculable. The organic significance of the cerebrum is that its paths have not been indelibly stamped by heredity into a mechanism functioning with pre-ordained inevitability. It is still a mechanism, and completely reflex in action, but so exquisitely contrived that the muscular reactions of the organism become, in increasing measure, modified by the past experience of the individual. The benefit to the organism of this development, the gain in its power of adaptability to environment, and therefore of its chance of survival, are obvious.[3] . . . The cerebrum may therefore be regarded, not as a modification necessitated by increase of sensory perception, but as primarily an adventitious adjunct —an elaboration of the pre-existing main centre of co-ordination, the thalamus, which gradually comes to occupy a subordinate position in its base. From this starting-point the cerebrum has gradually evolved into a highly complex organic instrument, undertaking, with increasing efficiency, the control and co-ordination of a receptor and an effector mechanism which in lower animals can function perfectly well without it. The outcome of this development is to provide reflex reactions with a choice of routes ; they may pass from the receptor organ across the primeval beaten tracks directly to the appropriate effector

[1] Brain and Strauss, l.c., pp. 115–18.
[2] Douglas, l.c., p. 64.   [3] Ibid.

organs, or they may arrive at the same destination via the more recently established cerebral loop-line.

" This conception of cerebral structure, that it consists of a highly organised and complex system of such loop-lines, justified as it is by the facts of evolution, receives also striking support from physiological experiment." [1]

Voluntary movements.—In our last example we have got one step farther in the hierarchy of patterns. It suggests that the contradiction voluntary-involuntary is a mere verbal one. In reality all movements of whatever kind are superimposed on lower, i.e. older patterns, which therefore supply an efficient postural activity. " We are not aware of the actual muscles involved in any movement ; we simply notice the end result, which is displacement of joints or segments of the body in a certain direction and to a certain extent. Many of the component parts of a ' voluntary ' movement are entirely outside consciousness, and have little of a voluntary character about them." [2] What distinguishes voluntary movements from emotional ones is simply and solely the choice of routes.

Our friend's ultimate intention is to avert the imminent danger which threatens him. He may, to achieve this, adopt different attitudes, (1) a fugitive one, or (2) an aggressive one. It is clear that both these attitudes may produce different postures, and that the ways and forms of action may differ too. All of them are based on well-established sets of adjusting actions. This being the case, movements should be described only as being more or less voluntary or more or less automatic. How this is to be understood will be explained in the chapter on the general principles in the evolution of the nervous system. [3]

Prevalence of one cerebral hemisphere.—The cerebrum is divided by a median fissure into two ' hemispheres.' They appear to be equal in form, dimension, and structure. Activities are directed from either hemisphere, but we have reason to believe that one of them has been given precedence in the carrying out of an action, so that, e.g., one of our hands as a rule possesses greater skill than the other.

This is what we understand by handedness. Right- or left-handedness seems to be largely inherited. As right-handedness is practically the rule in human beings, left-handedness is sometimes regarded as an inferiority. We cannot, however, accept this somewhat superstitious view.

Effort.—Let us now consider what would happen if the man threatened by the wasp were prevented from taking or preparing to take action, because we were holding his hands. He would instinctively make an effort. We are at once made aware of an increase of energy in the muscles of his arm, opposing the resistance applied by ours. This energy, in its primary, pure and free condition, we have

---

[1] Douglas, l.c., pp. 65–6. [2] Wright, l.c., pp. 76–8.
[3] The author is well aware of the intricacies of this subject. But its importance for the understanding of deviating tonicity in stammering renders it necessary to give at least a brief account of the structure of tonus. For full and detailed explanations the reader is referred to the textbooks.

already met in the simple spinal reflexes, and also in those super-imposed by the loop going through the striatal system. (It re-appears in the pathological condition of Parkinsonism, in which the striatal system gains the upper hand.)

But when we speak of ' energy,' ' force,' ' strength,' we are actually naming an abstraction which we have deduced from our observations, for we recognise it only through reactions of a particular kind, such as grinding the teeth, frowning, pursing the lips, and many gestures which remind us strongly of primitive evolutionary traits.

We may therefore infer that the conscious effort does not imply that strength is sent from the cortex into the muscles ; on the contrary, it means that a more primitive pattern of action which we have met with several times has gained control.

Attention.—Our considerations lead us easily to other psychological terms.

Efforts and actions will be prepared as long as there is awareness of the danger, in other words, as long as ' attention ' is drawn to it.

It is obvious that ' attention ' is a mere implication of what we have already seen. This is indicated by the word itself, which is derived from the Latin *ad,* ' to,' and *tendere,* ' to stretch,' which again is allied to *tenere,* ' to hold.'

Attention is thus the activity of holding a motor and sensory adjustment, which itself arose in evolutionary time.

It does not therefore surprise us to find at this juncture that terms referring to the concept of tightening and straining, such as *tension, tense,* and *tensive,* are derived from the same stem as *attention.*

Interest.—If our friend sees a flying insect of some as yet undefined configuration approaching, he shows his ' interest.' The clearer his perception becomes, the more his interest grows, and vice versa. The behaviourist would easily recognise it, because the attitude would change in the sense described.

Interest then, physiologically expressed, is merely a measure of the capacity of the incoming stimulus to arouse the attention-reflex, and varies with that capacity, and with the intensity of the consequent cortical reaction.[1]

Recognition.—If this experience repeats itself several times, the approaching insect will be ' recognised ' more quickly by our friend, and his readiness to respond adequately will grow. This is due to sensitisation (see p. 7). But it must be borne in mind that what has been canalised comprises the *whole* of the previously modified reflex.[2]

Thus in recognition the perceptive and the motor parts of the reflex arc are equally concerned.

Practice.—Someone who lives under the conditions described will also become ' practised ' or acquire ' skill ' in avoiding or killing wasps. It is obvious why these two terms are either used promiscuously or to enhance their mutual significance. Everyday life has taught people that by repetition they can on the one hand discern the units of perception more easily, and on the other hand respond (accomplish the

[1] Douglas, l.c., pp. 88–9.   [2] Ibid., p. 91.

necessary aim) more efficiently, that is to say, "there is no conscious effort for each of the distinct movements which go to form the complex whole. There is, however, a controlling receptor stimulus for each separate link in the effector chain. As we walk, for instance, each step we take gives rise to impulses from the kineaesthetic receptors, and these impulses, passing through the spinal cord to the motor-neurones, set in action the next step. All automatic, or semi-automatic, series of co-ordinated muscular movements depend for their perfect execution upon this parallel accompaniment of receptor impulses from the organs of locomotion." [1]

If our friend lives in a district swarming with wasps his actions will finally become 'habit'; this is the result of "sensitisation, by functional repetition, of the neural paths in question, and the degree of constancy in the response varies with the degree of that sensitisation." [2]

Terms such as practice, skill, recognition, memory, and learning refer to this process.

To continue with our example, suppose our friend hears a buzzing noise, produced by the alternating currents of his wireless set, he would be reminded to be on his guard against a possible attack by a wasp.

He could not do so without memory. This is simply the expression of the fact that previous reflex processes aroused by the visual perception of a wasp have become so well canalised that the 'channell' through which the original function ran is now so deep that actions produced by other stimuli, especially such as are similar to those accompanying the original process, can easily slip into it. [3]

Image.—The sensory phenomena implied in such attitudes are called 'images.' The word expresses the same idea as that contained in the word 'picture,' except that we do not actually see the object but perceive it more or less vividly in our mind.

Intelligence.—The mental activities of thinking, judging, and knowing, generally included under the category of 'intelligence,' are the most highly developed and relatively recent acquisitions of man. The word 'intelligence' is composed of the Latin words *inter*, 'between,' and *legere*, 'to choose.' The connotation derived from the concrete meaning of the original constituents fits well into our present knowledge. It means simply the process of choosing between various possible activities. How has this power of choice arisen, and how does it handle a given situation? There can be no doubt that it was and is biologically determined by the necessity of adjusting those more instinctive or emotional forms of action which developed when lower cerebral levels were still dominant, to peculiar conditions found in man's further endeavours to extend his mastery of the surround. The interaction between subcortical levels and the newly developed cortex has brought about a more effective attitude. The primary step towards this goal is "stopping to think," i.e. "the inhibition or arrest of the natural impulse to react at once." [4] Expressed in

[1] Douglas, l.c., p. 53.   [2] Ibid., p. 128. See also p. 7.
[3] Cf. ibid., pp. 94, 104.
[4] Schiller, F. C. (1929). *Logic for Use*, Bell & Sons, London, p. 198.

physiological terms, thinking is the result of a most complex inter-action between numerous reflexes. As a corollary it follows that thinking may take its course more or less without motion or speech, according to the extent to which impulsive movements with all their implications, such as tonicity, posture, form, and so on, are checked or modified. It may ultimately manifest itself in action, which, however, varies in conformity with the effectiveness and modes of the processes just mentioned. (See also Conditioned Reflexes, p. 17.)

Thought and action are, therefore, essentially *one whole*, a fact which, though almost a truism, the speech therapist will do well to bear in mind when dealing with the readjustment of certain modes and forms of speech action.

" The general theory that intelligence has evolved fits in well enough, however, with actual observations. It is generally true that the physically simplest organisms have also the most rudimentary forms of intelligence. Indeed, if we define intelligent behaviour as successful adaptation to new conditions, then we must conclude that large groups of organisms are without intelligence. The moth which flutters towards a candle flame is responding reflexly to a stimulus; it is not displaying intelligence. These tropisms, as they are called, which cause an organism to behave in an invariable way without any regard to its personal advantage, cannot be classed as intelligent, although in the creature's normal environment they may be of advantage to it. The same may be said of reflex actions, such as coughing, blinking, sneezing. Such reactions may be of advantage to their possessor, but they are not intelligent. It is characteristic of all these reactions that they are completely rigid and invariable. Instincts belong to a higher level of development, and although they can manifest a great degree of fixity they are, in the higher organisms, much more variable." [1]

. . . " We see that the question of the Evolution of Intelligence bristles with unsolved problems. We are not yet clear as to whether certain types of behaviour are to be classed as intelligent, nor can we draw any clear line of demarcation between the conscious and the non-conscious. The connection between physical structure and mental characteristics is still very largely hypothetical ; and we do not know whether consciousness arises only at a certain stage of complexity or whether it must be postulated of all living matter—or even of all matter. Thus the theory of evolution, though it can tell us a great deal about the development of our bodies, can tell us very little about the development of our minds. It may be that the structure of our minds is completely conditioned by the structure of our nervous systems, but researches on the nervous system, at present, throw practically no light on our mental processes. For the understanding of these we have to appeal to different methods." [2]

The processes of feeling, willing and thinking, in themselves ultimate introspective data, have already been elucidated by way of analogy, or rather by translating the neuro-physiological aspect into the psychological. It now remains to show—again by analogy and trans-lation—in what manner stabilised functions of old-standing come to

[1] Sullivan, l.c., p. 132.　　　　[2] Ibid., p. 140.

form the nucleus of newly emerging action patterns, generally referred to by terms, such as, learning and symbolisation.

Conditioned reflexes.—Here we touch the pith of the matter, viz. how stimuli other than the original ones can produce the same effects. This problem has been investigated with much care by Pavlov, the Russian physiologist. It is well known that the flow of saliva in dogs as well as in man is a reflex response caused by the stimulus of the sight of food. In one of his fundamental experiments a dog's salivary gland was connected with a tube through which the saliva could be secured and measured.

Whenever the hungry dog was shown his food an electric bell was rung. After several repetitions of this procedure, an increase of saliva flow could be observed when the bell was rung, though no food was visible. Thus the natural reflex of salivation had developed into a *conditioned reflex* which could be trained and modified in many ways. Conditioned reflexes can be graded and differentiated by using more and more varied stimuli, e.g. bells of a particular sound, pitch, etc. ' Learning ' can easily be explained on this basis.

The improved efficiency and speed of saliva production after the application of formerly concomitant stimuli need not be explained in detail, as they are obviously due to canalisation.

" In the learning of a performance, the action pattern is at first a mere framework—an orientation towards the goal—but it develops by incorporating parts into this framework. There is first a rather vague adjustment to the situation as a whole, and later, one by one, the various parts of the situation are found and located within the whole." [1] It must be remembered that the process of conditioning necessarily applies to the whole reaction, both impressive and expressive. In this way the perception of an outside event as well as the response can be brought to extreme perfection. " The skilfully learned movements which he (viz. the baby) develops a little later are not built up out of the definite reflexes but are differentiated out of his miscellaneous motor activity." [2] " The general body movements, then, are not combinations of small local reflexes. The smaller movements appear to differentiate out of the larger." [3]

Inhibition.—Conditioning may take place in such a way as to take the form of repression, e.g. if the bell were rung several times in succession and not followed by the presentation of food, salivation would cease. This led Pavlov to the conclusion that ' inhibition,' i.e. the checking of a ' habitual reaction,' is nothing but a negatively conditioned reflex.

In comparing natural reflexes with conditioned ones we may find that the difference is one of degree and of time. Reflexes which in our day are inherent in the new-born individual have been conditioned, canalised, and stabilised through long evolutionary periods.

The structural changes involved may be established while learning is taking place during a lifetime. Learning is activity which develops or modifies ' structure.' [4]

[1] Woodworth, l.c., p. 258. [2] Ibid., p. 218.
[3] Ibid., p. 218; Coghill (1929). *Anatomy and the Problem of Behaviour.*
[4] Woodworth, l.c., p. 224.

2

" For if those paths of nerve-reaction more frequently thrown into action become more highly organised, and more stable, there we have the key to structural differentiation. In a simple organism at an early stage of evolution the architecture of its nervous system would be determined by its shape and by its essential reactions to environment ; the nerve-paths most frequently stimulated would acquire a character of stability and permanence, and as evolution proceeded this primitive nervous system would undergo modifications strictly governed by morphological changes and external conditions." [1]

Learning is dependent on the existence of the cortex ; as this is, from the evolutionary standpoint, the youngest part of the nervous system, its cells are more likely to undergo conditioning, whereas the firmly established structure of tissues, such as the spinal cord or thalamus, opposes the process of learning.

The unconscious.—Up to this point we have followed the development of several mental functions as exhibited by our friend. In describing them he may have used such words as—" I did it quite unconsciously," " I was not aware of what was going to happen," " I did not want to do it, it just happened," " I do not know how it happened," and so on. Such phrases depict the fact that according to the stratification of functional patterns which has been described, we can observe a scale ranging from fully conscious action to the wholly unconscious. But here we must be careful to avoid the trap laid for us in the contradiction ' conscious-unconscious.'

Every one fancies he has a clear idea of the meaning of ' conscious ' so far as he himself is concerned, and all further definitions would be mere circumlocutions. But the denial of consciousness expressed by the prefix ' un ' does not necessarily indicate the absence of mental phenomena. The shifting of the notion on these grounds from the realm of psychology to that of physiology is in this case merely a matter of convenience, and we shall do well to bear this in mind.

If our friend is engaged in a violent discussion with us and afterwards cannot remember having brushed away a wasp, was his action merely reflex or was it in a way slightly psychic ? We might recapitulate various stages in our discussion and at a certain moment our friend might perhaps exclaim, ' Oh yes, now I remember it.' How has he become conscious of the experience ? These and other considerations seem to indicate that conscious human actions can be submerged until they fall below the level of awareness. Both the contra-distinctions ' voluntary-involuntary ' and ' conscious-unconscious ' should be understood as pointing to more or less of volition or awareness respectively.

Sociability.—We have so far not given up our assumption that behaviour is strongly influenced by the stimulation of the outside world. It makes no difference what kind of object we encounter. Our friend would make a gesture of self-protection if the irritation were caused not by a wasp but by a tickling sensation originating in himself or caused by some dust in the air. But in both cases his activity would have a distinctive character. The nature of the stimulating objects certainly causes a difference of interaction.

[1] Douglas, l.c., pp. 45–6.

When living beings are merged into a new unit the group which emerges is labelled ' society.' It is necessary, therefore, to distinguish between reactions observed, (1) in the individual responding to outside material stimuli ; (2) in the individual in interaction with other living beings (animals, persons) ; (3) in the group of individuals surrounding him.

It is evident, therefore, that all biological and psychological considerations are partly sociological. To the extent that the group activities, taken as a whole, " are rather different from the sum of the individual activities," they need special study, but must not lead us to the fallacious assumption of a " group mind as a mystical entity." [1]

Retrospective glance.—In retrospect, what have we discovered about the relations between psychological processes and the nerve units ?

The spinal cord, in co-operation with the sympathetic nervous system, is concerned with the lowest functions of man, which exhibit the highest degree of automatisation. In normal conditions they are so much under the control of superimposed centres that they hardly come into play independently. The spinal functions are integrated by the reflexes called up by the sense organs which have their nuclei in the spinal bulb and higher brain layers.

At the time of birth the nerve connections with the strio-pallidar system are not yet mature. Later on the thalamus is the first mass of brain ganglia which is occupied with the incoming messages. It is likely that this part of the nervous system at this level has, as it were, to put the question, ' What is to be done ? ' This results in a general attitude of attending to what is going on, which is accomplished via the thalamus-strio-pallidum-extrapyramidal tract. The striatum represents, as it were, the rein which the globus pallidus holds, producing and ensuring a firm posture. The mesencephalic grey masses and the thalamus may be regarded as the organs of character and temperament inasmuch as these are manifest in attitudes endowed with a certain tonicity. On a higher level of development the question as to how to respond is forwarded to the cortex, while the individual is turning his attention towards the given situation. The response is made over the loop from the thalamus via the cortex and the pyramidal tract. The cortex grades and distributes the impulses. In this sense the cortex is certainly the fount of reason and higher intelligence. It is superimposed on the centre of the ' self ' in the globular nucleus.[2]

Evolution of nervous functions.—The mere description of the elements of the central nervous system is like that of the various parts (screws, axles, etc.) of an engine. This enumeration involves a certain classification which proves useful, but it obviously does not, and cannot serve the purpose of attaining that knowledge of its construction which is fundamental to the understanding of the functioning of the engine. The description of the nervous system, given from the

[1] Mannheim, K. *The Psychological and Sociological Approach to the Understanding of Man.* Paper read at the Meeting of the Medical Staff of the Tavistock Clinic, 13/3/39.

[2] Küppers, E. (1923). " Weiteres zur Lokalisation des Psychischen," *Zeitschr. f. d. ges. Neurol. u. Psychiatr.,* **83,** pp. 263–76.

purely anatomical angle, could not avoid following the evolutionary line ; and as function can scarcely be disconnected from structure, it was inevitable to incorporate therein physiological terms.

We are now going to single out certain general principles which can be found if we pursue the evolutionary and developmental stratification of 'personality.'

Structure.—In view of its history the structure of the central nervous system might well be compared with a factory, succeeding owners of which have been compelled to build on more storeys and to alter the existing ones. Differences of design and style will change the aspect of the building, but the expert architect will always be able to single them out. The general plan of the building remains unchanged though the service is now carried out under the supervision of people in the upper storey ; and the products, say cars, are still of the same make though much more elaborate.

In the new-born we already find a rather elaborate building, in which we can distinguish, as it were, a ground floor where a mechanism is at work for the proper support of the essential life functions. It has superimposed on it various storeys concerned with reflex actions manifesting the rudiments of responses to the environment acquired during man's evolution.

Building up more and more storeys will, from the architectural point of view, require strong foundations if the building is to be safe, whereas the upper walls must be less substantial.

The addition of more influence from the upper storeys will modify and refine the resulting activity. But the original plan will always be recognisable, though not easily, as 'emergent evolution' might have concealed it, as it were, with stucco or decoration. A similar process can also be observed, with certain restrictions, in development and evolution.

"We have traced an ascending hierarchy of nerve centres, the controlling mechanism of which is strictly correlated to that fundamental necessity of every organism—the conservation of its own structural and functional integrity. In this conservation the rôle played by the sympathetic nervous system is of overwhelming importance, and to the adequate performance of the activities which that division represents the organism's power of movement is merely contributory. When in the course of evolution the spinal type of movement is developed, those fundamental stimuli (e.g. hunger and sex desire), transmitted from the organic factor, are provided with a path whereby they may pass to the voluntary muscles, and institute movements calculated to increase the chances of appeasing that hunger, or of satisfying that desire. To these two activities, self-preservation and the propagation of the species, which are the essential conditions of survival, is next subordinated the cranial (spatial-sense controlled) type of movement. And these three divisions function in reciprocal integration in such a way that the fact that the sympathetic represents the essential atomic activities upon which the continued existence of the organism depends is apt to be lost sight of. The other divisions of the nervous system, which from their size and distribution would appear to be of paramount importance, represent in reality nothing more than the control of spatial movement, grafted on to the sympathetic co-ordination of the molecular interactions which constitute the *sine qua non* of Life." [1]

As to the trend of the process we cannot do better than delineate the rules by Hughlings Jackson's concise words, with some explanatory comments. This will serve as terminology.

(1) " The doctrine of evolution implies the passage from the most organised to the least organised." [2]

When a certain degree of stability is achieved, *new* kinds of interaction emerge, which again result in the development of new functions and structures. The interplay of the old and the new mechanisms narrows the range of the former. " We say that there is a gradual ' adding on ' of the more and more special, a continual adding on of the new organisations. But this ' adding on ' is at the same time a ' keeping down.' The higher nervous arrangements evolved out of the lower keep down those lower just as a government evolved out of a nation controls as well as directs that nation." [3]

As to the structure of the nervous system, the passage from the ' most ' to the ' least organised ' means also ' from the lowest, well-organised centres up to the highest, least-organised centres.' [4] The progress proceeds from centres comparatively well organised at birth, up to the highest centres which organise continuously through life. "' Highly organised ' is frequently used synonymously with ' very complex ' ; but by degrees of organisation I mean degrees of perfection of union and certainty of action of nervous elements with one another. . . . The highest cerebral centres are the least organised (the ' most helpless centres ') although they are the most complex. . . ." [5]

(2) " Evolution is a passage from the most simple to the most complex ; again, from the lowest to the highest centres. There is no inconsistency whatever in speaking of centres being at the same time complex and least organised. Suppose a centre to consist of but two sensory and two motor elements ; if the sensory and motor elements be well joined, so that ' currents flow ' easily from the sensory into the motor elements, then that centre, although a very simple one, is highly organised. On the other hand, we can conceive a centre consisting of four sensory and four motor elements in which, however, the junctions between the sensory and motor elements are so imperfect that the nerve-currents meet with much resistance. Here is a centre twice as complex as the one previously spoken of, but of which we may say that it is only half as well organised." [6]

(3) Evolution is a passage from the most automatic to the most voluntary. The last remark, already used in our psychological survey, is not a mere question of words. The substituted expression does not imply " an abrupt division into the voluntary and the automatic, but implies degrees from most to least automatic, and that a

[1] Douglas, l.c., pp. 63–4.
[2] Jackson, J. H. (1932). *Selected Writings*, Hodder & Stoughton, London, ii, p. 58.
[3] Jackson, ibid., p. 58. [4] Jackson, ibid., p. 46.
[5] Jackson, ibid., p. 395. [6] Jackson, ibid., p. 46.

man, physically regarded, is an automaton, the highest parts of his
nervous system (highest centres) being least automatic ; the substituted term does not bring the will, a psychical state, into a purely
physical sphere." [1]

"A perfect automaton is a thing that goes on by itself. There are
degrees from those nervous arrangements which almost go on by
themselves, to those which come into activity by the aid of other,
lower, more organised nervous arrangements. To say that nervous
arrangements go on by themselves means that they are well organised ; and to say that nervous arrangements go on with difficulty,
if at all, by themselves, is to say that they are little organised.
Hence degrees from most to least automatic are, from another aspect,
degrees of organisation from the most to the least. Repeating what
has already been said in effect, if the highest centres were perfectly
automatic there would be no such thing as ' voluntary ' operation :
all being organised, there would be no possibility for correct adjustments in new circumstances ; we should be already adapted to particular external conditions, but no fresh adaptations to new conditions
could occur.[2] The becoming more perfectly organised, and the
becoming more automatic, are only different sides of one thing ; a
commonplace illustration is learning to write. There are degrees of
automaticity from those operations inherited comparatively perfect,
through the secondary automatic (writing, for example), up to the
activities of those least automatic nervous arrangements which are at
work during one's present thinkings and doings. We may say that
there are degrees from most organised and most automatic nervous
arrangements up to nervous arrangements just begun—nerve-stuff
being travelled by nerve currents for the first time." The triple conclusion come to is that the highest centres, which are the climax of
nervous evolution, and which make up the ' organ of mind ' (or physical
basis of consciousness) are the least organised, the most complex, and
the most voluntary.

Jackson, following Spencer, points to four factors which can be
observed in the evolutionary ascent : [3] (1) differentiation, i.e. the
growth of fresh characteristics. It is strongly connected with increasing complexity and provides new and more numerous movements.
This also involves division of labour. (2) Specialisation, i.e. increasing
definiteness. The functions have first a more general or indefinite
use which by degrees is restricted to special, i.e. to *definite* purposes.
(3) Integration, i.e. increasing width of representation by centres on
the higher level. This much-used term requires elucidation. The
Latin integer means ' untouched,' implying ' whole,' ' entire.' The
verb *integrare* means ' to make whole,' ' to renew,' ' to refresh.' Inte-

---

[1] Jackson, l.c., p. 68.

[2] The becoming more automatic is not dissolution, as I believe some think
it to be, but is, on the contrary, evolution becoming complete. The highest
centres are the most complexly evolving, but are also the least perfectly evolved.
In other words, the highest centres are " the ravelled end." In them evolution
is most actively going on, whilst in some lowest centres, e.g. the respiratory,
evolution is probably nearly completed (Jackson).

[3] Jackson, l.c., pp. 46, 68–9, 346 ff., 432 ff.

gration, therefore, not only implies ' to make into a whole ' by adding and putting together constituent parts, but it includes the idea of the originating of a fresh, new emergent phenomenon, and this is undoubtedly due to the manifold intercommunications between the ' centres ' concerned. (4) Co-operation. The centres are not merely connected with each other, but they work together. From that we can assume that each of them has given up something of its sovereign independence acquired during its evolution, in order to be proficient in the execution of its tasks.

It need not be explicitly remarked that the characteristics or functions mentioned extend far beyond the individual, and thus influence a group of beings which can also be considered as one whole.

This gives us an idea of the endless complexity and variability of human functions and traditions.

Localisation.—We have been speaking of ' layers,' ' levels,' anatomical units, ' patterns,' functions, processes, etc. It has become clear that functions as units or patterns of action are strongly connected with certain anatomical areas of more or less extensive magnitude. The principle of localising consists in assigning a function to a particular area.

Every activity is influenced by various layers. The higher strata (this has to be taken from the evolutionary point of view) become the leading ones ; but this must not mislead us into neglecting those areas which formerly had the leadership and are now more or less under the control of higher levels. They have not ceased but continue to be active, though they have given up a good deal of their sovereignty.

When we are faced with a particular form of action, say of speech or voice, it appears to us at first sight as a uniform whole ; but we must bear in mind that this ' form ' or ' kind ' or ' manner ' is only the outcome of the integration of several patterns each of which is localised.

If we want to modify a particular manner of speech we must take into consideration all its minor units. Only if we can isolate the layers concerned will it be possible to succeed in altering a peculiarity of form.

In localising, the speech therapist will be well advised to form a very clear picture of the various strata and their interrelations. For he is not only concerned with the mere problem speech or not speech, but with the hierarchy of its pattern. These elucidations have shown how much the ' tuning ' of the speech pattern as regards its cognitive and emotional meaning and its execution depends on those anatomical, physiological, psychological, and, last but not least, evolutionary structures.

Much has been said about the localisation of speech as a special kind of human behaviour. We will delineate presently the boundaries of the cortical area of speech. Here we must remind the reader that there is no such thing as speech, but only various methods of uttering communications.

The anatomical areas usually described as the ' speech centres ' control only the highest patterns of expression of ideas, thoughts, feelings, emotions, etc.

The cells of the dominant co-operating neurons are situated in a region of the cortex which " is limited above by the posterior limb of the Sylvian fissure, occupies probably the tip and the whole external convexity of the left temporal lobe, and spreads backwards into the supramarginal and angular gyri, while it extends forwards over all the convolutions of the insula and possibly to the posterior ends of the second and third pre-frontal gyri of the left side. . . . This ' speech region of the brain ' comprises not only the cortex but also the sub-cortical white matter which carries the paths of communication between the speech region and other parts of the brain.[1]

It seems that the speech areas are mainly established in the prevailing hemisphere. As most people are right-handed the speech area is usually found in the left hemisphere. In left-handed people it is usually located, therefore, in the right hemisphere.[2]

The task of localisation must be directed finally to the nerve-paths leading the stimuli out of the central nervous system (the ' nerves,' i.e. the offshoots of the neuron) to the effector organs.

On this path we shall meet with parts of the nervous system already described, such as the mesencephalic ganglia, spinal bulb, etc.

Finally we must search for the limitations of the speech and voice function in the structure of the effector organs.

The speech therapist might rightly ask, " What is the use of knowing in what area a specific speech function is located ? " We must admit that he is right if he says that he can often manage very well without this knowledge and that he could not do better if he possessed it, for those anatomical areas cannot be reached except by the knife of the surgeon or by organic means (drugs, etc.).

Here we must refer to later chapters where it will be made clear that speech therapists may well co-operate with the consultant neurologist, laryngologist, aurist, etc., in certain cases. It may be that the patient would be sent to the speech therapist who, though refusing to carry out the treatment, helps by indicating organic therapy. This will be the case in certain types of Aphasia (caused by tumours, abscess of the brain), spastic speech disturbances, hoarseness after encephalitis, sigmatism in high-frequeney deafness, dysphony, and so forth.

But what about the functional cases which definitely require the care of the speech therapist ? Here localisation should help to picture the particular integration or disintegration of the speech faculty, the economy and harmony of interaction between the different patterns, etc., which defines our plans of treatment and our prognosis.

A fine example is offered in the interpretation of types of stammering. Our elucidation will show that the particular feature of a stammer refers clearly to developmental stages of the disorder, which stages again reflect certain patterns of action in the stratification of speech. This method of approach will prove useful also in the explanation of disorders of articulate speech, especially of Dyslalia.

[1] Collier, J. (1933). *A Textbook of the Practice of Medicine*, Oxford University Press, p. 1555.
[2] It must be noted that owing to the crossing of certain nerve tracts the left hemisphere governs the right side of the body, and vice versa.

CHAPTER III

DEVELOPMENT OF SPEECH AND LANGUAGE

PERIODS OF SPEECH DEVELOPMENT

In accordance with our evolutionary considerations, we will now proceed to follow the track on which the tendencies described contribute to the development of speech in the growing human being. .

Speaking of periods, stages, etc., it must, of course, be borne in mind that, as elsewhere, they show no distinct but only approximate and often overlapping demarcations. General considerations justify us in speaking of stages though they in no way can be clearly separated.

CRYING PERIOD (SCREAMING TIME [1])

Id cries.[2]—The new-born baby has a long history behind him. Small as he is, the complexity of his structure is great. It reminds us of some old cathedral, such as Worcester or Mont St. Michel, which at first sight seems a fine, well-planned, harmonious building, yet reveals various stages of architecture to the trained observer, who also discerns what has as yet been left unaccomplished.

At the time of birth all the peripheral organs have achieved their development and are waiting to be used. They have been supplied with their nervous connections which, however, are not yet entirely capable of working.

With birth the first and not least important period of development has been completed. The speed of this development is comparatively fast. The parts of the nervous system, as far as they recapitulate those chiefly used by the ancestors of the animal kingdom (low layers), are therefore highly developed, and their functions well canalised.

Thus in a baby we find already in existence certain behavioural patterns. It is impossible to use any psychological terms for this stage. What we know is merely the baby's reactions. They serve his vegetative ' needs ' as far as the preservation of life (metabolism) is concerned.

The activities of breathing, sucking, and crying which are of extreme importance in the maintenance of life, require the co-ordination of many muscles. Being of great evolutionary age, they are ruled by older, i.e. lower parts of the nervous system. Accordingly they exhibit a high degree of automatisation.

Life in this period is mainly dependent on the activity of the spinal cord with its continuation, the medulla oblongata. The ganglia at

---

[1] Jespersen, O. (1922). *Language, Its Nature, Development and Origin*, Allen & Unwin, London.

[2] I have adopted here the psycho-analytic term ' id ' to indicate the ' unknown and unconscious ' (Freud) and little co-ordinated character of the first cries.

the base of the brain, and some of their connections with the cortical layers, are not yet mature.

The sympathetic nervous system plays its part in the regulation of the organs of digestion, respiration, etc.

To indicate the behavioural pattern of this level in evolutionary terms, note the following characteristic features :

The whole of the body and its reactions form *one* indivisible unit. In comparison with the pre-natal level, the condition is altered inasmuch as stimuli of the outside world replace the weaker stimuli of the womb (the mother's body) and further development of the responses takes place.

In so far as manifestations which form the basis of the future speech are concerned, it has to be emphasised that they do not form a *separate unit* but are strongly integrated with all the other movements referred to. The baby performs movements of its arms and legs, trunk, and head. It breathes, sneezes, swallows, sucks, and cries. Its cries are, compared with those of later periods, fairly weak and short, 60 per minute, and without a definitely individual, articulate, or modulated character. The pitch of this undifferentiated cry [1] is from fa[2]-fa[3].[2]

Its attack [3] is said to be soft [4] in spite of the fact that all other movements, including that of the soft palate, are performed with excessive discharge of nervous energy. It will be shown how very important this is for pathological considerations.

Two questions now call for explanation. First, What conditions determined the genesis of voice ? Second, Why is the attack soft ?

The question as to the ultimate reason for voice (manifested in the first cry) has at all times aroused the greatest speculation. Many philosophers have racked their brains as to the significance of the first cries. They were interpreted as a kind of protest against entering this rotten world. When some old observers pretended they could hear the sounds o-ah in boys, and in girls o-eh, which they interpreted as the abbreviation of " Ó Adam (Eve) cur peccavisti," [Oh Adam (Eve) why hast thou sinned ?], they proved a certain sense of phylogeny. But alas ! they did not go far enough back.

The right explanation seems to be found in a vital vegetative need. For if the glottal aperture of the glottis is narrowed, too sudden deflation of the lung is prevented ; the compressive action of the chest walls can distribute the air by squeezing some backwards into the lungs. The glottis can thus correlate the flow of air with the flow of blood in the lungs, and so keep the percentage of carbon dioxide in the blood constant.[5]

[1] O'Shea (1907). *Linguistic Development and Education,* Macmillan, New York.

[2] Garbini, A. (1892). Evoluzione della voce nell' infanzia. Verona.

[3] S.p. 27.

[4] Gutzmann, Sprachheilkunde (1912). *Fischer's Medizinische Buchhandlung,* Berlin, p. 94.

[5] Negus, V. E. (1929). *The Mechanism of the Larynx,* Heinemann, London, pp. 178–9 ; Curry, R. (1940). *The Mechanism of the Human Voice,* Churchill, London, p. 30.

It appears from this that the very pattern of natural voice is based on the approximation of the vocal chords as a means of preventing the air from escaping too fast ; and this merely requires a more or less narrow space between the vocal chords.

If the vocal chords are approximated so far that they meet in the midline, the escaping air puts them into vibration. The initiation of the voice, termed the Attack, is in this case ' soft.'

This pattern is fundamentally different from another mechanism by which voice may be started, viz. the glottal stop, or hard attack.

The movements of the chords cutting short the respiratory phases are controlled from the nucleus ambiguus of the vagus nerve. The impulses which put this nucleus into activity come from centres in the pons and in the spinal bulb. The nucleus ambiguus maintains also the habitual tonus of the laryngeal muscles.[1]

Quiet respiration shows approximately equal inspiratory and expiratory phases, and at the same time also shows the rhythmic repetition which can be observed in most primitive movements. The same type of respiration is noticeable in crying, but this will soon be altered, the rhythm of this vital function being superseded more and more by influences of a higher order.

The sucking movements are, during the first two weeks, mute.

Instinctive cries.—At the end of the first month of the baby's life his cries become stronger and longer—40 per minute. Respiration acquires another character when used for phonation, in that the inspiratory phase is shorter, while the expiratory phase is prolonged.

It is usually said that the baby is ' learning ' to master his respiration, thus recapitulating the respiration pattern evolved by the race. But strong emphasis must be laid on the fact that the type of respiration used in crying is actually a new type which does not replace that observed during the early days. In fact it takes its place beside quiet respiration which will always show practically the same curve though the rate of respiration in adults is on the average 17 a minute.

What characterises its newness is that the inspiration is short and rapid, and is actuated through the mouth, and with more effort, while expiration takes place either through the mouth or through the nose, is much longer and smoother, and is either silent or loud.

The quick inspiratory act recalls a similar feature in other movements, such as vestibular nystagmus,[2] which is primarily actuated by lower nervous areas.

We have pointed out (see Evolution of the Nervous System, p. 11) that it is the extra-pyramidal system which plays its part in creating postural reflexes in answer to environmental necessities. We encounter here a modification of an ancient metabolic process, which results in a specific motor adjustment. The gradual prolonged expiratory act seems to indicate the growing influence of the cortex, which harmonises the energy of posture.

---

[1] Negus, l.c., pp. 175–80.

[2] Involuntary rhythmical movements of the eyeballs, consisting of a slow component in one direction and a rapid component in the opposite direction. Produced by irritation of the vestibular organ.

In view of its great evolutionary age this kind of respiration is naturally highly sensitised. It may be added that it strongly resembles the kind of breathing performed in working.

The development of the respiration in crying, fits in well with the appearance of a new type of voice initiation, viz. the glottal stop.

The glottal stop requires closure of the glottis as does the soft attack ; but the two vocal chords are so strongly pressed against each other that the valve between the upper. and the lower air passages is practically impassable. The closure is then forced open with a concomitant sound of explosive character.

It is a postural reflex grafted on voice production in psychological states which, it can be inferred, are vaguely disturbing the baby's well-being. Observation of its appearance in later years and biological considerations explain its being of a tense 'and attentive character.

This process takes place, of course, in connection with other infantile movements. It should therefore by no means be regarded as a pathological process. Whether it will give rise to the latter is a matter of quantity.[1]

The glottal stop is a sign of instinctive orientation of the baby in conditions concerning self-preservation and related behaviours, for it protects the lungs against penetrating foreign bodies, particularly food particles, which would cause serious damage. Both its evolutionary pattern, shown in the chapter on the Evolution of Speech (see p. 48), and its use in later phases of development seem to suggest that it is a symbol of awareness of danger, thus a sign of displeasure. Soon the cries begin to be differentiated slightly in tone and timbre. They are still rather indistinct. Their timbre is now 'nasal.' This does not indicate that the nasopharynx is open, since nasal twang can also be produced by the constriction of the pharynx.[2]

We may add that the nasal resonance of the voice has been preserved in the languages, and particularly in the songs of most of the primitive peoples.

The sucking movements change into a labial noise.[3] Here we find the root of the labial sounds, which all observers agree to be ' early sounds ' if not the ' earliest ' beside voice.[4]

To draw a picture of the mentality of this period we may describe it in W. James's words that " the baby, assailed by eyes, ears, nose, skin and entrails at once, feels it all as one great blooming, buzzing confusion." [5] It has also to be borne in mind that " . . . sounds and pains, every shade of colour and every degree of heat that enter into experience has a character of its own which sets it off from everything else. But to be different and to be distinguished are not the same. . . . In the experience of the infant, however dim and indiscriminate its sensations may be, those sensations are still different. But they

---

[1] See *Development of the Tonic Stage of Stammering*, p. 120.
[2] Curry, l.c., § 25, 6.
[3] Allaire, quot. by Chamberlain, A. F. (1900). *The Child*, Scott, London, p. 96.
[4] Jespersen, l.c., p. 106.
[5] James, W. *Principles of Psychology*, i, 488. Quot. by Blanshard, l.c., i, p. 61.

are certainly not distinct in the sense of being distinguished." [1]
" Accordingly during the first two months there is no proper discrimination of speech-sounds." [2] There occur innumerable random
variations of sounds, timbre, degree, etc., but Blanton stresses the
fact that no one was used in response to " one set of circumstances
that was not at the same time used to others." [3] Thus they have no
meaning to *us* and for this reason *we* do not usually discriminate them.

This period may be characterised as a time of developing patterns
of behaviour, but definite utterance sets can scarcely be observed,
except for the soft and hard attacks. Since little can be said about
the psychological background, it is necessary to emphasise some
negative features. Utterances are not yet articulate because they are
not significant ; nor can they be labelled communicative, since we
know nothing about what should be specially expressed.

It will serve our understanding to regard this stage as ' fringed '
with rudimentary instinctive patterns. The fringe may be regarded
as instinctive, because " An instinct may be taken to be a pattern of
behaviour ; that is a set, automatic mode of response to a given
stimulus." [4] As such the child's ' language ' is, at this stage, natural
and common to all times and all peoples. It forms a unit with other
behavioural patterns.[5]

Emotional cries.—At the age of about 8 weeks the child's behaviour indicates that the stimuli received by the organs of the
higher senses are better differentiated, and thus integrate and specialise
the child's original behaviour. The child's eyes follow a moving
person (2nd month) or things (3rd month), and the head turns freely
in inspection (3rd month).[6]

Darwin observed the first smile by this time, but others place it
in the 3rd month.[7] Such smiles seem to be mere expressive patterns,
but are not intended as communications of an emotional state.

During the 3rd and 4th months the canalisation of the auditory
and visual pathways increases, and so prepares the way for further
adaptation of vocal utterance.

The two modes of initiating voice are now well established. The
soft attack is used in states of ' gratification ' or pleasure, while the
glottal stop manifests states of ' frustration ' or displeasure.

The relation between the suckling and its mother may be regarded
as the primitive form of a vocal unit. It is, therefore, at first only
the experienced mother who ' understands ' these sounds, that is to
say, who knows their import.

[1] Blanshard, l.c,, i, p. 64.
[2] Seth, G. and Guthrie, D. (1935). *Speech in Childhood*, Oxford University
Press, p. 83.
[3] Blanton (1917). " The Behaviour of the Human Infant during the first
thirty days of Life," *Psychol. Rev.*, 24, pp. 456–83.
[4] MacCurdy, J. T. (1928). *Common Principles in Psychology and Physiology*,
Cambridge University Press, p. 9.
[5] Egger, quot. by Chamberlain,
[6] Gesell, A. (1929). *Infancy and Human Growth*, Macmillan, New York,
p. 129.
[7] Gesell, ibid.

The timbres of the voice and the facial response correspond with these emotional states.

To separate emotional cries from instinctive ones is justified by the appearance of the first *definite* sets of reactions in speech and voice. Now the foundation of emotional utterance is laid. But these manifestations do not seem to be significant, i.e. they are not intended as signs by the child, nor are we so far justified or compelled to assume there being a cognitive element in the baby's consciousness.

Whether they should be labelled instinctive or emotional is a matter of definition. The behaviourist will call them instinctive because of the observable definite sets of motor response. The psychologist's introspection infers the emotional accompaniment "which is so marked a feature of instinctive response." [1] "It is the muscular constituent (comprising *either excitation or inhibition*,[2] the same qualification applying to the organic constituent) which differentiates one emotion from another, the organic elements, circulatory and glandular being in various forms of emotion practically the same." [3]

And it is the definite muscular sets in infantile voice which characterise this phase.

As for the neurological aspect of this level, we may assume that the subcortical areas of the brain (thalamus, striatum, etc.) play their part ; but it seems likely that the cortex begins to differentiate sensory stimuli. We also notice that the differentiation of the expressive part of the reflex arc does not keep pace with the impressive, a disproportion which will be seen to be of importance also in later life.

In this way at the completion of the screaming stage the fundamentals of emotional utterance are laid. There is not yet any considerable sound differentiation to be noticed, but definite variations in the *tonus* and pitch of vocal utterance can be recognised.

BABBLING PERIOD (CROWING OR BABBLING TIME) [4]

Prelinguistic differentiation.—From the age of about 2 to 3 months up to 6 months the baby's cries grow still longer and steadier, about 27 per minute. Their pitch declines to the octave do²-do³.

Towards the end of the first half-year the voice of the child becomes more and more differentiated by an increasing variety of mouth shapes. Soon an enormous, uncountable number of sound shades (vowels) is to be heard.

Sucking movements.—At the age of 2 or 3 months the baby already begins to produce the movements of suction, chewing, etc., independently from actual drinking. The resulting noises, the first of a consonantal character, are termed ' clicks.' In sucking as well as in ' clicking,' the buccal canal is divided into three chambers, (1) the labial chamber ; (2) the palatal chamber ; (3) the velar or laryngeal chamber. The air is rarefied by the rounding of the lips, the curving

---

[1] Douglas, l.c., p. 132.   [2] My italics.
[3] Douglas, ibid.   [4] Jespersen, l.c.

of the tongue, and the lowering of the larynx.[1] Clicks are thus independent from respiration.[2]

The study of the clicks has proved to be of the utmost importance in elucidating the evolution and the history of language. We must deny ourselves any attempt to give a more exact explanation of the nature of these sounds, however attractive that might be. For references to this subject the reader is advised to consult the proceedings of the Third International Congress of Phonetic Sciences.

The evolutionary importance of the clicks will make it necessary to refer to them again in various chapters (see Chapter XII, Stammering, p. 122; Laryngektomy, p. 195; Lateral Sigmatism, p. 154; Evolution of Language, p. 49).

Suffice it to mention that suction involves roughly a sequence of three clicks, namely, a labial, a medial, and a velar one, which can be well discriminated acoustically.[3] These clicks, in course of development and of evolution (see p. 49), differentiate into uncountable variations which are described as dental, palatal, cerebral,[4] lateral, and so forth.

Soon the processes of digestion and of respiration, i.e. phonatory activity and sucking movements, come to be integrated. As a result the voice-stream is interrupted by clicks inserted in rhythmic succession, thus giving rise to an intimate union of sounds of both consonant and vowel character.

The amalgamation of two essentially antagonistic functions necessitates in its course the abandonment of impeding characteristics. Thus for the sake of a unified pattern the rarefaction of air implied in the clicks gradually comes to be replaced by expulsion of air. At first the sounds so produced are half clicked and half explosive, until in the end they are entirely expiratory. This process can also be traced in the evolution of primitive languages (see p. 50).

The sound sequences which have come into existence in the way described above impose as reiterated syllables, and phenomenally do not differ from them.

At a certain stage we may find, in addition to the clicks, many shades of consonants and vowels. Some may be familiar to us owing to their resemblance to the sounds of our mother-tongue. The philologists may recognise other speech-sounds which normally occur in other languages at a different evolutionary level.

Gesell was able to count 75 sounds and combinations of sounds during one day in a child of 6 months.[5] It is in this sense that we

---

[1] Ginneken, J. van (1939). *Les clics, les consonnes et les voyelles dans l'histoire de l'humanité.* 3rd Congr. of Phonetic Sciences, Laboratory of Phonetics of the University, Ghent, pp. 321-6.

[2] Pancoucelli-Calzia, G. (1921). *Ueber im Munde und im Kehlkopf synchronisch erfolgende, aber von einander unabhängige Phonationsvorgänge,* Vox No. 3, pp. 79-84.

[3] Ginneken, J. van, l.c., p. 322.

[4] This term is due to a misunderstanding of a word used by Indian grammarians, and applied in Sanscrit philology to consonants formed by inversion of the tip of the tongue; such sounds should rather be called point-inverted consonants. Wyld, *Dictionary,* s.v. cerebral.

[5] Gesell, A. (1925). *The Mental Growth of the Pre-School Child,* Macmillan, New York.

are to understand the remarks of some observers who assert that the infant at the age of about 4 months is able to produce every sound.

Reiterated syllables.—Our examination of the rise and integration of the primitive speech-noises explains why almost every worker in the field of child psychology has found *reiteration of syllables* during the period from the 2nd to the 6th months.

According to Miss Shinn, a " long series of nonsense syllables would be chanted in a kind of recitative with increasing variety of pitch and rhythm and with much more evident enjoyment " up to the 3rd year.[1]

The term ' reiterated syllables ' has certainly been coined from the adult's point of view. As such it is misleading, for it would lead us to assume that the syllable was the prototype which afterwards had been iterated. This is certainly not the case. The common idea that single ' speech-sounds ' are primitive units which, when arranged in sequences result in ' syllables ' or ' words,' is due to an abstraction induced by the operations of reading and writing. It does not seem to have any onto- or phylogenetic basis.

Consonants are originally not produced as separate units. They have been inserted into voice like bricks into the pre-formed framework of a Tudor house. The noises which the educated adult conceives as and calls iterated syllables are in reality *one* stream of voice interrupted by rhythmically recurring noises which originated from suction. The original unit is not the syllable but the continuous stream of voice integrated by movements which result in noises such as ' clicks ' or ' consonants.' Before this the noises concerned constituted vegetative random noises on the one hand and cries on the other.

Reiteration of syllables is a new emergent mode of sound production. As such it appears to obey one of the general principles on which all movements are based, viz. rhythm.

We know that many infantile movements are at first rhythmic, i.e. iterated, for instance the fidgeting, kicking, and struggling movements in babies.

The primitive nature of reiteration is evidenced by the following observations :

It has been stated by many child psychologists [2] that little children utter reiterated syllables more easily than non-iterated ones. Recognition is facilitated in children who are just growing out of the babbling stage if iterated monosyllables are presented. A child might, for example, render the syllable ' fa ' as ' pa ' but would correctly iterate ' fafafa.'

Even when children appear to recognise a non-iterated syllable presented to them, they seem to be embarrassed or even reluctant to make any attempt to reproduce it if asked to do so. The high grade of sensitisation is also proved by the appearance of reiteration in deaf and in blind babies who have had no chance of *imitating* speech.

[1] Quot. by Seth and Guthrie, l.c., p. 89.
[2] Perez (1894). *La psychologie de l'enfant*, Alcan, Paris ; Preyer, W. (1889). *The Soul of the Child*, Heath, Boston ; Shinn (1900). *The Biography of a Baby*, Houghton, Mifflin, Boston ; Hall (1896–7). *The First 500 Days of a Child's Life*, Child Stud., No. 2 ; Kroeber (1916). *The Speech of a Zuni Child*, Amer. Anthropol., **18**, pp. 529–34.

As to the psychological aspect of reiteration, we have reasons to infer from the child's general behaviour that iterated syllables are produced only in states of well-being, comfort or pleasure. They can scarcely be observed in states of discomfort, such as anger, sadness, etc.

We shall have many opportunities of showing how well sensitised this mode of utterance has been in evolutionary time, and how great a rôle it plays in the individual's further development, normal and abnormal.

This kind of speech, characterised by an overflowing amount of unstable sounds produced in iterated ' syllables,' is called ' babbling.' The word is plainly onomatopoeic. It means originally ' to keep on saying ba-ba ' and so imitates a child's attempts to utter sounds. Its illustrative strength is augmented by the frequentative suffix ' -le.' Kindred words can be found in other germanic languages, e.g. Dutch *babbelen*, Danish *bable*, Icel. *babbla*, German *bappelen*. The corresponding French expression is *babiller*. To indicate the primitiveness of these utterances Sully speaks of primordial babbling; Kussmaul [1] called this time the stage of primitive sounds. To emphasise also the fact that in no way do they represent the beginnings of language as communication of thoughts, though they constitute one of its basic factors, one might—in accordance with McCarthy—call it ' prelinguistic babbling ' in contrast to the subsequent stage which I term ' linguistic babbling.'

This biological explanation plays an important part in the treatment of stammerers who in the course of their development have misconceived the structure of speech (see p. 128).

Conditioned speech.—The patterns of speech response to outward stimuli so far described are of great evolutionary age, and therefore highly sensitised.

Up to the age of about 5 months both the perception of speech in detail, and utterance remain unaffected by incoming speech stimuli.

As soon as the child forms a social group with his mother, she becomes the outstanding factor in the *conditioning* of the natural speech reflexes.

A simple example : when the baby gets food which it likes, it is eager to suck it in ; but it is not only the food itself that the baby is aware of—the mother's approach, her voice, her gesticulations, etc., are additional stimuli. On succeeding occasions such events will again arouse the same motor response. Thus the baby will give a hearty smack, perhaps, when the mother comes, or her steps are heard, or when food is shown, and so on. This explains the use of clicks and timbres of voice under certain conditions ; but it does not necessarily imply their purposive use.

Gesell notes vocalisation of displeasure on withdrawal of a coveted object (5 months), of pleasure (6 months), and satisfaction in attaining an object (7 months). [2] This need by no means involve any consciousness of the special articulatory or acoustic feature of the utterances ; but it represents perhaps the rudimentary beginnings of

[1] Kussmaul, A. (1877). *Störungen der Sprache*, F. C. W. Vogel, Leipzig.
[2] Gesell (1929), l.c., pp. 130–1.

3

'meaning.' "Meaning may be called a conditioned response to the sign." [1]

The struggle for the fulfilment of desires will then serve in the further specification of the response. More and more functions will be singled out. In this way certain responses or parts of a response will disappear. In view of the fact that they had been performed originally, unconditionally, or naturally, we now speak of 'inhibition.' Take the example of the begging dog. The untrained dog leaps at the food shown to him. This is an inherited, unconditioned reflex, serving the striving after gratification of the food desire. If the food is held above the dog's head it is forced to rise up on the hind legs and to make rhythmic movements of the forefeet in an effort at balance.

These measures condition and modify the natural reflex, so that there emerges a new attitude, which then 'means begging.'

Other actions of the experimenter, such as the way of holding up the arm, involuntary 'teaching' attitudes, etc., will eventually also constitute conditioning (i.e. 'inhibiting') influences.

It is an old circus trick to restrict the begging response in such a way that the dog will not beg if certain sounds or sayings (e.g. 'it comes from Hitler') are used, and conversely. Conditioning thus furthers the specialisation of positive or negative responses to particular sounds.

Speech attention.—Owing to the constant canalisation, vocal utterances produced by those around the child will also find well-prepared channels and will strengthen the link between the baby and the environment. These influences manifest themselves normally at the end of the first six months.

In the same way the child applies his inherited vocal response to conditions in making it serve the fulfilment of its desires. We now say that the child has had the 'experience' that certain muscular responses connected with noises are useful. This term is synonymous with the "modification of the original reactionary course and effector response to an external stimulus, due to the intercurrent sensitisation of some localised portion of its cortical path." [2] The child's previous experiences as to speech have—naturally—aroused its attention, interest, and recognition (see Chapter II), so that certain sounds become *dominant stimuli*.

Meaning.—Many times the child has found himself in a situation where certain events (bringing food, a toy, the voice of those in charge of him) have formed the impressive unit, whereas his adaptive behaviour as well as his utterance have constituted the reactive part of the reflex arc.

The same adaptive behaviour will soon emerge as a response to the concomitant sound, even when not accompanied by action—a further conditioning of the set of reflexes. Thus to the child's mind the sounds heard 'mean' something. Speech acquires meaning.

In general, 'meaning' is an expression denoting our being aware in some way that a given thing refers to another given thing. The latter may be the individual himself.

[1] Woodworth, l.c., p. 452.   [2] Douglas, l.c., p. 98.

In this sense meaning may be conceived as a ' social act.' Sociality again may be manifest on different developmental levels. The level we are concerned with here is one which is predominantly emotional. Thus meaning as described hitherto is feeling-meaning, directed by the interests of this period. In so far as the appropriate interests are concerned feeling-meanings cannot possibly be mistaken.[1] (It may be remarked, by the way, that the word expresses an *act*, namely, of mistaking, that is, taking wrongly.)

We have hinted at the integration of natural reflexes into a more complex reflex chain, whose psychological aspect is characterised by interest. The latter "is largely unconscious in its operation and, therefore, meaning must rest frequently on mental processes that are not exposed to the consciousness of the subject. This kind of meaning then appears as an affect attached to the object. Symbols, which bulk so largely in the mental life of human beings, fall into this class, the special meaning which they enjoy being derived almost entirely from the emotional reaction which they engender." [2] The setting of the object determines psychological meaning. " The associated reactions are not serving to orient the central reaction, but determine its very nature, while the object itself is determining the orientation." [3] " The study of meaning is, then, the study of associated reactions." [4]

' Significance' is a term reserved by MacCurdy [5] for an unconscious setting of an object, different from the conscious meaning ; ". . . the former is betrayed by the behaviour of the patient."

Emotional Expression.—The features of the associated reactions, viz. utterances bearing ' significance,' are now no different from some of those discussed in earlier stages. According to their emotional character in the sense of purely adjusting attitude without regard to the analysis of the outer world, the earliest utterances seem to be of the character of emotional ejaculations, i.e. interjections.[6]

Interjections.—In accordance with their above-mentioned derivation and essence they constitute a form of speech which on the one hand conceals within itself the roots of articulation and intonation, but on the other hand is not grammatical [7] nor capable of becoming so without losing its original character.

Nearly all sounds, including clicks, may assume an interjectional character (see Hearing-Mutism, p. 96 ; Stammering, p. 122). So far as my observations go, interjectional expression becomes attached to clicks very early, roughly two months after their first performance. They express especially emotional meanings, such as disgust, admiration, pain, pleasure, reluctance, agreement, and so forth. Sometimes they are accompanied by facial movements and gesticulation. If emotional utterances jut out of cognitive expression, the former appear ' interjected' into the structure of language proper.[8]

---

[1] Blanshard, l.c., pp. 70–1.   [2] MacCurdy, l.c., pp. 110–11.
[3] Ibid., p. 106.   [4] Ibid., p. 107.   [5] Ibid., p. 110.
[6] Moore, K. C. *The Mental Development of a Child;* Gesell (1929). *Infancy and Human Growth,* p. 131.
[7] Earle, quot. in *Shorter Oxford Dict.,* s.v. interjection..
[8] Wilson, R. A. (1937). *The Birth of Language,* Dent, London, p. 54.

Apart from that, intonation has been playing its part as correlated in the emotional pattern for several months. From 9 months its rôle as a means of true emotional expression begins to be obvious.[1]

Summary.—At this stage the child's utterance can be regarded as still partly instinctive and emotional in so far as the persisting pre-linguistic babbling indicates *definite* pattern-sets and adjustments to the outer world. These sounds are not yet intentional symbolic signs; therefore they are only slightly social and articulate.

Heard speech and other noises possess as large units 'meaning' based chiefly on their specific intonation.

It is in this respect, i.e. on the impressive side, that social adaptation of speech begins. The communicative character of developed speech is impressed on the child by those around him, while the child's expressions are communicative only to a small extent.

We can thus certainly accept the generally adopted opinion that " in earlier stages of an infant's language-learning, speaker's meaning and hearer's meaning may be imperfectly correlated," [2] so that " long before he has learnt more than the mere rudiments of communication by speech, the child can grasp the meaning of relatively long and complicated sentences." [3]

This disproportion will to a certain extent persist up to the adult age.

When children begin to play actively, to exploit their surroundings, to manipulate toys and so on, that is to say, from 5 to 8 months,[4] ' concepts ' originate in their minds as a further integration of conditioned responses. " The child's behaviour, even before he starts to talk, strongly suggests that he is already building up concepts. The child's concept of a thing centres around what he does with the thing and what it does to him." [5]

IMITATION PERIOD

Self-imitation.—So far the child's utterances have been a kind of motor reaction to external stimuli, like smiling and other facial responses, crawling, head-raising, etc. Gradually the situation unit was divided into several smaller units by further development of the perceptive faculties.

Staring at windows, etc., or at conspicuous moving objects, for example (1 month), develops into following with the eyes a moving pencil, varied inspection of environment (3 months), regarding a cube (4 months), or a pellet on a table surface (6 months).[6]

The audible part of the influencing unit may now also influence the flow of reflexes.

By progressive conditioning the speech reactions to the sounds heard now operate as stimuli.

What we call playful self-imitation seems to be nothing else than

[1] Woodworth, l.c., p. 175.   [2] Bloomfield, l.c., p. 18.
[3] Seth and Guthrie, l.c., p. 92.   [4] Gesell (1929), l.c., pp. 130-1.
[5] Woodworth, l.c., p. 480.   [6] Gesell, l.c., pp. 128 ff.

" an outlet for weak excitations set up by weak visceral disturbances," facilitating the integration of new patterns.[1]

It has been observed that the child's babble occurs at special times of day, obviously when digestion, etc., have brought the body into equilibrium.

By the end of the first year the number of sounds which the little babbler has mastered is considerable. He loves to combine long series of the same syllables, dadadada . . . , nenenene . . . , bygnbygnbygn . . . , etc., and this game need not even cease when the child is able to talk actual language.[2]

Imitation.—From 9 months active imitation,[3] particularly as to " intonation when a word or sentence was repeated several times," [4] is recorded by many authors. This goes hand-in-hand with the imitation of scribble [5] (10 months), and utilising various objects.

It is apparently a new kind of play. It in no way implies any necessary understanding of what the imitated sounds 'mean.' It is the final integration of the cause and effect game the child has been playing before, when banging a spoon or patting the table (6 months [6]) or showing interest in throwing and sound-production play (8 months [2]). These imitated utterances remind us of the speech of parrots. Though they may be divided into distinct parts, they cannot be regarded as ' articulate ' since they do not ' signify ' anything (see p. 39).

Listening.—The part imitation plays is obviously of great value, as it helps ' hearing ' to develop into ' listening.' In this way auditory complexes are being distinguished in their parts, the hearing perceptions are integrated and connected with the persons or objects causing them, and are thus gradually endowed with more specific ' meaning.'

Types of imagery.—There seem to be various constitutional types of imagery. That is to say, that from the onset the same sense stimuli will have different effects on different children.

Thus the final motor impulse may be pre-eminently excited by either visual, auditory, tactile, gustatory, or olfactory stimuli. Even the proprioceptive reflexes, i.e. those motor impulses which are effected by stimuli coming from the muscles themselves, may be differently developed. They are apparently based on certain as yet undefined structural patterns which, however, as experience shows, can be altered to a certain extent by function. The influence of these peculiarities on speech and voice has been emphasised by many workers, especially by Fröschels and S. Stinchfield.[7] We shall have to return to this subject in various chapters (Retarded Speech, Phonasthenia, Dyslalia, etc.).

Adaptive expression.—Conditioned speech (see above, p. 33) is now ready for further integration. Voice has for long been used as a means to obtain fulfilment of desires. It has meanwhile developed into speech through differentiation into separate sound units.

[1] MacCurdy, l.c., p. 83.   [2] Jespersen, l.c., p. 106.
[3] Whipple and Whipple (1909). " The Vocabulary of a Three Year Old Boy," *Ped. Sem.*, 16, pp.1–22.
[4] Champneys (1881). "Notes on an Infant," *Mind*, 6, pp. 104-7.
[5] Gesell (1929), l.c., p. 132.   [6] Ibid., pp. 331-2.
[7] Stinchfield, S. M. (1933). *Speech Disorders*, Kegan Paul, London, p. 21.

When the child recognises—first perhaps by chance—that any of his playful utterances are followed by changes of the environment which minister to his own needs, speech is on its way to become *purposive*. Meumann has rightly labelled it "emotional-volitional" speech.

The number of random variations of sounds decreases through conditioning (inhibition) if certain sounds only reach the ear of the child, and if the emission only of these same sounds leads to the fulfilment of the child's desires. This quite conforms with Taine's opinion [1] that children do not learn new sounds by new co-ordinations for the purpose of imitating those heard in their environment, but only by further practice, i.e. sensitisation of the sounds which have already emerged in the period of differentiation (prelinguistic babbling).

From the age of 14 months [2] or thereabouts, utterances can be observed which, though not of a 'standard' type, more or less allow us to recognise that they are based on adult speech. They are 'imitated,' and are by many authors [3] regarded as 'words.' Darwin's boy used from the age of 11 months the form '*mum*' when he wanted food. It was later integrated by combining it with imitated words to '*shu-mum*' for sugar. [4] The sound sequence 'ndobbin,' arising during the eating act, was then used for things concerned with food by O'Shea's niece. [5] As her environment responded to it, she used it for objects distantly referring to food, such as dining-room, high chair, kitchen, apple and plum trees. These examples show the integration of original instinctive utterances by adjustment to growing needs.

Some authors, such as Bühler, Seth and Guthrie, [6] and others, admit an utterance to be linguistic only when and if it is the result of a judgment. This is merely a matter of classification. I should prefer to agree with Bloomfield [7] who defines a word as a 'free form,' i.e. "a form which can be uttered alone with meaning." . . . "A form ('form' always means 'meaningful form') which cannot be uttered alone with meaning is a *bound* form. Examples of bound forms are the suffix '-ish' in 'boyish,' 'girlish,' 'childish,' or the suffix '-s' in 'hats,' 'caps,' 'books.' . . . 'Boy,' which admits of no further analysis into meaningful parts, is a word; 'boyish,' although capable of such analysis, is a word, because one of the constituents, the suffix '-ish,' is a bound form." According to these definitions the examples given above are 'words.' A sentence is a linguistic form, i.e. a meaningful segment of speech which is not a constituent of any larger form. [8] As the child does, at this stage, not possess any larger form, his words are also sentences. The terms 'sentence-words' (Pelsma, Lukens) and

[1] Taine, H. (1877). "Acquisition of Language by Children," *Mind*, **2**, pp. 252–9.
[2] Woodworth, l.c., p. 175.
[3] Bateman (1917). "Papers on Language Development. I, The First Word," *Ped. Sem.*, **24**, pp. 391–8; O'Shea, l.c.; Smith (1926). "An Investigation of the Development of the Sentence," *Univ. Iowa Stud., Stud. Child Welfare*, III, No. 5; Gesell, l.c., p. 132.
[4] Quot. by Seth and Guthrie, l.c., p. 92.
[5] O'Shea, quot. by Jespersen, and Seth and Guthrie, l.c., p. 93.
[6] Seth and Guthrie, l.c., p. 92.
[7] Bloomfield, l.c., pp. 23–5.　　　　　　　　[8] Ibid., p. 27.

'one-word sentence' (Koffka) indicate that such forms are used in circumstances when adults would use a sentence. The stage of sentence-words coincides with the period of imitation, i.e. roughly from the second to the third half-year.[1]

Linguistic Babbling.—Since acoustic phenomena are fugitive, it is difficult to focus their details in perception. How far the child's perception of words equals ours we cannot say ; but our introspection, when dealing with a language not yet heard, suggests that it might be somewhat inadequate and imperfect. So far as observation goes, "the understanding of what is said always precedes the power of saying the same thing oneself—often precedes it for an extraordinarily long time. One father notes that his little daughter of a year and seven months brings what is wanted and understands questions while she cannot say a word." [2] The beginnings of this process appear at the level of 12 months.

As far as I was able to observe this stage, the first recognisable utterances which we are inclined to regard as words correspond not only to words but very often also to entire sentences, which are to a great extent distorted through elisions, assimilations, and so forth. The utterances are said to be distorted, but in so far as they are divided into distinct and significant parts, they should be considered as articulate.

What is articulate speech ? The word 'articulate' is of Latin origin—articulus is the diminutive of artus ; this again is related to arm, art ; the stem is AR 'to join.' The adjective 'articulate' means (1) united by a joint, composed of jointed segments, (2) distinctly jointed or marked, (3) of sound : divided into distinct [3] and significant parts ; speaking intelligibly. The verb 'to articulate' means the action that leads to the state expressed by the adjective. Thus : to attach by a joint, to form a joint with, and, finally, to divide (vocal sound) into distinct and significant parts, to pronounce distinctly,[3] express in words, utter.[4]

Other characteristics of speech, such as stress, intonation, etc., do not belong strictly to articulation, but they are so closely connected with it that they should be mentioned so as not to disturb the structure of our argument.

I call this kind of infantile speech, for the above reasons and in antithesis to prelinguistic babbling, *linguistic babbling*. In labelling it thus I want to indicate that two manners of speech are now overlapping and becoming integrated, namely : (1) natural, and (2) conventional.

The former is maintained first by the babbling character which manifests itself predominantly in primitive sounds and reiterations. These continue to be largely used, and only give way gradually to non-iterated utterances.

Examples are : *tumtum* = stomach, *shooshoo* = fly (Jespersen),[5]

---

[1] Seth and Guthrie, l.c., p. 106.   [2] Jespersen, l.c., p. 113.
[3] I.e. possessing differentiating characteristics, clearly perceptible or discernible by the senses or the mind (*Shorter Oxford Dict.*).
[4] *Shorter Oxford Dictionary* (1933), s.v.   [5] Jespersen, l.c., p. 179.

boom-boom = book, *nana* = naughty. Similar examples are, of course, found in other languages, e.g. French *peau-peau*, ' chapeau' (Sully), or Germ. *guch-guch*, ' Kuchen' (Ament), [akabaka], ' Onkel Jakob'.

In such variations the sounds change in accordance with certain rules which have to be regarded as fundamental, since they can be observed in all peoples and at all times. The underlying processes, such as elision, substitution, assimilation and others, will be met with in the phylogeny of languages and in speech disorders (see *Evolution of Language*, and *Disorders of Articulate Speech*).

Mentally, this type of speech is characterised by its emotional-volitional character.

As a result of further conditioning reiterations are gradually suppressed, particularly in conversation with adults. They may be used among other children until the age of about three. How are we to understand the disappearance of these infantile speech features ?

The child's mind has gone through many experiences which have caused him to realise that he lives in a group the members of which are expected to behave alike. Speech is so important a social link as to make the child adopt the group speech, or else speech loses its *raison d'être*. Thus whenever natural utterances crop up, they are opposed by conventional speech. If, for example, the child, expecting his mother to relieve his pain in the stomach says, ' tumtum ' and is not understood, he must feel induced to suppress the reiteration and so comes to say ' tum,' which makes the mother realise that something is wrong with the child's tummy.

With the first appearance of linguistic babbling, the cultural history of speech overlaps its natural history. The child will gradually give up being a linguistic individualist.[1]

The language peculiar to each child and adjusted to its needs is, when used for communication, enforced upon those around him. Its fringes will project into cultural, conventional language. They will gradually become smaller but will never disappear in the ontogeny and phylogeny of language (see pp. 50 ff.).

Natural language is from the age of about 12 months subjected to a continuous adaptation to the speech forms used in the child's environment. But we must never forget that natural characteristics, no matter whether they are innate or acquired in the first period of life, may ' disappear ' only phenomenally. In fact they are simply *overlaid* by other features. Being strongly canalised, however, they will always be ready to reappear should the circumstances be favourable.

Vocabulary.—Until the age of about 1½ years the growth of vocabulary is scarcely noticeable.

At the age of 18 months children have been observed to use 12 to 22 words.[2] There are, however, records of extraordinarily premature development. Jespersen[3] quotes the exact report on an American child who had in the tenth month 3 words, in the eleventh 12, in the twelfth 24, in the thirteenth 38, in the fourteenth 48, in the fifteenth 106, in the sixteenth 199, and in the seventeenth 232 words.

---

[1] Jespersen, l.c., p. 103.   [2] Seth and Guthrie, l.c., p. 99.
[3] Jespersen, l.c., p. 125.

The features of the child's speech undergo a decisive change at the age of 2, when it enters the ' naming stage,' W. Stern's ' stage of substance.' This is due to ' things ' being brought into relief out of the confusing medley of the environment. Accordingly everything gets a name, and the vocabulary therefore contains mostly substantives.

McCarthy's investigations [1] as to the various grammatical kinds of words correspond fairly well with those of others such as Zyve, Day, Smith. They all hold the view that at first the child's vocabulary contains 50 per cent. nouns, i.e. words which are used by the observers as the name of a ' person or thing.' [2]

Another considerable and sudden increase takes place when " at the close of the third year questions with ' Why ' crop up : these are of the utmost importance for the child's understanding of the whole world and its manifold occurrences, and, however tiresome they may be when they come in long strings, no one who wishes well to his child will venture to discourage them. Questions about time, such as ' When ? How long ?,' appear much later, owing to the child's difficulty in acquiring exact ideas about time." [3]

From 4½ to 5½ years the vocabulary grows again enormously and rapidly.[4]

Syntax.—Having realised the details of the outside world as units to which definite vocal expressions are attached, the child at the age of about 2 years or earlier [5] begins to ' put them together.' His speech becomes syntactic.[6] When two words are joined together they become ' *constituents* ' [7] of a new ' *resultant form* ' which we call ' *construction* ' (see Glossary). A syntactic construction results if the constituents are phrases.

The following instances quoted by Jespersen may illustrate the way in which ' sentences ' are being formed : " A Danish child of 2, 1 said the Danish words (imperfectly pronounced, of course) corresponding to ' Oh papa lamp mother boom ' when his mother had struck his father's lamp with a bang." . . . " Another child said, ' Papa hen corn cap ' when he saw his father give corn to the hens out of his cap." [8]

The various substantives have certainly not always got the ' meaning' which we attribute to them. They might well take the place of a whole sentence. Each of the constituents is rather a symbol of a peculiar concatenation of thoughts.

Sentence constructions originate also in another way, viz. by drawing ready-made groups of words out of sentences heard. An Austrian child's first ' sentence ' of this kind, uttered at the age of 1, 11, was: (piʃtame:dal). Only after numerous guesses was it possible to find the right meaning. It referred to the question : " Bist du ein Mäderl " (are you a girl ?) which the boy, still wearing girl's clothes, had been asked very often in fun. The boy's behaviour showed that this sentence implied to his mind the following meanings : (1) that the

---

[1] McCarthy, D. *Handbook of Child Psychology*, Clark University Press, Worcester, Massachusetts.

[2] Wyld, *Dictionary*.   [3] Jespersen, l.c., p. 137.
[4] Seth and Guthrie, l.c., p. 99.   [5] Gesell (1929), l.c., p. 134.
[6] Greek *syn*, ' together,' *tassein*, ' to put.'
[7] Bloomfield, l.c., p. 25.   [8] Jespersen, l.c., p. 135.

assertion concerned himself, (2) that he was called a girl (gesture), (3) that he agreed (intonation). The utterance represents *one unit* in every respect, though ' etymologically ' it can be proved to be derived from three words of different grammatical categories (substantive, verb, article). It is thus obvious that the acquisition of such conventional constructions is just a further step of sound-differentiation.

The little speaker has now become able to discriminate larger sound-units as being divided into smaller ones ; but the latter are not recognised as being capable of separation, however long the sentence may be. The smaller units (sounds, syllables, words) will not be recognised as such until the child learns to read and write.

This analytic process is active at all times. Every adult may observe it when picking up a foreign language. This language at first impresses him as a conglomerate of noises not divided into units (words),[1] which is similar to the above-mentioned experience of a baby. By careful observation of the behaviour of those around him, he gradually finds out to what these noises refer.[2] If he is ever going to classify words as nouns, verbs, etc., it takes a considerable time. Some languages will not bear such procrustean ' classification ' (see pp. 53, 58).

Thus ' real ' sentences, i.e. sentences conforming to those conventionally used, are at first nothing more than the outcome of further integration of acoustic patterns. The motor achievement is the easier, since speech sound production has already been practised, i.e. canalised for a considerable time.

Thus the child's ' natural ' syntax may greatly differ from the conventional one owing to what peculiar relations he establishes between himself and the things around him. The construction of sentences by deliberate ' putting together ' of speech-units gained by analysis is learned with considerable strain. It is only much later, generally at school, that the child comes to know the meaning of grammatical orders.

National language.—Only a relatively small step is required for a family language to grow into a national one. The infant-society's membership is open to the mother who must and does temporarily accept the rules of the group, manifest in linguistic babbling. This obviously distinguishes a social group with special mental and emotional characters. It is easily understood by members of this group who will respond to it and will use it so as to influence the other members of the group in the same way.

With the appearance of true and comprehensible syntax the transformation of speech into *language* is well under way, i.e. natural means of utterance are now used in accordance with the needs of an ever-increasing group, which uses a code combining all words by certain methods.[3] The process is, to be sure, not yet complete, as language involves also " the conventional use of vocal sound in communities."[4] The range of sounds is narrowed down to the number allowed by the code.

---

[1] Cf. Aphasia, pp. 85 ff.
[2] Cf. Reports of missionaries in savage countries.
[3] See *Shorter Oxford Dictionary*, s.v. Language.   [4] Bloomfield, l.c., p. 6.

Thus " the acquisition of language is not only an extension of the child's dominion over the world, but also an extension of society's dominion over him." [1]

We have abundant opportunity for observing that every speaker, every group, every nation, lives in a world of its own. This world is to be comprehended as a *structure* which finds and always strives to find its expression in language. We shall see later (pp. 105 f.) that this natural process eventually finds its limitation.

Dissociation of thought and utterance.—Our examination of the substrata of human activities, their development and evolution, has hitherto made it plain that any type of speech consists of a number of stratified patterns. This hierarchy involves all the characteristics mentioned, such as sensitisation, specialisation, conditioning, and inhibition, and so on.

In the course of specialisation the constituent mental and linguistic patterns acquire a certain independence as well as rigidity. More and more minute facts and concatenations of circumstances in the stimulating world are focused ; but the verbal expressions which refer to them are not always certain of being handed on. Thus the world is, as it were, pressed into pre-existing sets of words.

History and everyday life show that at any time these means may prove insufficient. When the individual comes to rebuild his world out of the parts gained by analysis, he uses words and all methods of grammar as acting forces, or tools to dominate the world. They are subjected to constant improvement if they do not come up to his requirements. Thus a constant re-creation of both the impressive and the expressive side of the world takes place. The world is perceived, as it were, as a mosaic, and an attempt is made to reshuffle the pieces, and to reconstruct the picture ; but because of their very shape they resist being rearranged, and compromises are enforced. ' Thought leapt out to wed with thought ere thought could wed itself with speech.[2] And now thought and speech must go along separate pathways ; mentation comes to be *dissociated* from verbalisation.

Verbal expression must, naturally, always lag behind, for ' Thought is deeper than all speech ; Feeling deeper than all thought ; Souls to souls can never teach What unto themselves was taught.[3] Verbal utterances learned from those around the speaker never correspond entirely to the speaker's thoughts. From the angle of evolution and development speech and language are more recent acquisitions than mentation. We must therefore presume a gulf between the latter and utterance ; a gulf which persists to a certain extent during the whole of the individual's life. The minimum of disproportion between thought and expression is to be found in poets ; we will consider this later under the heading of ' Diction.'

The kind and rate of this disproportion depends on the development of the more differentiated and independent faculties. There are periods of rapid growth and of inactivity. They differ in various individuals, sexes, and races and at various times. Sometimes

---

[1] Ogden, C. K. (1930). *ABC of Psychology*, Kegan Paul, London, p. 127.
[2] Tennyson, *The Princess*, xxiii.   [3] Cranch, C. P., *Stanzas*.

linguistic development keeps pace with mentation, sometimes it lags behind, sometimes it hurries on in advance.[1] The difficulties which handicap the speaker could be compared with the training of two fresh horses, harnessed to a carriage. They both may have the qualities which may fit them to pull the vehicle singly ; but when they have to co-operate, their peculiarities are constantly interfering with each other. It requires a skilful trainer to impose enough inhibition to ensure harmony of action.

Standard speech.—The child finally suppresses many traces of his natural mode of speech. These traces have by no means been lost, but have merely become submerged by new modes.

We have seen that child and mother form an at first indivisible unit which persists after birth as a unit of two separate individuals. It should now be stressed that to the child's mind the mother is obviously the other member of *his* group ; she is, therefore, a decisive factor in speech development.

This rôle of a group member is later on transferred by the child to other adults (the family in its broadest sense : parents, adult brothers and sisters, nurse, etc.), whereas young children under 4 " do not at first constitute a *group* in the psychological sense. They behave simply as a number of independent persons." . . . A child " will not look upon the other children as ends in themselves, but always as a means to serve or an obstacle to hinder his own particular interests." " . . . under the stress of a strong desire or a vividly conceived purpose, any young child may fall into this attitude on occasion. In itself it seems to constitute the primary matrix of social feeling, out of which all others are developed by experience of one sort and another." [2]

Psycho-analysis of children has shown that " for a large part of the time the children implicitly accept the grown-up as the natural leader of the group." [3] " There is indeed nothing that a child under five or six enjoys more than having a group of adults pliant to his will, doing what he suggests and admiring what he says and does." [4]

The development of standard speech will thus predominantly depend on the extent to which the child acknowledges the leadership of the adults around him. The growing individual will pick up from them as many means of communication as he is in need of to serve him for the rest of his life.

This process is in due time facilitated—and in some ways perhaps endangered—by learning to read and write.

The ideal language which man more or less consciously seeks would, according to Ogden, be characterised by the following canons : " (1) One symbol stands for one and only one referent. (2) Symbols which can be substituted one for another symbolise the same reference. (3) A symbol refers to what it is actually used to refer to." [5]

[1] This fact will show itself as of great influence in the formation of speech disorders, such as Cluttering and Stammering.
[2] Isaacs, S. (1933). *Social Development in Young Children*, Routledge, London, p. 213.
[3] Ibid., p. 267. [4] Ibid., p. 239.
[5] Ogden, quot. by Chase, S. (1938). *The Tyranny of Words*. Methuen, London, p. 72.

These statements seem to be mere truisms ; but history has shown in all its aspects that this goal has by no means been reached as yet. Many traps have been and still are laid on the way which make the speaker overlook (1) that words ' are ' not things ; (2) that words mean nothing in themselves ; they are as much symbols as X or Y ; (3) that meaning in words arises from context of situation ; (4) that abstract words and terms are especially liable to spurious identification. The higher the abstraction, the greater the danger ; (5) that things have meaning to us only as they have been experienced before ; (6) that no two events are exactly similar ; (7) that finding relations and orders between things gives more dependable meanings than trying to deal in absolute substances and properties ; (8) that to improve communication new words are not needed, but a better use of the words we have. (Structural improvements in ordinary language, however, should be made) ; (9) that the test of valid meaning is first, survival of the individual and the species ; second, enjoyment of living during the period of survival.[1]

Chase also stresses " that internal ideas, whether spontaneous or not, are felt before they are verbalised. The feeling is often vivid. I do know that meanings of this nature are charged with dynamite—brilliant, noisy, dangerous." [2]

The need for adequate verbalisation increases with the growing insight into the nature of the world. The gap between our ' ideas ' and their verbalisation manifests itself in the more or less conspicuous ambiguity of our utterances. We can only hope that man will be able to restrict linguistic ambiguity to the lowest possible degree, but it will never be possible to abolish it altogether. For " the growth of our understanding is among other things an increase in our discrimination, by which the big blooming, buzzing confusion from which we start is gradually distinguished into its components. Now our words must reflect the extent to which we have carried this process, the extent to which we have detected differences in things. They discriminate what we have discriminated, and confuse what we are still confusing. But, since we shall never have done clearing up confusions, our words will always be concealing differences, and there lies . an eternal possibility of ambiguity. . . . Whether an argument is ambiguous depends on what the facts are ; and our only way of knowing what the facts are is by argument and words." [3]

[1] Chase, l.c., pp. 116–17.   [2] Ibid., p. 122.
[3] Robinson, R. (1941). " Ambiguity," *Mind*, **50**, 198, pp. 145, 155.

CHAPTER IV

EVOLUTION OF SPEECH AND LANGUAGE

In accordance with Haeckel's Biogenetic Law, the development of speech and language which we have followed in the child may in principle be regarded as a recapitulation of human speech which must naturally have been going on for many thousands of years. We may therefore expect to find some traces of the basic features of the development of speech in evolutionary time.

Comparative Philology, Anthropology, Archaeology, and Biology furnish us with many parallels which have, of course, to be most carefully considered in order to avoid deception.

One of the outstanding difficulties is the fact that the state of evolution of peoples believed to show an earlier evolutionary level than, say, the peoples of Western civilisation, is not necessarily primitive. Those peoples have certainly gone through stages of evolution which have not yet been sufficiently explored, and perhaps never will be, because of lack of documents or other records.

But some features universally found may be believed to be real signs of earlier development. In comparing these and inferring from certain biological phenomena, we assume that the realms of phylogenetic evolution and history have something in common, an assumption which has been often denied. But recently E. Zilsel [1] has subjected this question to a philosophical examination, the result of which seems to justify our procedure.

Zilsel finds that "the realm of history comprehends human occurrences and their causes which are slower by one degree than the reactions of the individuals and faster by one degree than biological evolution." This definition deliberately neglects mental phenomena. It points only to the changes in the reactions of man, and thus avoids the gulf between the concepts of natural and 'mental' sciences. Furthermore, it gives "its due to the peculiarity of history by a quantitative criterion only and without involving metaphysics."

Introducing the criterion of velocity enables us to discover essential points in phylogenetic and historical development. Their "peculiar laws and causes correspond to the peculiar order of magnitude," and "it is the difference between tradition and heredity that corresponds to the different velocities of historical and biological evolution." . . . "Phylogenetic evolution goes on much slower than historical evolution, because, and only because, heredity is a much more powerful brake than tradition is." We have shown the rules of these developments in the respective chapters.

The age of 'homo sapiens' has been estimated at 25,000–40,000 years.[2] That of rudimentary speech might well be estimated as the

[1] Zilsel, E. (1940). "History and Biological Evolution," *Philosophy of Science*, vii, 1, pp. 121–8, Baltimore.
[2] Ritchie, J. (1939). "Perspectives in Evolution," *Nature*, pp. 534–8.

same. But let it be borne in mind that speech as intended for communication of symbols referring to mental states must naturally be
younger than biopsychological processes ; for the former is based on
the latter. We could imagine that, when the first representative of the
genus *homo* developed, he could already make use of basic patterns of
sound production which had developed during the evolution of animals.
The primary reflex pattern originated when animals had developed
auditory organs and were thus given the power of perceiving certain
vibrations as a special entity.[1]

Animal language.—We will not dwell on the production of noises
in insects which for example produce sounds by friction of the hard
parts of the integument,[2] but will only point to those animals which
produce voice by using the larynx, such as some hissing lizards, snakes,
birds,[3] and finally mammals. The latter have undoubtedly integrated
phonation to the purposive level. They have put the acquisition of
voice to the use of the survival of the individual or of the species.
Intimidation or want of help or food, sexual desires, keeping touch,
etc., are expressed in this way. To achieve this aim, dogs can bark
" in at least four or five distinct sounds." [4] " In Paraguay the *Cebus
Azarae* when excited utters at least six distinct sounds, which excite in
other monkeys similar emotions." [5] These utterances are so highly
canalised that " the animals do not increase the number of their few
natural sounds, nor do they show any impulse or tendency or need to
increase them as time goes on, except where man deliberately interferes
in order to effect a temporary increase in the imitative vocabulary, say,
of the parrot. The few instinctive natural sounds without increase
seem to satisfy the needs and capacities of the animal's mind, and to
correspond with its nature." [6]

We have seen that the production of noises is originally a random
emergence which occurs while the upper organs of digestion and of
respiration are operating. Thus we might infer the possibility of
noise production (1) through penetration of air into the tubes representing the respiratory or digestive tracts ; (2) during the escape of air
through these tubes. (Cf. Pseudo-voice, p. 195.)

It is therefore not impossible that both the lungs and the stomach
may be used as air-chambers for the production of noises, performed in
the mouth and throat, which are common to both systems. Thus
" animals can make sounds by expelling air out of the gullet, the
orifice of which is closed by muscular contraction. The Deathshead
Moth, for example, produces noises by forcing air out of its stomach." [7]

It is not to be wondered at that this primitive method of noise
production has not developed any further. As the degree of elasticity
of the orifice of the oesophagus cannot be altered appreciably, the
range of sounds and their loudness have certainly proved to be of
inferior value as compared with phonation by means of mechanisms
associated with breathing, which will be dealt with presently. But if

[1] Negus, l.c., chapter ix.   [2] Ibid., p. 297.
[3] Ibid., p. 299.   [4] Darwin, *Descent of Man.*
[5] Ibid.   [6] Wilson, l.c., p. 54.
[7] Landois, *Textbook of Human Physiology.* Quot. by Negus, l.c., p. 348.

the use of the respiratory tract is through disease made impossible for phonation, stomach-voice reappears and can be highly differentiated (see Laryngectomy, p. 196).

Voice.—The effector organ which serves phonation, the larynx, was originally a protective device for the lungs. It is essentially a valve which prevents foreign bodies of any kind from entering the lower air-tracts, especially the lungs, as has been thoroughly explained by Marshall, Stuart, and Negus.[1] It is, by the way, of interest to note that the aforementioned muscular band around the orifice of the gullet also has, in Negus's opinion, " the function of preventing entrance of air into the oesophagus during inspiration." [2]

The protective closure of the glottis has been retraced by Negus as far back as to the lung fish, axolotl salamanders, frogs, crocodiles, turtles, and birds.[3] It can thus be seen that the primordial structure of the laryngeal mechanism reaches far down the scale of evolution. This supports the view that the particular explosive noise produced by tight closure of the glottis appearing as the glottal stop in babyhood (see p. 28) is connected with instinctive attitudes towards events causing *danger*, which, seen from the introspective angle, amounts to *fear.*

Voice and its different attacks have been so thoroughly canalised that the new-born baby produces voice involuntarily by way of the medulla.

The glottal stop may be regarded as one of the most automatic patterns serving as symbols. The process of symbolisation may be illustrated by the following example: If some one unexpectedly throws a large piece of wood towards you, you will, among other smaller movements of the body, certainly also raise your hands, as a protective measure. Let us now give another example : If you are on good terms with your friend, and if he suddenly suggests you should do something entirely dishonest or immoral, you would, of course, refuse but would probably accompany your utterances by the above-mentioned movements of your arms. Your friend would thus recognise more fully your genuine reluctance ; even if you did not say a word he would still know.

Reading only the foregoing paragraph would not make it clear why raising the arms ' means,' I do not want, I reject your proposal, and so on. The two examples together make the explanation easy. Men have for many thousands of years raised their arms in circumstances similar to those in the first example, so that this pattern is now highly automatic. Its inherited aim is to parry a blow which affects the self. As this aim is involved in our latter instance, its reappearance is not to be wondered at, there being a coincidence of similar ideas. Thus two events have one thing in common, viz. the idea of keeping away something undesirable and are consequently ' thrown together,' i.e. symbolised.[4]

---

[1] Marshall, J. (1867). *Outlines of Physiology*, Human & Co., i.; Stuart, T. P. A. (1892). " On the Mechanism of the Closure of the Larynx," *Proc. Roy. Soc.*, **50**, p. 323 ; Negus, l.c., chapter ii.

[2] Ibid., p. 347.   [3] Ibid., pp. 122–3.

[4] Greek *symballein*, from *syn*, ' together,' *ballein*, ' to throw ;' hence a symbol is something which represents another thing. See Wyld, *Dictionary*.

As this movement like many others has been canalised in all human beings its meaning is easily understood. Likewise the closing of the glottis, resulting in the glottal stop, which was originally designed to protect the body from material danger, has in the course of time become a symbolic attitude towards any danger and consequently a symptom of fearful anticipation.

The foregoing considerations are in accordance with the over-whelming influence which the oral zone exerts in the early development of children, as elucidated especially by psycho-analysis.[1]

Speech-sounds.—Sounds other than those produced in the larynx are not known to be generally used by animals. Lips, tongue, and palate, which play their part in the development of speech-sounds, thus seem to have been utilised first by mankind. Their function may therefore be considered as evolutionarily younger, that is to say, less highly organised, less automatic and less rigid, therefore more adjustable but also more vulnerable.

As we descend the scale of language, i.e. pass from advanced linguistic systems to primitive languages, the sound table exhibits more varieties of speech-sounds.

Clicks.—Among the primitive sounds the clicks are particularly notable. They are highly primitive, and can be retraced to the apes. Man often addresses these by means of clicks, which implies the assumption that the expressive value of clicks is familiar to apes.[2]

In certain living languages, e.g. in the Namagua (Hottentot) language, in Bushman dialects, and Bantu dialects, clicks still consti-tute distinct and definite phonological patterns. They occur in almost every word in Hottentot, where they often precede other consonants, such as *n, h,* and all vowels.[3]

Clicks may undergo phonetic changes just as other speech-sounds ; they may become lateralised, palatalised, velarised, and so forth [4] (see p. 31, and Sigmatisms, p. 154).

Clicks also play their part among civilised people as emotional expressions. The dental click expresses impatience, pain, and so on, the alveolar click manifests approval or pleasure, the palatal expresses admiration, the labial is a decoying sound and a symbol for kissing,[5] the lateral is used in encouraging horses.[6] "When a Chinese drinks a mouthful of good soup, he gives a hearty smack." [7]

It is perhaps worth remarking that 'smack' means "a smart explosive sound in kissing or tasting anything," [8] and that the word

[1] Cf. Isaacs, S., l.c.

[2] Stopa, R. (1939). *Die Schnalzlaute,* 3rd Int. Congr. of Phonetic Sciences, Laboratory of Phonetics of the University, Ghent, p. 331.

[3] Havelacque, A. (1877). *Science of Language,* translated by A. H. Keane, Chapman & Hall, London, pp. 49.

[4] Van Ginneken, l.c., pp. 322–3.

[5] Chatterji, Suniti Kumar (1939). *Evolution in Speech Sounds,* 3rd Int. Congr. of Phonetic Sciences, Laboratory of Phonetics of the University, Ghent, p. 340.

[6] Stopa, R., l.c., p. 331.

[7] Liu Yutang (1938). *The Importance of Living,* Heinemann, London, p. 49.

[8] Wyld, s.v. smack (III).

4

probably originated by introducing the imitation of a natural sound in word building.[1]

It characterises the emotional mentality (though highly developed) of the Chinese, when Liu Yutang says : " As for the so-called table manners, I feel sure that the child gets his first initiation into the sorrows of this life when his mother forbids him to smack his lips."[2] When he suggests that " one ought to imitate the French and sigh ' Ah ' when the waiter brings a good veal cutlet, and make a sheer animal grunt like ' Ummm ' after tasting the first mouthful,"[3] he furnishes a nice example of the use of primitive hummed sounds.

Clicks have become rare in the languages of to-day, being transformed into expiratory consonants. In South Africa and in the Caucasus the first part of the initial sound in most words is still 'clicked,' whereas the second part has already become an expiratory consonant.[4]

One would not like to go quite as far as Van Ginneken who believes that apparently there were no vowels in the archetypes of language. Interjections, such as [ps : t, s : t], are according to him still persisting examples of those very first phases of speech ; this explains also the otherwise unintelligible fact that Old Egyptian has no vowels, and that Old Semitic and Old Ouralo-Altaic orthographies use characters for consonants only. It can tentatively be assumed that in primordial speech, expressions containing clicks alone and voiced utterances coexisted, and that later the two became integrated (see also **p. 31**).

The amount of clicks and other primitive sounds was presumably very large on primitive levels of language. But on higher levels also, such as that of the presupposed Indo-European common tongue, the diversity of speech-sounds was much wider than was believed by those who reconstructed its sound system in the last century.

Reiteration.—The reiteration tendency which plays so great a part in the child's period of primitive sounds can also be traced in the languages of primitive peoples. We find words consisting of mere reiterations in languages of every evolutionary stage up to Greek and even modern languages. In languages of a relatively primitive kind they possess either no special meaning, or they have developed into expressions of emphasis, plurality, etc., for example, the vernacular name of the Hottentots *khoikhoib*, ' man of men ' or ' friend of friends,' indicating plurality or gradation,[5] *pow-wow* ' palavar ' (Algonkin-Indian).

Lubbock[6] has shown us that in descending the scale of evolution, reiterated syllables become increasingly conspicuous in the vocabularies concerned. Phylogenetically young languages, such as English, French, German, and Greek, exhibit only about two or three words, consisting of reiterated syllables, per thousand words, whereas the Brazilian Tupi contains 66, Hottentot 75, Tonga 166, and Maori 169 of these.

---

[1] Skeat (1887). *A Concise Etymological Dictionary of the English Language*, Clarendon Press, Oxford, s.v. smack (2).
[2] Liu Yutang, l.c.   [3] Ibid.
[4] Van Ginneken, l.c., p. 323.   [5] See Havelacque, l.c., p. 48.
[6] Lubbock, J. (1889). *Origin of Civilisation*, Longmans, Green & Co., London, pp. 523-5.

We can often trace their course from baby talk into standard languages, e.g. English *gee-gee,* ' horse.' Lat. *Turtur* is an iteration of ' tur,' which is itself an onomatopoeic imitation of the dove's cooing. Engl. *turtle,* Germ. *Turtel,* Ital. *tortora, tortola.*[1] Talkee-talkee : (1) broken English, esp. of negroes, (2) incessant, futile, idle chatter ; useless, empty loquacity.[2]

Phonetic changes.—The times of Voltaire, who could sarcastically assert that in etymology the vowels mean nothing, and the consonants scarcely anything (" où les voyelles ne font rien et les consonnes fort peu de chose "), have long been superseded. It is now common knowledge that words have ancestries, and that certain words in the same or different languages are kindred with each other. The rules which indicate the development of sounds, words, morphological structure, syntax and so on are now fairly well worked out. No one who has traced the historical development of languages would, for example, doubt that the English word ' cheer ' [tʃiə] is kindred with French ' chère ' [ʃer] which, again, is the offspring of Latin ' cara ' [kara]. It is also agreed that the Indo-European velar plosive [k] has developed into the palatal sound [t] in Greek, and into [kŭ] in Latin before palatal vowels (Greek, tis ; Lat. quis ; cf. Engl. wh- as in what). Every etymological dictionary provides many similar examples, but we may consider one in some detail.

How has Lat. *cara* changed into Engl. *cheer ?* It is, first, recorded that Lat. [a] was at a later date pronounced with elevation of the front of the tongue, which led to a change of resonance resembling [e]. In every succession of movements one pattern influences the neighbouring one. Thus in anticipation of the following elevation of the blade of the tongue towards the palate for [e], the articulation of [k] was slightly altered, the place of contact between tongue and palate being brought forward. This again produced a change of resonance in the direction of [t]. Later the vowel [e] was differentiated into the diphthong [ie], which becomes by a further rise of the front tongue [je]. The [j] then led to the development of [ʃ] or [tʃ].

This was the state of things in the Middle Ages, both in France and in England, when the word was introduced. In France the [j] was then incorporated into the [ʃ], which was probably ' mouillé ' (cf. *Filia*—fille [fij], that is to say, palatalised. Finally the [t] disappeared.

This example shows the interaction between motor tendencies and acoustic stimulation. ' Random ' variations may at first produce very slight changes ; in the course of development the resonances become perceptible to the ear, which in its turn influences the motor pattern.

There are many other tendencies, such as velarisation, assimilation, labialisation, etc., which play their part at a given time and in given social groups (families, societies, nations).

The phonetic changes are certainly to be regarded as natural, and manifesting universal tendencies. If, on the other hand, we can state that one and the same word adopts differing features in different people, races, and at different times, it is due to the interaction of these

---

[1] Skeat, l.c., s.v. turtle.   [2] Wyld, *Eng. Dict.,* s.v.

tendencies with particular social influences, which on their part shape a given language.

To attempt an examination of the psychological and social factors would lead us too far afield. Suffice it to quote Jespersen, who ascribes the fertility in linguistic changes of some particular period to the diminished influence of parents and grown-up people generally; he also thinks that " there may be periods in which the ordinary restraints on linguistic change make themselves less felt than usual, because the whole community is animated by a strong feeling of independence and wants to break loose from social ties of many kinds, . . ." [1]

Phonetic factors manifesting in assimilation, elision, etc., tend, if allowed to exert their influence, to change the course of development from extreme multiplicity of sounds and long words towards unifying the sound table and shortening the words. The Gospel of St. Matthew contains in Greek about 39,000 syllables, in Swedish about 35,000, in German 33,000, in Danish, 32,500, in English 29,000, and in Chinese only 17,000.

But let it be borne in mind that phonetic tendencies do not signify anything of themselves; they have to be considered in connection with the meaning they convey.

Vocabulary.—The strong unity of thought and action at the onset of human development manifests itself clearly in the extremely rich vocabulary of primitive tribes, such as the Pygmies, the Australian natives, the Eskimos, and others. A multitude of subordinate notions can and must be expressed by special words. [2] In Tasmanian there is no word for ' tree,' but each species of tree is named. The Mohicans have special terms for cutting various objects, but they have no word to express the idea of cutting.

All these observations seem to indicate that verbal expression is always strongly dependent on the individual's needs. The same applies to the classification of words. In Tasmanian there are no adjectives, similes being used in their stead; the reason is, no doubt, that it is easier to observe a concrete object which can be used in comparison than to abstract the notion of an attribute. [3] Moreover, the fact that the Tasmanians have not separated qualities such as hard, long, etc., from the object, suggests that to their mind there was no social or any other necessity to do so.

The same considerations have to be applied to other categories of words. In primitive languages, " conjunctions of a purely formal or logical significance, such as our copula, are rare or entirely wanting. They are obviously a very late product of linguistic development, and appear only when thought has reached a high level of abstraction." [4]

Morphology.—Inflexional forms seem to have sprung from a compact flow of sounds referring to highly individual situations. States and qualities which the classifying mind of man includes under the cate-

---

[1] Jespersen, l.c., p. 260. [2] Ibid., p. 427.
[3] Jones, E. (1918). *Papers on Psycho-Analysis*, Bailliere, Tindall & Cox, London.
[4] Werkmeister, W. H. (1939). " Natural Languages as Cultural Indices," *Philosophy of Science*, 6, 3, p. 360. See also *Paragrammatism*, p. 79.

gories of gender, number, tense, etc., vary frequently and in many ways ; we can therefore quite easily see the enormous multiplicity of grammatical forms which occur in certain primitive languages and which are very difficult to understand. This accounts also for the rigid use of ' irregular ' forms in those languages.

The more man has been induced to master the outside world and to adjust himself to it, the more he has tried to divide the original units into significant smaller units, which can then be attached where needed. These represent grammatical categories for which European languages have sometimes no analogy or equivalent. Take as an example the Wintu language phrase ' pom oltikalulesunikilake,' which would, somewhat inadequately translated, read ' the land flashed-*like*,' that is, the land was covered with bright flame-coloured poppies. The construction not only shows the length of the word, but also hints at the vagueness of the distinction between word, inflexion, and syntax in the present sense.

Some progress is shown in that the Wintu unit ' ulesuni ' (which the reader will see in the above phrase) has become an *infix* [1] indicating that the speaker " likens something unknown to something within his experience. The burden of proof is left, then, to the event itself, not to the speaker ; or the speaker gets out of all responsibility for the truth or falsity of his statement by implying that something has the appearance, only, of being such-and-such, so far as he knows." [2]

Languages gradually develop into " analytical languages, which have the power of kaleidoscopically arranging and rearranging the elements." [3] " The direction of movement is towards flexionless languages (such as Chinese, or to a certain extent Modern English) with freely combinable elements ; the starting-point was flexional language (such as Latin or Greek) ; at a still earlier stage we must suppose a language in which a verbal form might indicate not only six things, like ' cantavisset,' but a still larger number, in which verbs were perhaps modified according to the gender (or sex) of the subject, as they are in Semitic languages, or according to the object, as in some Amerindian languages, or according to whether a man, a woman, or a person who commands respect is spoken to, as in Basque. But that amounts to the same thing as saying that the border-line between word and sentence was not so clearly defined as in more recent times : cantavisset is really nothing but a sentence-word, and the same holds good to a still greater extent of the sound conglomerations of Eskimo and some other North American languages. Primitive linguistic units must have been much more complicated in point of meaning, as well as much longer in point of sound, than those with which we are most familiar." [4] " Now, it is not only the forms themselves that are irregular in the early languages, but also their uses : logical simplicity prevails much more in Modern English syntax than in either Old English or Latin or Greek." [5]

---

[1] A modifying element inserted in the body of a word (*Oxford Dict.*).
[2] Lee, D. D. (1938). " Conceptual Implications of an Indian Language," *Philosophy of Science*, 5, 1, pp. 101–2.
[3] Jespersen, l.c., p. 334.   [4] Ibid., p. 425.   [5] Ibid., p. 333.

Syntax.—" In historical times we see a gradual evolution of strict rules for word order, while our general impression of the older stages of our languages is that words were often placed more or less at random. This is what we should naturally expect from primitive man, whose thoughts and words are most likely to have come to him rushing helter-skelter, in wild confusion. One cannot, of course, apply so strong an expression to languages such as Sanskrit, Greek, or Gothic ; but, compared with our modern languages, it cannot be denied that there is in them much more of what from one point of view is disorder, and from another freedom." [1]

Retrospective survey.—" The sum total of these changes, when we compare a remote period with the present time, shows a surplus of progressive over retrogressive or indifferent changes." [2] " That language ranks highest which goes farthest in the art of accomplishing much with little means, or, in other words, which is able to express the greatest amount of meaning with the simplest mechanism." [3] It is still true that " thus all languages are, like us, imperfect. . . . They have all been made successively and by degrees according to our needs." [4] But certainly some languages and some speakers have succeeded in making verbalisation a powerful instrument in mastering the world. This is achieved by cleverly maintaining the happy medium between the structure of language and that of the facts as they appear at a given moment. " Language as it has developed is less influenced by reflection than thought is influenced by the accepted structure of language." [5] What we regard as the outside world has been constantly subjected to our efforts to define its structure. Its pattern has been, is, and will always be changing, and thus " there can be but little doubt that the difference between the older and the more recent linguistic forms corresponds to a difference in the ways of thinking." [6]

The unity of linguistic and mental patterns is in a constant train of separation, differentiation, and stabilisation, thus giving rise to fresh units which in their turn are always interacting. It is obvious that there must be innumerable possibilities of moulding and shaping both linguistic and mentation patterns. Thus every individual, every group lives in a world of its own, in accordance with the evolutionary level. ' Things,' ' actions,' ' states,' ' qualities,' ' modes ' and so forth owe their existence to this.[7]

Language creates new words whenever the speakers are in need of them, so that the growth of language is marked by the appearance of neologisms. Once they are established they tyrannise over our minds in such a way that older ways of expression are suppressed ; they become ' awkward,' ' queer,' ' abnormal,' and even ' unintelligible.' Linguistic means in a given group at a given time are thought to be the only possible and adequate expressions, and are then ' valued ' accordingly.

[1] Jespersen, l.c., p. 356.   [2] Ibid., p. 326.   [3] Ibid., p. 324.
[4] Voltaire's *Philosophical Dictionary*, selected and translated by H. I. Wolf (1929), Allen & Unwin, London.
[5] Chase, l.c., p. 43.   [6] Werkmeister, l.c., p. 360.
[7] Cf. ibid., p. 361.

A few examples may illustrate this. If you want something from another place, you will simply 'fetch' it. Not so in China. "In Chinese . . . one does not 'fetch' me something, but one 'goes takes comes gives me.'"[1] You would then express your gratification by saying "I am happy"; but an Eskimo could only say, "Happy being me."[2]

"The more advanced a language is, the more developed is its power of expressing abstract or general ideas. Everywhere language has first achieved expressions for the concrete and special."[3]

Language and speech.—There are no utterances, no languages, no kinds of speech, but only *beings* using certain kinds of communication, such as sounds, letters, gestures, gramophone records, etc., which ensure their sustenance and other needs.

We have now indicated how living creatures have developed into speaking and language-gifted beings. In other words, we have studied the integration of the constituent units in the course of emergent evolution. (The careful reader will notice that the 'integration of the constituents' *is* 'emergent evolution'!) But we find that the 'parts' of speech, such as sounds, voice, etc., have been isolated by linguists after the event, by dissection as it were. That does not mean that these artificial units do not play a useful rôle in preserving language, especially in the hands of the poet, who is able to subordinate stress, melody, rhythm, sound, to emotional motives.

Speech is said to be a function, that is to say, activity; but it might also be regarded as a function in a more mathematical sense. In so far as any of its particular features vary in conformity with the variation of the many stimulating external and internal factors, it resembles a mathematical function.

Over and over again our minds are impressed by the comparison of speech with some noble old cathedral, say Mont St. Michel, in the architecture of which centuries have co-operated. The finished structure gives a glorious unified impression; on closer inspection, however, one discovers variety of style. In just the same way speech as a whole shows a superimposing of structures which represent categories derived from practical "attitudes of the child and of primitive or natural man to the surrounding world."[4]

The same simile may well be applied to mental functions. They likewise show a stratification which, under certain conditions and at certain levels of development, may overlap with speech patterns. But it should be borne in mind that, though speech can be the expressive side of psychic processes, we are not entitled to conclude that the essential nature of thought must necessarily consist in speech. The latter is only one of the possible behaviours which betray mentation.

Having examined the 'unfolding' of the means of communication, we are now in a position to establish the references between the words we use and the facts. There are two words, viz. 'speech' and 'language,'

---

[1] Werkmeister, l.c., p. 358.   [2] Ibid., p. 359.
[3] Jespersen, l.c., p. 429.
[4] Malinowski in Ogden, C. K. and Richards, I. A. (1923). *The Meaning of Meaning*, Kegan Paul, London, p. 497.

which seem to be equivalent at first sight ; and this is apparently
confirmed by the definitions given in the dictionaries. But the ordinary
man would admit without hesitation that ' speech ' is the wider concept.
and ' language ' the narrower one. Language involves speech, whereas
not all speech is language.

If we take speech and language as phenomena which have become
what they ' are,' according to our evolutionary examinations, it appears
that language is the *more recent differentiation* of utterance.

From a certain level on, language becomes more and more independent ; that is to say, it follows its own particular track, developing
its own rules, though resting on the well-canalised mechanisms of
speech. The latter are handed on by inheritance as automatisms
which are, on higher levels still, modifiable in the individual's development. Linguistic rules are imposed on the speaker through tradition ;
being very young they are apt to undergo comparatively rapid and
manifold changes (cf. pp. 59 f.).

Aspects of voice and speech.—Speech and Language can be looked
upon from different viewpoints. These are : (1) the physical aspect ;
(2) the neuro-physiological aspect ; (3) the biological aspect ; (4) the
philological aspect ; (5) the psychological aspect ; (6) the artistic
aspect. It will not be possible, however, to avoid overlapping in
describing these aspects.

The physical aspect allows two points of view, viz. (1) the motor,
and (2) the acoustic. These two constitute the most superficial view,
for they are regarded merely as movements and noises performed in
the material realm. The moving articulatory organs appear like
marionettes ; but the puppet-man and his wire-pulling remain in-
visible.

It is important, however, to understand the construction of our
marionettes in order to know what we can expect of them.

Our marionettes are distinguished by their accidental ability to
produce noises. If we regard these noises as independent entities we
can subject them to an investigation of their physical structure.

The neuro-physiological point of view deals with the wires moving
the marionettes, through instigating the contraction and relaxation of
the muscles.

The psychologist acknowledges speech as a means of expression of
our thoughts, emotions, etc. Considering that man is only a unit of
that greater unit the social group, it must be looked into as to what
extent it serves the purpose of linking the members of the group
together.

The biologist sees in speech just one of the many adaptive
mechanisms which characterise life.

Philology may be said to start where biology stops. It deals with
the nature and evolution of speech from the time when it acquired
a degree of specialisation and differentiation of sounds which are
codified in the languages of peoples.

Phonology studies the sound system of a given language and the
laws governing their changes.

It has been given considerable support by a younger branch,

Phonetics, which is concerned with the physical and physiological rules involved in the mechanisms for the production of voice and speech.

Phonetic alphabets.—It is well known that spelling is often an inadequate means of conveying accurately the features of a given sound. Phonetic sciences therefore have produced systems of transcription in order to make good this deficiency. They are based on different classifications : (1) on the motor aspect of speaking ; (2) on the sensory aspect.

(1) Jespersen [1] has suggested a system by which any sound can be represented by symbols and figures indicating the organs of articulation, their particular position, shape, and the degree of narrowness of the articulating chamber. The transcription thus effected resembles a long chemical formula.

The sounds [p], [b], and [m] can in concordance with Diagram No. 1 be represented by formulas : [p] = βbo, $v$lo, μ2 ; [b] = βbo, $v$lo, μo ; [m] = βbo, vl2, μo.

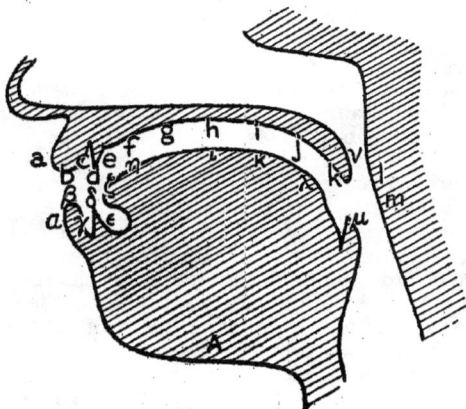

Diagram No. 1.
9–0 degrees of decreasing aperture.

(2) The Alphabet of the International Phonetic Association employs the symbols used in the spelling of the sounds of the European languages, as far as they indicate sounds by *one* symbol. Where this is not the case new symbols have been introduced. Thus the initial sound heard in the English word ' shoe,' being represented by two symbols, is phonetically spelled [ʃ]. Many other symbols are required for variations of vowel shades (cf. Engl. vowels in father, cow, fly, cab, etc.) or in cases of ambiguity (Engl. thin, than).

Other systems use diacritic signs, indicating variations or deviations from a given sound. When, e.g., the original [l] in the Latin word *filia* in some French dialects becomes ' mouillé ' (palatalised), this change is indicated by ' (l').

[1] Jespersen, O. (1904). *Phonetische Grundfragen*, Leipzig.

The spelling system of some European languages (Czech, Serb) is based on this method.

It is necessary to be acquainted with these systems of transcription, for in many speech disorders we find peculiar articulations which deserve the minutest description, if we are to find out the nature of the deviation. It will depend on the specific purpose which of the systems of transcription may be found useful.

Peculiarities of some languages.—Everything in the evolution of mankind and its behaviour seems to suggest that the primordial utterances of our ancestors were long sets of sounds of immense variability. These must, as comparative philology shows, have developed into certain types of language which still had " a superabundance of irregularities and anomalies." " They were capricious and fanciful and displayed a luxuriant growth of forms." [1]

As far as meaning and articulate expression were brought into systems, we can in the rough discriminate three types ; these have been termed by philologists, inflexional, agglutinating, and isolating languages.

Agglutinating languages express relations by simply placing significant elements in close association. This system is used in the majority of the known languages : to give only a few examples, in the Hottentot and Bushman dialects, Bantu and many other African languages, in Australian and Malyo-Polynesian idioms, in Japanese, the Finno-Tartaric languages such as Finnish, Hungarian, and Turkish, the languages of the American Indians, and Basque.

A Hungarian example may illustrate the principle : *vár*, ' he waits;' *várja*, ' he awaits him;' *várják*, 'they await him,' where *ja* denotes the direct pronominal object, and *k* the plural.

In Turkish a number of suffixes are added to the leading word, whereby various shades of the manner of being of the same action are expressed. " Thus *ma, me* being the negative particle, the infinitive *sevmek*, to love, will yield *sevmemek*, not to love ; *dir* denotes causality, *il* the passive, and *in* the reflex idea ; hence *sevdirmek*, to cause to love ; *sevilmek*, to be loved ; and *sevinmek*, to love oneself. But these and other such suffixes may be combined together, resulting in such forms as *sevinmemek*, not to love oneself. In this way every root might furnish some fifty derived forms." [2]

Inflexional languages, such as the Semitic and Indo-German, express relations not only by combining the word conveying the leading notion with suffixes or prefixes, but also by modifying the sound-structure of the leading word itself ; e.g. English sing, sang, song, sung ; Greek derkomai, dedorka, edrakon.

Unlike the suffixes in agglutinative languages, those of inflexional languages cannot be separated from the stem and cannot exist as independent words ; e.g. Greek oikoi, ' at home,' cannot be divided into oiko, ' home ' and i, ' at,' though probably at some prehistoric period such a division was possible. [3]

[1] Jespersen, l.c., p. 428.   [2] Havelacque, l.c., pp. 97, 102.
[3] Giles, P. (1895). *A Short Manual of Comparative Philology*, Macmillan, London and New York, p. 33.

In the isolating languages such as Chinese, Tibetan, Annamese, words essentially correspond with general conceptions, and are not modified into forms denoting person, gender, number, time, mood, etc. The relational meanings are determined by their mutual position in a phrase, and by intonation ; e.g. *Yu tê chih jên,* ' have virtue's man,' i.e. ' a man of virtue,' the genitive being expressed by the juxtaposition of *chih,* the original meaning of which was ' go to.'

There can be found gradual transitions from one type to another in many languages. In English, for example, all types are found.

We are far from recognising the exact evolutionary scale into which these and other systems may be placed, but it seems that " the evolution of language shows a progressive tendency from inseparable irregular conglomerations to freely and regularly combinable short elements." [1]

It may perhaps not be superfluous to say a few words as to why we have dwelt on this subject which is seemingly a purely philological one. The reason is this : our examples show that the methods of conceiving the world and of expressing how we live and experience it are manifold. Comparing sound units, grammatical and syntactical forms found on evolutionary levels with similar ones occurring in a given pathological case, will give us a clue as to the nature of the latter's personality both as regards his mentality and his speech.

This will become clear in our explanation of disorders of articulate speech, where phonetic changes (see Dyslalia) or deviations of sentence formation (see Paragrammatism) will appear in a new light.

Peculiarities of the English language.—The comparative philologist notices several characteristics of the English language which distinguish it from other highly developed languages. These peculiarities have given rise to misunderstandings among English people and among foreigners. The foreigner who attempts to acquire this language finds it at first sight ' easy,' easier indeed than most other languages he happens to have learned. How does this come about ? It is due first and foremost to its simplicity of grammar, i.e. the comparatively small number of inflexional forms. Sound changes of all kinds have more or less blurred the phonetic character of all languages descending from the Indo-European mother-tongue. There are still a great number of forms for tenses, modes, and declensions in the languages cognate with English (Greek, Latin, Slavonic, Albanian, etc.). Progress in the English language has abolished almost all forms of inflexional forms. Consequently many words can act, to speak in terms applicable to more inflexional languages, as verbs, nouns, adjectives, and so on, without altering their forms ; e.g. *fast* signifies ' firmly fixed,' ' rapid ' (adjective), ' to go without food ' (verb), ' the period appointed for fasting ' (substantive) ; *round* may indicate ' the property of having a circular outline ' (adjective), ' a circle ' (substantive), ' to make round ' (verb), or express direction (preposition).

Influenced by this development, English syntactical construction is most free in the arrangement of its constituents. So great is this

[1] Jespersen, l.c., p. 429.

flexibility that relations can be expressed in much greater variety and precision than in other languages, a fact mostly overlooked by the foreigner who naturally, being bound by the rules of his own language, cannot readily adjust his mind to a more subtle world-view and its outward expression. Note, e.g., the difference of meaning between ' I am being extravagant ' and ' I am extravagant.' [1] Such characteristics induced the German philologist Jacob Grimm [2] to point out that " in wealth, good sense, and closeness of structure, no other of the languages of to-day deserve to be compared with it, not even our German, which is rent, even as we are rent, and must first rid itself of many defects, before it can enter boldly into the lists as a competitor with the English."

We will now glance at the speed with which the English language has grown. Up to the time of King Alfred (871-900), Celtic was spoken in the West and North of the island, while in the South, East and Centre the Teutonic or Saxon dialects were predominant. Latin, which had hitherto been the official language, was during Alfred's reign replaced by Anglo-Saxon.

Through the Norman Conquest (1066) the development of Anglo-Saxon was led into other pathways, Norman French being exclusively spoken by the upper classes. The lower and middle classes, particularly in towns, gradually learned this foreign language and thus became bilingual.

The infiltration of French during the 300 years from 1048-1348, ten generations, was very slow and gentle. Many local dialects of Anglo-Saxon were spoken in the small and compact units of the populace, which constituted the manorial system.

The most profound change was probably caused by the Black Death in 1348. Among its many effects, the break-up of the old manorial system is perhaps the most remarkable. The shortage of servants forced the well-to-do classes to allow their children to be nursed by people speaking Saxon. This caused a much closer and compulsory contact between French and Saxon-speaking people and ' English ' could now be formed as the last vernacular integration. " Before the end of the first third of the 15th century English . . . . [is] the universal tongue, because . . . [it was] the end of the longest lifetime of those who were brought up as children after the Black Death." [3] " Chaucer's English is no longer the dialect of a particular geographical area, but rather a fully developed literary or official form of speech which shows considerable dialectal mixture." [4] It is already characterised by the French order of words and a simplified, freer syntax, and seems like modern English.

The Black Death also cut England off from the general culture of the Western Continent. And so under the Stuarts at the beginning of

---

[1] For more details see Jespersen, O. (1924). *Philosophy of Grammar*, Allen & Unwin, London.
[2] Quot. by Keane, A. H. (1878). *Handbook of the History of the English Language*, Longmans, Green & Co., London, p. 170.
[3] Belloc, H. (1934). *A Shorter History of England*, Harrap, London, p. 189.
[4] Wyld, *The Historical Study of the Mother Tongue*, p. 212.

the seventeenth century English "was always the same language, ignorant of scientific terms, and instinct with a poetical feeling about life that was native to the whole generation of those who used it. Its fault, corresponding to the state of thought in that age, is·want of exactness and of complexity in ideas, that renders it unfit for psychology or for close analysis of things either material or spiritual." [1] In modern time it has again undergone an enormous improvement as to its vocabulary which renders it superior to most languages.

Estimating the period from the Indo-German mother-tongue until modern English tentatively at about 10,000 years, we can follow up a relatively slow development which was interrupted by a growth of relatively immense velocity between the middle of the fourteenth and the beginning of the fifteenth centuries.[2]

Behaviouristic peculiarities.—It is evident that, as language and thought through their very nature originally form one unit, a correlation between the means of expression and the mentality of those using them must be assumed. Evolutionary considerations show that our behaviour constantly tends towards the checking of primordial responses, and it seems that through this very process the emergence of new characters, especially of a more cognitive nature, is activated.

Throughout the whole world we can trace a scale of inhibitory achievements. At the one end stand certain primitive peoples who exhibit expressive movements of practically the whole body. The Polynesians, for example, use even their back muscles in expression. In Europe, the nations of Slav and of Roman origin are highly demonstrative in expression, whereas those of Teutonic stock have developed towards better behavioural control. Thus Slav and Roman nations are "determined really to 'live' their lives; they yield to their emotions and give outward expression to them; when they love or hate, they feel happy or sad; they consider it the right thing to yield to these emotions and, so to speak, enjoy their flavour to the full. In doing this the Latin shows moderation and the Slav shows none, while the Englishman avoids it as far as he can and the German oscillates between the two ideals. To one type the suppression of the emotions seems unnatural and gives a feeling of hypocrisy; the other type regards the uncontrolled expression of emotion as undignified, ill-bred, vulgar, almost bestial."

A somewhat similar outlook is characterised by the immobile and smiling attitude of some oriental peoples, especially the Chinese and Japanese.[3]

Almost all characteristics of small and big groups or social classes can be reduced to this formula. Disregarding it leads to misconception which the speech therapist, having to deal with the whole of this

[1] Trevelyan, G. M. (1919). *England under the Stuarts*, Methuen, London, p. 54.
[2] This rapid achievement of comparative perfection may still be playing its part in the peculiar features of some speech disorders in English-speaking countries, but I am as yet unable to give more than a mere surmise.
[3] See Cohen-Portheim, P. (1936). *England, the Unknown Isle*, Duckworth, London, pp. 41 ff.

complex, must carefully avoid. Taking into consideration the aforementioned formula, he will not be misled by what he might regard as
qualities such as false modesty, silence, cynicism, puritanism, senti-
mentalism, concealed ambition, passion for liberty, conventionality,
shyness, etc.[1]

[1] As to the English, cf. also Maurois' charming *Conseils à un jeune français
partant pour l'Angleterre* (1938), Grasset, Paris.

CHAPTER V

PATHOLOGY

Dissolution.—In the foregoing chapters we have been trying to follow the development and evolution of speech up to its present stage, in answer to the question already put by Herbert Spencer : " How came it to be thus conditioned ? " This question must naturally be followed by : " How will it cease to be thus conditioned ? " [1]

The consideration of cosmic, geological, chemical, and biological facts convinced Spencer that events cease to be what they are by some antagonistic process which may lead to the disintegration of matter. This negative process, the 'taking to pieces,' he called Dissolution.[2] The more appropriate term would, in fact, be Devolution, though it would seem from the connotations given in Wyld's *Dictionary*, that the two terms are almost equivalent. But the former term is so commonly used, particularly through Hughlings Jackson who introduced it into medicine, that we must adhere to it. Jackson characterises dissolution as " being the reverse of evolution. . . . It is a process of undevelopment; it is a ' taking to pieces ' in order from the least organised, from the most complex and most voluntary, towards the most organised, most simple, and most automatic. I have used the word ' towards,' for, if dissolution were up to and inclusive of the most organised, etc., if, in other words, dissolution were total, the result would be death. . . . Dissolution being partial, the condition in every case of it is duplex. The symptomatology of nervous diseases is a double condition ; there is a negative and there is a positive element in every case. Evolution not being entirely reversed, some level of evolution is left. Hence the statement ' to undergo dissolution ' is rigidly the equivalent of the statement ' to be reduced to a lower level of evolution.' In more detail : loss of the least organised, most complex, and most voluntary, implies the retention of the more organised, and the less complex, and the more automatic. This is not a mere truism, or, if it be, it is one that is often neglected. Disease is said to ' cause ' the symptoms of insanity. I submit that disease only produces negative mental symptoms answering to the dissolution, and that all elaborate positive mental symptoms (illusions, hallucinations, delusions, and extravagant conduct) are the outcome of activity of nervous elements untouched by any pathological process ; that they arise during activity on the lower level of evolution remaining. The principle may be illustrated in another way, without undue recapitulation. Starting this time with health, the assertion is that each person's normal thought and conduct are, or signify, survivals of the fittest states of what we may call the topmost ' layer ' of his highest centres : the normal highest level of evolution. Now, suppose that from disease the normal highest level of evolution (topmost layer) is rendered functionless. This is the dissolution to which answer the negative

---

[1] Spencer, *First Principles*, p. 235.   [2] Ibid., pp. 241–2.

symptoms of the patient's insanity. I contend that his positive mental symptoms are still the survivals of his fittest states, are survivals on the lower, but *then* highest, level of evolution. The most absurd mentation; and most extravagant actions in insane people are the survivals of their fittest states. I say ' fittest ' not ' best ' ; in this connection the evolutionist has nothing to do with good or bad. We need not wonder that an insane man believes in what we call his illusions ; they are his perceptions. His illusions, etc., are not caused by disease, but are the outcome of activity of what is left of him (of what disease has spared), of all there then is of him. His illusions, etc., are his mind." [1] " . . . The reverse process of dissolution is not only ' a taking off ' of the higher, but is at the very same time a ' letting go ' of the lower. If the governing body of this country were destroyed suddenly, we should have two causes for lamentation : (1) the loss of services of eminent men ; and (2) the anarchy of the now uncontrolled people. The loss of the governing body answers to the dissolution of our patient (the exhaustion of the highest two layers of his highest centres) ; the anarchy answers to the no longer controlled activity of the next lower level of evolution (third layer)." [2] It has also to be remembered that " dissolution from disease is rarely if ever the exact reverse of Evolution. . . . We have to bear in mind not only the Dissolution, that which is effected by disease in the sense of pathological change, but also the Evolution going on in the undamaged, healthy, remainder." [3]

H. Jackson discriminates two kinds of dissolution, Uniform and Local Dissolution. (1) " In Uniform Dissolution the whole nervous system is under the same conditions of evil influence . . . but the different centres are not equally affected." The comparatively lower, i.e. more organised, centres resist longer. (2) Dissolution may affect only one part of the nervous system (e.g. the cortex, the striatal system, etc.), and thus cause a local reversal of evolution, in the same sense as in Uniform Dissolution, i.e. from voluntary towards automatic.[4]

Functional and organic disorders.—We now pass on to consider two chemical examples so as to illustrate the *degrees of stability* which are inherent in the processes described.

If, for example, carbonmonoxide (CO) comes into contact with steam (H_2O) there arise carbondioxide (CO_2) and hydrogen

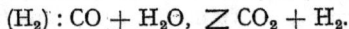

$$(H_2) : CO + H_2O, \; \rlap{\diagup} Z \; CO_2 + H_2.$$

This goes so far that $\dfrac{CO_2 \times H_2}{CO \times H_2O} = k$ (a constant dependent on the temperature). Adding more steam makes the reaction go back, so that we regain CO and H_2O. The reaction is thus *reversible*.

The explosive substance ammonium nitrate, on the other hand, tends to disintegrate into N_2O and $2H_2O$, which cannot be reintegrated. This reaction is an instance of an *irreversible* process.

In both processes structural changes take place, similar to those

---

[1] Jackson, l.c., ii, pp. 46–7.   [2] Ibid., p. 58.
[3] Ibid., p. 436.   [4] Ibid., p. 47.

produced in the body. The chemical reactions taking their course in the organs of the body determine the ' function ' of the organs.

It is customary to speak of functional disorders, as long as we cannot, by means of the methods of investigation at present in use, detect any stabilised structural change of the tissues concerned. More or less stabilised structural changes caused by more or less irreversible reactions constitute disorders commonly named organic.

We have been surveying the natural tendencies which have given rise to what is called the standard of any given language, and which always foreshadow further developments. We are now in a position to make an attempt to deal with those modes of utterance which deviate from the given standard.

In doing so we must obviously adhere to the same general principles and pursue the course which led them eventually into what is called a disorder. The speciality concerned with these aims is Pathology. It will prove useful to make a few preliminary remarks on the concepts and terms used in Pathology.

Diagnosis.—The immediate aim is to establish the Diagnosis. The word is derived from the Greek verb *gnonai*, ' to know,' and the prefix *dia*, ' between,' hence the meaning ' to distinguish.' [1] It may be noted that Diagnosis consists of a mass of perceptions all having a meaning. But it is more than a mere collection of notions. Diagnosis thus means the act and result of identifying a disease through the knowledge of its history, symptoms, and signs, and their relation. It certainly involves a definite structure and organisation like any other true knowledge, and this stratification of knowledge is assumed to represent in some way the processes which have caused the disorder to emerge.

Disposition.—All influences act upon already existing, firmly joined structural and functional arrangements, the sum of which, peculiar to each individual, constitutes his disposition.

Disease.—A disease represents any impairment of a well-established and firmly cemented pattern. The structures are either too weak for what is asked of them, or else they become damaged by extraordinary demands. Disease may therefore be regarded as the permanently or temporarily unsuccessful attempts of a living being to combat noxious influences. These are noxious inasmuch as the individual is not or not yet adjusted to them. [2]

According to the evolutionary rules elucidated above, we must also take into account the level on which the morbid factor operates. Going down the scale of evolution we find increasing automatisation and stabilisation. We must therefore, given the same influences, expect greater vulnerability on higher levels of evolution. On the other hand, the structure of the pattern will be more severely impaired if morbid factors succeed in affecting the lower levels, which constitute the framework of the pattern.

Psychopathology.—It has been noted (see p. 30) that we speak of physical or psychic phenomena, according to the angle from which we

---

[1] Cf. Wyld, *Dictionary* ; *Encyclopaedia Britannica*, s.v.
[2] Cf. Schleich, C. L. (1916). " Aus Asklepios' Werkstatt," *Deutsche Verlag-sanstalt*, Stuttgart and Berlin, pp. 27-31.

look at the same process. Thus processes which for convenience are spoken of as psychic follow the analogous rules of change to those of physical processes.

Psychopathology is the science which deals with disordered psychological processes, always bearing in mind that we use a *term of convenience*. From the pragmatist's standpoint, we often convince ourselves in daily life that reactions, movements, functions of living creatures change when we influence them through words, gestures, or other stimuli. These are themselves the outcome of some chemico-physical reactions which can only be detected by special means. As long as we cannot or need not think in chemico-physical terms, we say that the reactions in question are psychically brought about, and the phenomena themselves are *psychogenic*.[1]

It has often been said that functional and mental processes are *interwoven*, as though they were two separated and clearly distinguishable entities. Thus, for example, Core says : " The emotional factor in the formation of functional disorders is of fundamental importance, and as such is to be included in any definition of them that is based upon a pathogenic conception. . . . Functional nervous disorders are inherently associated with defective emotional control." [2]

This can certainly be agreed with, but we must still ask ourselves whether it is expressed correctly. Is it not perhaps an amalgamation of classification concepts which, if not perceived, might cause confusion ? It seems to me that here again language imposes its yoke on us, which we then gladly bear, feeling quite at ease in this slavery.

We speak, for instance, of Sigmatism as a functional disorder, whereas Stammering is grouped with psychogenic disorders. The reason is that as a rule we cannot detect any decisive psychological factors causing the disordered articulation of the hissing sounds, whereas in stammering the emotional factors are in the foreground. In the chapters concerned we will endeavour to show that this by no means strictly holds good in any case. Thus we will regard the distinction between functional and psychic disorders as a matter of convenience, viz. as labels corresponding to the most noticeable characteristic in the deranged evolutionary pattern.

From the point of view of development and evolution, it is hardly possible to discriminate between psychogenic and ' purely ' functional disorders. Psychological factors may not be easily observable, but not to assume its presence would render our task of rebuilding all the harder, since we should be fighting an unknown enemy.

Therapy.—Upon a clear perception of a given pathological state, we can then rest our hopes of restoring the desirable pattern ; we can, in fact, carry out therapy.[3]

We have put forward the view that all human actions have developed out of more general attitudes principally through basic ' conditioning.' It has been considered " very rash to describe the mind as wholly built up of conditioned reflexes," . . . " so that, by

[1] psyche, ' soul ' ; genēs, ' born of, derived,' from gignein, ' to bring forth.'
[2] Core, D. E. (1922). *Functional Nervous Disorders*, Bristol, p. 7.
[3] Greek therapeuein, ' to serve,' ' to attend upon.' Wyld, *Dict.*

proper conditioning and environment, a baby can be turned into any kind of man." [1]

What is particularly objected to is the ignoring of the fact that constitution plays a part, and that the latter is inherited. But Jennings describes as a "fallacy that what is hereditary is certain, fixed, unchangeable." ". . . To assert that a thing is hereditary signifies merely that the organism has received such a constitution as to produce it under given conditions." It will be easily understood that ". . . this does not deprive of significance recognition of the part played by heredity in medicine ; which is but recognition of constitutional differences that have origin in diversities of the germ cells. The individual who may produce an inherited defect under certain conditions need not produce it under others." [2]

Thus in view of the amazingly subtle changes which could be established by proper conditioning, we do not hesitate to hold an optimistic view. If we succeed in reaching a level that has remained intact—and this is what all theories of psychopathology ultimately attempt to do—we may hope that by proper means we shall be able to help nature in rebuilding the hierarchy of patterns which would satisfy the needs both of the patient and of his social environment.

As far as the means of the material world (medicaments, diet, etc.) are applied, we are tackling restitution of a disintegrated mechanism physically and ignoring the reverse side, viz. the psychological.

Psychotherapy.—In endeavouring to influence the disordered mechanism by primarily psychological factors, we are using psychotherapy.

In the chapter on development, we emphasised the overwhelming influence and the stratification of ' meaning ' in behaviour. " Effective psychotherapy," therefore, as MacCurdy rightly points out, " often or always rests on producing a change in meanings."

Re-creative treatment.—As to the technique of psychological treatment we must refer to the textbooks (see Bibliography). But we shall expound such particular procedures as are indicated by the special character of some speech disorders. Here it may be pointed out that in dealing with disorders in which actions are predominantly affected the technique must—apart from other aetiological methods—avail itself of such methods as involve action. An action is by no means a simple unit, but the offspring of a hierarchy of behavioural (i.e. mental and motor in one) patterns. Our efforts must, therefore, consist at first in consciously and deliberately leading the patient back to such levels as allow him to find a firm foothold. Only then can we try to help him forward again. His and our efforts will be constructive in so far as a pathological pattern is first split into parts which then serve as building stones for the re-creation of such patterns as render the individual fit to meet environmental needs. Emphasis must be laid on this statement, for it stands in contrast to the common belief that actions, and speech activity in particular, can be corrected (literally ' led straight ') by mere exemplification. If this were possible,

[1] Sullivan, l.c., p. 149.   [2] Jennings, l.c., pp. 63-4.

our patients would not exist as such, being as a rule constantly surrounded by correct patterns !

Anyone who has taken the trouble to observe carefully nature's way of building up motor patterns will realise how delicate this task is. He will also assuredly appreciate the gain from such studies.

Prognosis.—Prognosis [1] is the process of judging the further development of a pattern in the course of disintegration, or of reintegration.

Our opinions naturally rest on previous experiences and observations which, in their turn, become true cognition if they are based on the knowledge of the natural tendencies in evolution and dissolution.

The degree of stability implied in structural change (see pp. 64 f.) which constitutes a given disorder, must be carefully assessed. On this assessment depend the line of treatment and the results obtained. It will prevent the therapist from being too optimistic, expecting and requiring too much at a time of his patients, and will save him disappointment and discouragement.

[1] pro, ' beforehand ' ; gnōsis, ' knowing.'

CHAPTER VI

SPEECH DISORDERS. GENERAL

Diagnostic examination.—By taking the point of view of dissolution, the speech therapist finds himself in a favourable position when he has to face a special disorder for the first time. Bearing in mind the sequence of levels through which ' standard ' speech has been developed, he has but to go back from it until he finds characteristic evolutionary symptoms by which the patient's speech can be determined.

Since we are dealing with disorders of speech, i.e. deviations concerning a *function,* we must first and foremost endeavour to analyse the latter. Further investigations will sometimes be necessary as to the anatomical state of the organs which are involved in a speech disorder, because they may also be diseased.

The speech function is examined by listening to the speech and by observation of the movements of the patient.

In some cases it seems advisable to aid the eyes and ears by various recording apparatus which will be mentioned in the respective chapters.

The first task is to find out whether speech can be used by the patient as a social link at all. At the first interview we should try to get in contact with the patient, child or adult, as we do when we meet a person in daily life. We observe his general attitude, manner of walking, sitting down, facial expression, etc.

We greet him in a friendly manner and observe his responses. We engage him in ordinary conversation. During this we shall be in a position to note deviations as to syntax, morphology, semantics, vocabulary, articulation, and voice. Indications as to what special signs and symptoms are to be paid attention to will be given in the chapters concerned. Short stories secure a basis for judging the patient's power of understanding the meaning of a verbal statement which he hears, and of reproducing it.

The following story, which I commonly use, may easily be altered as to the words, sentences, etc., according to our particular purpose and to the peculiarities of the patient. In the following version it is put in the simplest way :—

The Sick Lion

Once upon a time there was a lion. This lion was ill. While he was ill all the animals came to see him.

The first was the wolf. As the wolf came into the den, the lion asked him : " Don't you think there is a bad smell in my den ? "

The wolf answered : " Yes, there is a bad smell in your den."
The lion became furious because the wolf was so rude, and he ate him up.

The hare was waiting outside. Being asked in, he thought he would be wiser.

Having greeted him, the lion asked the hare : " Don't you think there is a bad smell in my den ? "

The hare answered : " No, I think there is a lovely smell in your den."

The lion rose in rage, saying : " You are a liar," and ate him up.

Next came the fox. When he was asked the question : " Don't you think there is a bad smell in my den ? " he replied politely and excusingly : " Dear lion, I could not say, because I have got a bad cold in my nose and so I cannot smell anything."

This story has proved to be one which arouses the interest of nearly all patients.

Case history.—During the first interview with a grown-up patient we can often make inquiries as to the patient's history. If this is not possible, for reasons involved in the patient's ailment, age, or mental state, we should do it afterwards. There are two reasons for not doing it *before* the first conversation : (1) According to our dissolution principle we are able to deduce a great deal as to the possible or likely factors which have influenced the given disorder. It is then easier to lead the discussion on previous facts into the right track. (2) As speech is one of the outstanding social links, it must naturally be most painful and discouraging to the patient to submit to or to suspect a discussion about it, which he then regards as a ' secret tribunal.' This feeling must not be under-estimated even in little children.

The results thus found must now be brought into a certain order. Relying on our evolutionary considerations, we must fit them into our scheme of levels, layers, and so forth, as shown in Chapters I-V.

Tables of child development, such as given in Appendix II of *Abnormal Speech*,[1] prove useful guides.

General Remarks.—It is evident that we have got to proceed on different lines when interviewing a child or an adult patient. A case history must needs keep two main points in view : what we want to find out and how we are to set about it. The difference between the adult patient and the child in this respect mainly concerns the second point. As to what we want to find out, we know that information of a certain quantity and quality must be got in both cases, the child's and the adult's, to enable us to understand the patient ; the way to extract this information must necessarily somewhat vary with each case. But there is one important difference between interviewing a child and an adult : the greater part of the information about the child must be got from his parents, guardian, teacher, or relatives.

Let us first consider the way of eliciting information about a child. The child comes in, sometimes very much frightened at the idea of having to see the therapist, and is generally accompanied by mother or father, sometimes by both of them. Mostly the parents are only too ready to give information about their child. The more enlightened parents send their child out of the room before telling us about him, others do not mind speaking in front of the child. Both ways are to

[1] Publication No. 91, Children Bureau, U.S. Department of Labour, quot. by Boome, E. J., Baines, H. M. S. and Harries, D. G. (1939). *Abnormal Speech*, Methuen, London, pp. 119 ff.

be avoided. Children should never be made the topic of conversation when they are present, but neither should they be made to mistrust their parents as well as the therapist ; they inevitably imagine that what is going on behind the closed door is, in some way, to their disadvantage, else why should they have been sent away ?

Parents and children ought to be interviewed separately but not ostensibly so. The first interview had best be of a sort of general friendly conversation, by means of which we can make friends with the child and gather very essential impressions about the relations between parents and child and its social behaviour, quite apart from forming our opinion about his individual defect of speech. An appointment to see the parents alone is easily made without the child noticing it. This interview is very important. Quite apart from the knowledge we want to gain about the case, we must keep in view that children should only be asked questions about their pursuits and interests, friends, etc., and never about themselves. Not only do such questions about themselves tend to foster a morbid interest in their own personality, which is doubly dangerous in the case of neurotic children, but they also have the effect of making them self-conscious and unnatural, thus greatly impeding our observation.

The interview with the parents will give us a reasonable amount of information, not always so exact as to satisfy us completely, but generally enough to enable us to draw the necessary conclusions. Observation of the parents, of their relation to each other and to the child, of what questions are readily and openly answered and what are evaded, is of great assistance in forming our impressions.

Our next meetings with the child must be devoted to establishing friendly relations with him, gaining his complete confidence and eliciting the most important information he can give : the unconscious revelations about his personality made by his general behaviour. Needless to say, the symptoms of his particular defect of speech must be carefully observed.

In some cases the picture will be complete very quickly, sometimes we shall have to see the child quite a number of times to understand the case thoroughly. We may, now and then, have to make one or the other intelligence test, be it only to confirm the general impressions we have got.

The history of an adult has certainly got two things in common with that of a child : the winning of the patient's confidence and the gathering of the significant information given us unwittingly by what he says and what he leaves unsaid, and by his general behaviour.

It is obvious that we cannot, in general, get the material facts about adult patients from other sources of information than themselves, although that might sometimes be very desirable. So we must content ourselves with questioning them carefully to help our observation. It is, however, sometimes possible to get supplementary information from relatives or friends.

As to what kind of information we want to get, we must say that we want to know practically everything that there is to be known about him, his *milieu*, his family, ancestors, etc.

A questionnaire such as the following, based on that compiled by Dr. Boenheim,[1] may be of help in taking case histories :—

Name. Age. Sex. Age of parents. Status of parents before marriage. (Mother working ? Father's occupation. Was father or mother an only child, etc.) Are grandparents still living ? Do they live with their children and grandchildren ? Uncles and aunts ? Does family form sort of clan ? Diseases in family ? Hereditary diseases in family ? Alcohol ? Insanity ? " Nervousness ? " Left-handedness ? Peculiarities of speech, in family ? State of mother during pregnancy (bodily and mental) ? Delivery ? Health of child during stages of development up to present ? (Spasms in babyhood ? Diseases ?) Lazy sucker ? Put on weight and grew normally ? Normal periods of crying, or much given to whimpering ? First sitting up ? First attempts at walking ? First attempts at speaking ? Further development of speech ? First symptoms of speech disorder ? Development of the disorder ? Any striking changes after any illness ? When were parents first alarmed by symptoms of defect ? Was the child's speech corrected at home or at school ? Was he laughed at because of it ? Did anyone talk baby-talk to the child ? Did change of teeth seem to affect speech ? Did any of the other children speak particularly well ? Do parents or teachers or patient himself know under what conditions symptoms grow worse ? Is defect more marked at work, school, or at home ? Does patient apparently suffer in consequence of his defect ? Do the parents (or the patient) believe in any particular cause of the defect ? Sound sleep over normal periods ? Scared when left alone ? Systematic education from birth onward ? Clean within normal time ? Digestive trouble ? Subject to colds and catarrhs ? Pavor nocturnus ? Adenoids ? (If removed, when ?) Bed-wetting ? Development of teeth ? (family). Goes to school ? Went to Kindergarten ? Social status ? Standard of living ? Flat ? House (garden) ? Mother has complete charge of house and children ? Do children sleep with parents ? How many persons sleep in one room ? Does anyone in the home do night work ? Do children play in street much ? Are they sometimes kept up late ? Are hours of meals, sleep, play, and work regular ? Position in family : Only child ? Eldest child ? (if not, how many brothers and sisters, what rank ?) Spoilt ? (if so, by whom most ?) Tyrannical in nursery ? (At play ?) Subservient to any brother or sister ? Distinct predilection for any member of family ? Remarkable change of behaviour after some major illness ? Poor eater ? Has to be coaxed into taking food ? Slow eater ? Greedy ? Anxious to get proper share of everything ? Generous ? (Reverse ?) Fussy ? Difficulties when going to bed or rising ? Position in sleep ? Nightmares ? Dirty or clean ? Neat or untidy ? Special children's vices ? (picking of nose, etc.). Timid ? Bold ? Afraid of the dark ? Excessive imagination ? Given to ' story-telling ? ' If boy, likes to play with things boys usually like or prefers dolls, etc. ? (The reverse question for girl.) Has the child ever heard that a child of the other sex would have been

[1] Boenheim C. (1938). *Practical Child Psychotherapy*, John Bale, London, Appendix.

preferred ? Is the child or any other child of the family specially talented ? Any talent 'hereditary' in family ? Any virtue (e.g. to tell truth at all costs) specially appreciated and emphasised in family ? Relations between parents ? Did parents wish for children ? Did they wish for the patient ? Is there any 'black sheep' in the family ? If so, is it the patient ? Has either of the parents favourites among the children ? Is any member of family supposed to be an object of special consideration ? Did patient (or any member of family) ever gain anything by being ill ? Education severe ? Corporal punishment ? Is punishment meted out as in a court of justice, as it were ? Are younger children treated more leniently than the older ones ? Is (or was) patient fond of society of children ? Generally solitary or social ? If social, actively so ? Good mixer or leader ? Any tendency to bullying ? Tale bearer ? If at school, what subjects are preferred ? Games or studying preferred ? Bookworm ? Courageous at games and sport ? If so, naturally so or by fear of criticism ? Are team games or single games preferred ? Very ambitious ? Given to moods or merry disposition ? Specially obedient or disobedient ? Steady worker or by fits and starts ? Given to subterfuge and taking the easiest way ? Given to remorse ? Quick or slow ? Tendencies to pampering himself ? Self pity ?

CHAPTER VII

SPEECH DISORDERS. SPECIAL

The successive order in which we are now going to arrange deviations of speech and voice implies an evolutionary classification ; that is to say, we place every disorder on that phylo- or onto-genetic level, which provides a symptomatological parallel. We are aware of the fact that for didactic purposes this classification might cause inconvenience, for it disconnects disorders which, seen from other angles, would belong to the same group. We will take this disadvantage into account so far as it proves necessary by adding other classifications.

On the other hand, the evolutionary classification enables the speech therapist to answer the question as to the severity and the prospects of a given disorder. " Going down step by step, we get evidence that the forms of deviation are at the same time also degrees." [1] Be it recalled that " the meaning of ' step ' and ' degree ' was originally the same—stages in an ascending or descending scale or process." [2] We can thus " assess through the symptoms the severity of a disorder . . . and . . . become independent of the often unreliable history." [1]

This applies also to those cases where, on the one hand, the speech symptoms may represent useful and even the *only* hints to the neurologist, laryngologist, etc., if their clinical examination has been negative ; on the other, it may suggest additional treatment that would otherwise have been overlooked (see Addental Sigmatism, Hoarseness, Dysarthric Disorders).

We have seen that evolution in its differentiating and specialising tendencies never stops. On the other hand, there is a limit placed, which is determined by the conditions of the environment.

The individual as a communicating organism thus always forms a highly stratified, but little stabilised unit with its environment.

One of the most highly developed capacities of the speakers is to adapt speech and language to a special aspect of the world, the world they are living in.

This world may be focused in innumerable ways. Language has to follow our ever-fresh experiences of the interrelations which constitute the substratum of the ' world.'

Progress in language thus implies all the changes of syntax, grammar, vocabulary, articulation, phonation, etc., serving this purpose (see Chapter on Evolution of Language and Speech). The complex of such modes of speech, which we have already seen growing, constitutes *diction*.[3]

---

[1] Stein, L. (1940). " On Disorders of Articulate Speech," *Brit. Med. Journ.*, i, June 1.

[2] See *Oxford Dictionary*.   [3] See pp. 43, 105 f.

It is in this diction that we shall see some disharmony if conditions become pathological.[1]

What then can be done about an individual who has been building up his world during a series of years, thus acquiring certain modes of utterance, and who suddenly finds himself faced with a 'world' the description of which he cannot convey clearly to those with whom he is associating by the speech rules of this group ? He will obviously be only in a position to make use of the possibilities provided by this same speech.

A good example of such cases of disharmony is given by Dementia Praecox (Schizophrenia, Hebephrenia).

Judging by their utterances these patients often appear like ' scatterbrains.' The listener is extremely puzzled because the patient utters ' real ' sentences, but there seems to be no connection between the constituent parts of the sentence, or in a sequence of sentences.

One of MacCurdy's patients said, " He kicked the door and she had a baby." This sentence ceases to be meaningless " if it be known that forcing a door in any way is a symbol for sexual intercourse." [2]

This example shows how the patient is, so to speak, floating between two levels. In the first part he finds himself on the lower level, where concrete expressions replace more abstract ones. It can be seen that by dissolution this level has been freed so that it can act. The utterance, therefore, manifests a ' negative ' symptom in so far as it is seemingly nonsense ; on the other hand, it is the ' positive ' influence of a formerly lower level, now a top level, giving rise to a ' neologism.' The second part of the sentence requires no explanation, being a ' normal ' expression.

This kind of speech gives us the impression of a monster. It reminds us of those prehistoric animals which through their excessive ' progress ' were no longer adapted to their environment, and were doomed to extinction. The same destiny threatens the speech of the Schizophrene and those with similar diseases.

Nothing remains to be said about treatment. Nothing can be done as to the re-adaptation of this speech unless the environing world regains in the speaker's mind the aspect it has in the minds of those around the speaker.

Similar processes are continuously going on in the development of language, where they greatly contribute to its progress. And any given ' last stage ' of development presents us with words which carry in themselves the hierarchy of emotional and cognitive meanings grafted on successively through the ages.

Take the English word ' believe.' It expresses our approval of a thing which is thought to be true ; but it expresses more than thinking because it carries in itself the former more emotional meaning of being pleased with a thing, holding it dear ; it is kindred with Latin *libet*,

---

[1] " Diction is a mixed sensory and intellectual act by which the words are not only united with the idea but also linked with syntax and grammatical form, in order to give the thought its full expression. Disturbances of diction might be termed Dysphasia." Kussmaul, *Die Störungen der Sprache*, 4th ed. 1910. Quot. by Gutzmann, l.c., p. 258.

[2] MacCurdy, l.c., p. 27.

'it pleases,' Latin *libido*, ' desire,' Sanskrit *lobha*, ' desire,' which also survives in the word to love, i.e. to like.

The ways of semasiological growth are sometimes so twisted and obscure that the connections between several words can hardly be traced. Who would, for example, at first sight think that the English word *mild*, ' soft, gentle,' has derived its present meaning from an etymon [1] the offspring of which is *melt*, ' to make soft,' and that these words have their origin in common with Engl. *mallet*, Lat. *malleus*, ' hammer'; Engl. *mellow*; Old Slavonic *mladu*, ' young '; Engl. milk, mill, to mention only some of this extensive word family.[2]

What is it then that distinguishes the growth of meaning, the vicissitudes of the words of normal language, from those connotations which words acquire in abnormal speech ? Apart from the phonetic changes which are throughout the ages unavoidable, it is apparently at first the degree of velocity which matters.

In normal development the progress is very slow and gradual, continuously keeping pace with the requirements of the environment. In abnormal speech the development is more or less unbridled, because the higher levels have lost their control over the lower ones.

We shall have the opportunity of seeing this principle, already foreshadowed in our evolutionary considerations, at work in many speech disorders.

LACK AND LOSS OF SPEECH

So far we have merely glanced at an example in which speech patterns of a high order, i.e. well-divided constructions, are preserved ; but the world in which the speakers are living has a different aspect to ours, and is therefore represented by words whose meaning is no longer, or even not yet, familiar to us.

We will deal presently with a class of disorders in which the power of symbolic conception of the world and of its symbolic representation (Head's " Symbolic Formulation and Expression ") [3] is more seriously disordered.

Aphasia and Mutism.—The Greek term for the use of language is phēmi, ' I declare,' ' I clearly proclaim,' derived from a root BHA, to shine, to appear.

Patients who are incapable of symbolising verbally or are restricted in doing so, i.e. in showing by their speech what they live and experience, suffer from Aphasia or Dysphasia. The term answers the question as to the existence of speech in the negative and therefore presupposes its former existence ; thus the term points to a more or less complete *loss* of speech.

Children who have been prevented from acquiring this capacity of speech are said to be suffering from Mutism (*mutitas*).

---

[1] The primary word from which a derivative is formed (*Oxford Dict.*).

[2] See Müller, M. (1882). *The Science of Language*, Longmans, Green, London, ii, pp. 349–67.

[3] Head, H. (1926). *Aphasia and Kindred Disorders of Speech*, Cambridge University Press.

CHAPTER VIII

APHASIA

Let us, to begin with, bear in mind that patients who are roughly classed as speechless are nevertheless making some sort of response to the world by living in it ; but we must not forget that the kind of living represents a highly integrated pattern which we have seen developing from childhood onward.

Reviewing the development and evolution of speech, we recall that it has sprung out of many superimposed reflex loops. Thus there have emerged more and more integrated patterns of speech—and also of thought. They always strive to preserve the original shape, though many other reflex loops join in. In the course of development the 'fringes' of the pattern differentiate afresh ; they become outgrowths which tend to become independent. In the end speech and thought constitute a large whole in which many smaller units more or less co-operate. There is a constant process of analysis and synthesis culminating in harmonisation, co-ordination, etc., still going on, which is largely determined by environmental conditions. These influence the type and the degree of specialisation and canalisation of the units.

The area where all the pathways conveying the stimuli effecting speech and thought converge has already been described (see p. 24) ; but within this area there are fields where special pathways meet which, if blocked, obliterate special parts of the speech pattern, thus giving rise to Aphasia, i.e. the more or less complete loss of the conventional linguistic patterns. The types of Aphasia can be classified in accordance with the speech areas involved.

Motor forms of Aphasia are localised mostly in the anterior part of the speech area (chiefly the frontal lobe) and sensory forms in the posterior part (mainly the temporal lobe).[1]

It must, however, be emphasised that pure forms of motor or sensory Aphasia are practically never met with. Nor can reading be isolated from writing, so that mostly Alexia and Agraphia (lack of the faculty of reading and writing) are found combined.

This classification, therefore, can nowadays merely serve the purpose of clinical orientation.

Taking the view that these functions are in the process of dissolution, we are to expect deviations of behaviour similar to the normal behaviour in the building up period : *similar* and not equal, because the dissolution process does not affect all the well-differentiated and canalised patterns in the same way.

The dissolution point of view therefore enables us to adopt a method of classification, which in contrast to the anatomical one, *grades* pathological speech patterns according to their evolutionary order.

All pathological processes affecting the cerebral speech area, such

[1] Pick, A. (1925). "Aphasie." Bethe's *Handbuch der normalen und pathologischen Physiologie*, Berlin, xv.

as injuries, degeneration, tumours, inflammation, disturbances of the blood circulation, and intoxications, may cause Aphasia both in adults, and in children who have already acquired speech.

Psychological influences may also play their part in impairing verbal symbolisation and understanding.

AMNESTIC APHASIA

In this relatively mild type of Aphasia the patients' vocabulary is reduced in varying degrees. They have difficulty in naming readily, and in writing and drawing. Some cases appear to be quite all right, but, put in unfavourable circumstances, e.g. told to explain a somewhat unusual event, they get into obvious difficulties. Sometimes the difficulty is not apparent, but the patients themselves show or declare that they cannot find the appropriate word for, let us say, a given colour.

But strangely enough the power of naming is not really lost ; it sticks, as it were, to the environment ; that is to say, it has adopted a more primitive method which combines the object with its verbal property more firmly. One of Gelb and Goldstein's cases did not recognise or recall the conventional names of colours, but he could say ' cherry colour,' ' grass colour,' ' like an orange.' [1]

Patients are orientated in time but may fail to name the hour, which they describe correctly as " when you eat " or " when we went there." [2]

As in the growing child, the patient's responding behaviour is fairly intact. It shows that he understands and recognises the words said to him and their meaning ; he knows the use of all objects, he can handle them correctly, and so forth. This indicates that the patient is strongly connected with the outward world and its symbols. So far as objects and/or their names stimulate him, he can respond adequately.

This type of Aphasia is usually termed ' Amnestic,' as it appears that the patient cannot recall the words he had acquired before his illness. In view of the fact that thoughts cannot readily be put into words, though this capacity is, as it were, merely lying dormant, it may be termed ' Verbal Aphasia ' (Head).

In severer cases dissolution narrows the range of words considerably, but leaves well-canalised phrases and sayings less impaired. Oaths, interjections, simple formulas of response, especially emotional ones, such as ' Oh, yes,' ' thanks,' ' not a bit,' are often preserved.

PARAGRAMMATISM

The next lower level of speech disintegration is characterised by the more or less complete loss of grammatical and syntactical constructions.

Aetiology.—According to Pick, lesions of the temporal region of the cortex cause all kinds of syntactical and grammatical deviations.

---

[1] Gelb and Goldstein (1924). " Über Farbenamnesie nebst Bemerkungen über das Wesen der amnestischen Aphasie überhaupt und die Beziehung zwischen Sprache und dem Verhalten zur Umwelt," *Psycholog. Forschung,* 6, pp. 127–86.

[2] Head, l.c., i, p. 215.

Structural changes of the frontal lobe are especially characterised by the so-called telegram-style.[1]

Symptomatology.—The impression one gets at first sight from these patients is that they talk jargon. They often speak rapidly, their words are more or less correct, but the outstanding feature of their speech is the strange way in which they put the constituent parts of the phrases together, i.e. the syntactical and inflexional construction. Formularised utterances, i.e. thoroughly organised units of speech, such as 'come in,' 'thank you,' are not affected, having lost their syntactical significance.

Substantives, verbs, and adjectives are principally used. Auxiliary verbs, personal pronouns, prepositions, conjunctions, adverbs are more or less dropped. The arrangement of words is fairly free, and there is a very considerable lack of morphology.

Neologisms, e.g. 'blacklead' or 'blacking' for 'pencil' occur not infrequently. Inflexions, the copula, and prepositions are missing in the speech of Head's patient No. 15. " Asked what he had done since his admission into the London Hospital, said : ' To here, only washing, cups and plates. . . .' To the question whether he had played games he replied : ' Played games, yes, played one, daytime, garden.' " [2] The constructions " When it do go up, pain inside." " Here's lay, here handle, the man condukr, on the nines, shot seats on it, zee passengers, two man lady," stand for : " Here is the lady, she is at the handle ; the man conductor ; on the lines ; it's got seats on it ; three passengers, two men and a lady." [3] Note also the following examples : " Always chuck to a small white 'un ; try to hit it. Me and another try to play it (personal pronouns omitted ; morphology impaired). I afraid (I am afraid). I have not suffered headache " (I have not suffered from headache) (preposition missing).

The utterances of Head's patient No. 19 : " I been good. Then was going. Not enough (sc. money) me go there," show that the participle implies the past tense, and that the verb implies the personal pronoun. The last sentence shows an unusual mental grouping. The patient wished to say that there was not enough money to allow him to go there. He did not apparently see any need to express the time ; the first part of the sentence therefore lacks the verb (' was '). It may be remarked that words expressing merely the existence of a given object manifest a high level of abstraction. The concept of existence consequently finds no representation in the speech of primitive peoples, infantile persons, and paragrammatic patients.

The history of languages shows that all forms expressing mere ' existence,' such as the copula, i.e. a word acting as a connecting-link between the subject and the predicate of a sentence, e.g. ' is,' are relatively late phenomena.[4] In Indo-European languages they were originally words which conveyed the meaning of remaining, dwelling, staying, becoming, growing, breathing, living, and so on.[5] To the mind

---

[1] Pick, l.c.   [2] Head, l.c., i, p. 230.   [3] Ibid., p. 231.
[4] Wundt, W. (1901). *Sprachgeschichte und Sprachpsychologie*, Engelmann, Leipzig, pp. 77–9.
[5] Wyld's and Skeat's *Dict.*, s.v. be, was, am, are.

of the said patient ' not enough ' involved both the statement of
existence and of time.   In the second phrase, ' me go there,' the juxtaposition of the personal pronoun and the verb indicates the relation
of the action to the speaker in a somewhat possessive way.

Articulate speech is, in some perhaps not quite ' pure ' cases, more
or less affected.   Labials and dentals are slurred, so that, for example,
' past ' becomes ' pass,' ' black ' > ' back,' [1] ' lay ' < ' lady ' (later in
the same conversation correct !), ' mins ' < ' woman's,' ' bixet ' <
' victory.'

Head rightly stresses the similarity to baby language of utterances
like " tiff-rent from uffer 'um . . . kā tell ooh, know zis 'un seems
strong ; tittles for tickles." [2]

The phonetic changes are usually ascribed to the extreme rapidity
of utterance,[3] but it should be noted that such patients cannot be
induced to correct mispronounced words.   If told to do so they become
confused or angry.   The more they concentrate on articulation the
worse their speech becomes (cf. Cluttering, p. 107).   Finally, they stop
speaking altogether.   Thus it seems that they do not comprehend
what the hearer is talking about ; they apparently think their utterances are quite intelligible.   We shall have to revert to this point
later (see Dyslalia) when it will become clear that not only the childlike character of such speech has to be emphasised but also the appearance of tendencies found in the progress of all languages.   These are
recapitulated in ontogeny at the age of 2 or thereabout, when a child
for example says ' me go snow ' for ' I want to go into the snow.' [4]

The sensory aspect of single names and the grasping of their meaning are intact ; but orders given in a phrase, or the meaning of what
the patient reads, may not always be correctly understood.

In view of the fact that not only is the articulatory balance of
words or word-groups affected but also the structural form of the
phrase is disordered from want of those verbal elements which help
to knit it together, Head regards these defects as syntactical rather
than as agrammatic.[5]

We cannot but agree with Head's rejecting this term, though it
has been rightly suggested by Fröschels that the word Agrammatism
should be replaced by the term Paragrammatism.   It should not be
assumed that the language of an agrammatic patient does not possess
any grammar.   We can only assert that his grammar is another one,
a grammar of his own.   This is expressed by the prefix para-, which
means ' beside.'   The term Paragrammatism serves better as it does
not touch the question as to whether or not any grammar had existed
before the disorder arose.   It can therefore be used both in cases
which have lost grammar and in those which have not yet acquired it
(children).

It is obvious that we are facing here the borderland between purely
expressive speech and communicative language.   Consequently also

---

[1] The head of the arrow indicates that the word (or sound) behind the head,
whichever way it is facing, has changed into the form to which the arrow points.
[2] Head, l.c., i, p. 231.   [3] Ibid., i, p. 230.
[4] Jespersen, l.c., pp. 134–5.   [5] Head, l.c., i, p. 240.

the feature or character of the disorder must to a certain extent depend on the character of the patient's mother-tongue, as far as the special inflexions and syntax of a given language are concerned. The paragrammatic patient thus does not use the constructions used by the members of his group, no matter whether he had formerly possessed them or not.

Paragrammatism in children.—In some children the development of syntactical constructions has been inhibited. Their Paragrammatism corresponds fairly exactly to that in adults. Here also syntactical and grammatical deviations are found together with those of articulation. Words are arranged simply by juxtaposition. They are placed side by side without the use of separate relational words.

The majority of cases of Paragrammatism in children as well as of severe developmental Dyslalia are characterised by developmental arrest of the archicapillaries.[1] This indicates their being on a lower evolutionary level.

Aetiology.—In the history of these cases we find lesions of the brain acquired in early childhood, mental defectiveness,[2] and checked maturation, for example through Mongolism.

Dissolution.—It does not assist our understanding—and this is the most important factor for pragmatic purposes such as treatment—to state that the grammar of a given language differs from that of the investigator. Supposing the observer speaks a language of a similar kind, is Paragrammatism on that account to be regarded as 'disordered'?

It follows that Paragrammatism must be analysed with full consideration of the evolution of grammatical and syntactical constructions up to the highest level of construction in special national languages, as has been strongly advocated by Pick.[3]

It is a mistake to value languages only for their feature of utterance. If we are to value them, which implies comparing them, we must also take into account their relation to the mental background to which the particular mode of expression refers. That mental background in its turn must be of a kind which will secure the fullest mastery of the environment.

Such attempts can be clearly observed in primitive languages and their development. Striking similarities can be found in those languages which have arisen out of the contact of European speakers with natives.

Pidgin English and kindred languages.—In Beach-la-Mar English " words have only one form, and what is in our language expressed by flexional forms is either left unexpressed or else indicated by auxiliary words." [4] " Verbs have no tense-forms." [5]

In the Chinook jargon " the grammar is extremely simple. Nouns are invariable ; the plural generally is not distinguished from the

---

[1] Hoepfner, Th. (1929). Discussion. III, ' Kongr. d. Int. Ges. f. Logopädie u. Phoniatrie,' Deuticke, Leipzig-Wien, pp. 71–2.

[2] Tredgold, A. F. (1937). *A Textbook of Mental Deficiency,* Bailliere, Tindal & Cox, London, p. 428.

[3] Pick, A. (1913). *Die agrammatischen Sprachstörungen,* Springer, Berlin.

[4] Jespersen, l.c., p. 218.   [5] Ibid., p. 22.

singular. . . . The genitive is shown by position only. . . . Like the nouns, the verbs have only one form, the tense being left to be inferred from the context, or if strictly necessary, being indicated by an adverb. . . . The verb ' to be ' is not expressed." [1]

These languages owe their origin to the necessity for communication between natives and invading people. Such a process is not unknown in the history of language, an outstanding example being English. As a rule the vernacular language is not given up, but various peculiarities of the invaders' language, words and modes of expression, gradually pass as current in the natives' language. The relational elements are not absorbed, so that, for example, English, in spite of all foreign elements, has still preserved its Saxon character. Phonetic tendencies have also been allowed to take their course ; so that in the end there has emerged a highly developed language, distinguished by simplicity of form combined with freedom, variability, and complexity of sentence construction.'

In Pidgin English and kindred languages the outstanding difference is that the language of the *invaders* is adopted. The natives express the relation between the items of their experience by standardised linguistic patterns borrowed from the invaders. The latter, however, coined their linguistic symbols for modes of thought which are entirely strange to the natives.

Pidgin English supplies good examples. Two peoples endowed with highly developed languages have met. But Chinese thought and consequently verbalisation " does not summarise, it does not analyse, but it sees all things apart in never-ending variety. It accumulates one concrete simple image after another in the order in which they occur to the mind. It does not easily form comprehensive perceptions. To express these it has to recur to compounds ; e.g. to express the comprehensive idea ' to bring ' it is necessary to use an associate formation like ' to take—come.' . . . The Chinese mind has learnt to think by the way of analogies, not along lines of causality. The development of an idea is effected by the juxtaposition of the parts of a sentence in which each describes the different aspect of an idea. . . . Almost the only means of developing an idea is the use of rhythmical antithetical phrases. . . . Rhythmical interplay by its very nature belongs to the old Chinese conception of a harmonious universe, in which microcosm and macrocosm, in fact all things, were interrelated in some intimate way, which is quite different from the ' unity ' which a modern logical mind will sometimes discover in the universe." [2] The linguistic symbols to a great extent still convey subconsciously their original concrete meaning. An example may illustrate how difficult it is to correlate two kinds of expression. A simple phrase like " hsin chih so chih " (heart's what goes-to) translated by Giles as " what the heart desires," [3] shows the word *chih* twice. Once it

[1] Jespersen, l.c., pp. 230–1.
[2] Duyvendak, J. J. L. " A Literary Renaissance in China," *Acta Orientalia,* 1922–4. Quot. by Purcell, V. W. W. S. (1935). " The Language Problem in China," *Psyche,* 15, p. 90.
[3] Purcell, *ibid.,* p. 94.

renders the English genitive, once it means ' striving.' Both meanings can be understood by the sequence of meanings which, starting from ' go to ' conveys connotations such as ' arrive,' ' hence,' ' to,' ' he,' ' she,' ' it,' ' this,' ' that,' ' those,' a particle denoting that the action is finished.[1]

Phrases such as ' rope along ' (= belong), ' bush ' for ' liana,' ' me look him finish ' for ' I have seen him ' [2] manifest a similar development.

Owing to dissolution, or checked development, paragrammatic patients reach a lower level of mentation and verbalisation, while modes of expression are forced upon them which correspond to higher levels with more elaborate syntactical constructions.

It follows from this that formal simplicity need not and cannot be a reason for estimating a language as being on a lower level. On the contrary, as the dictionary meaning of English words shows, it may evidence a highly developed stage.

Or are we perhaps justified in assuming that Pidgin English and similar languages exceed the level of English which the natives had originally adopted ? And should this idea apply to Paragrammatism too ?

Certainly not. In regard to the arrangement of constituent parts, Paragrammatism certainly shows progressive traits which can be found in any language ; but we must not detach this attribute from the sum total of the other attributes.

In English certainly we find great simplicity of forms ; but this is combined with great versatility of sentence construction. And these possibilities have increased the co-ordination (i.e. harmony) between mentation and communicative expression, and subsequently the mastery of the surround.

Julian Huxley [3] has pointed out that it is certainly the degree of adaptation and complexity which indicates progress, if an increase of co-ordination, i.e. harmony, brings the fundamental task further towards a state of fulfilment.

Speech should serve mentation, and in turn should be served by mentation, so as to bring both thought and expression to higher levels, and to facilitate closer collaboration among speakers, i.e. social groups. It appears that none of these characteristics can be found in either Pidgin English and the like, or in Paragrammatism. This is why the latter must be considered a pathological phenomenon, brought about because a natural progressive tendency, being dissociated from its mental parallels, strives forward unchecked and so does not help to master the world. We shall meet this principle in the disorders of articulate speech which often accompany Paragrammatism and other disorders of symbolic expression.

MOTOR APHASIA

The classical form of motor Aphasia is pre-eminently characterised by the loss of the power of spontaneous communication by means of

---

[1] Purcell, l.c., p. 94.   [2] Jespersen, l.c., pp. 219–20.
[3] Huxley, J. (1923). *Essays of a Biologist,* Chatto & Windus, London, pp. 13–30.

language, spoken or written. The patient cannot utter anything except under the influence of emotion which would lead to swearing or expressions that have become automatic, such as ' yes,' ' no.' Therefore he cannot repeat what is said to him. Likewise he cannot write or reproduce the letters of the alphabet, but may be able to write well-canalised words, such as his name or the address of his house, in single letters. One of Head's patients (Case No. 19) " wrote his name and the address of his previous home in the country ; but he failed to complete that of the house in which his wife had lived for a year, although it was to this place that he returned every time he left the hospital on leave." [1] It is obvious that the latter address was less canalised than the former.

The patient's behavioural reaction to the objects of his environment and to their communicative symbols is correct, his gesticulations are so obvious that his fellows can with little difficulty recognise his ideas. He may be able to draw pictures or plans with all details ; he may play games well and put together jigsaw puzzles.[2]

But it has been stressed by Fröschels, Head, and others that it would be delusive to assume that these patients' power of understanding speech symbols has escaped dissolution. The partial loss of understanding of words becomes manifest in their inability to grasp the meaning of longer logical propositions, whether spoken, written, or printed. They can, however, appreciate, though slowly, names, heard or read. Head's patient No. 17 " could not read a book with ease or pleasure ; for although he understood each isolated sentence, he was obliged to go back, when he reached the middle of the paragraph, and to start again from the preceding full stop. He had forgotten or missed several of the words." [3] Copying, writing to dictation, yield better results, apparently owing to the pattern being presented.

This type of Aphasia reminds us of the phase in the child's speech development when it attends to conventional sound-symbols and has grasped their reference to the surrounding world, but is unable to use them. These children can likewise not be induced to repeat words. If they utter anything, it only happens when the emotional situation requires it strongly. When these children begin to talk, they often form strange ' neologisms.' A child of Otto Ernst, the poet, used, e.g., Maulbürste (mouth-brush) for moustache.[4]

Motor Aphasiacs, too, have difficulty in arranging the constituent parts of a word. Head's case No. 17 " described a person as ' strong-willed ' and ' strong-headed ' when he wanted to say ' head-strong.' " [5] Similar word formations are found in the speech of early childhood, e.g. güterei (derived from gut, ' good,' by means of the suffix -erei, which can only be joined with verb stems) for sweetshop.[6]

---

[1] Head, l.c., i, p. 172.   [2] Ibid., pp. 170–4.   [3] Ibid., p. 200.
[4] Stern, W. (1914). *Psychologie der frühen Kindheit*, Quelle & Meyer, Leipzig, p. 117.
[5] Head, l.c., p. 200.   [6] Ibid., p. 107.

SENSORY APHASIA

Severe cases of Sensory Aphasia cannot understand ordinary conversation at all, nor do what they are told, as they do not grasp the
meaning of words or phrases. Likewise the ability of mastering writing
and reading is impaired (Agraphia and Alexia). Here the same mistakes
occur as in speaking. What the patients read aloud, or write, is mispronounced or misspelt (Paralexia, Paragraphia). Written commands
are badly executed. The comprehension of single sounds is less
impaired. Letters have lost their symbolic value and have become
mere forms, which can be copied.

The positive characteristics are as follows : the patient can speak
spontaneously, mostly he is extraordinarily eager to chat. His loquacity
is as characteristic as the distortion of the phonetic structure of the
words. He seems to be subjected to constant ' slips of the tongue '
(paraphasia). Once the patient gets hold of a word he tends to use it
again and again, which makes his speech more like gibberish.

Sensory aphasiacs, even when they do understand a good deal,
have difficulty in grasping the exact meaning of relational words, such
as ' to ' and ' past,' ' high ' and ' low,' ' up ' and ' down,' ' back ' and
' front,' when contrasted with one another.[1]

Their general intelligence is, in spite of this, not considerably
impaired. They get on very well if everything that is said to them is
illustrated by a sketch.

These patients resemble children in the babbling stage or the
transition period from mere expression to communication.

AUDITORY IMPERCEPTION

A graver degree of dissolution is represented by patients who can
easily recognise acoustic phenomena, such as musical notes, their
pitch, their timbre, e.g. female and male voices, tapping, whistling, etc.
But a patient described by Déjerine and Sérieux [2] " had difficulty in
appreciating the difference between whistling, the song of birds, and
the human voice. She mistook the birds for the voices of women in
church, and complained that she did not hear the words. She could
neither recognise nor sing certain popular airs, and said ' Au clair de la
lune ' was a funeral march." That also explains why " she failed to
comprehend most of what was said to her, and was unable to carry
out oral commands. She complained that although she heard the
words, she could not understand them. Certain words in common use,
such as ' bottine,' ' chapeau,' ' table,' were, however, recognised, and
she frequently picked out some part of a phrase, appreciated its meaning,
and gave an answer, which bore some more or less appropriate relation
to the question." As for the rest, she showed the symptoms found in
Amnestic and Sensory Aphasia.

[1] Head, l.c., ii, p. 32.
[2] " Sur un cas de surdité verbale pure," *Rev. de Méd.* (1893), **13**, pp. 733–50.
Déjerine, J. and Sérieux, P. " Un cas de surdité verbale . . .," *Comptes rend.
de la Soc. de Biol.* (1897), **4**, pp. 1074–7, quot. by Head, l.c., i, pp. 112–13.

This picture readily recalls that period of childhood when the infant heeds to sound, and attends to the speaking voice (Gesell's 2 months' level), up to the time when he listens with selective interest to familiar words (Gesell's 9 months' level).[1]

That emissive speech is, on the other hand, preserved is due to the persisting stimulation of the motor pattern from other (visual, etc.) sources.

We shall meet a similar syndrome again in childhood, when the resemblance between auditory imperception and the afore-mentioned period of speech development will disclose itself more clearly.

SEMANTIC APHASIA

Some patients are described as able to talk without difficulty in pronunciation, and with correct syntax and intonation. Verbal repetition and naming are not affected. But there is in these cases of Semantic [2] Aphasia " a want of recognition of relative significance and intention. Everything tends to be appreciated in detail, but the general significance is lacking." [3] This crude mode of grasping meaningful relations between the objects perceived corresponds roughly to a child's 5 years' level.

Head rightly points out that the patient looks, for example, at a picture "like a child, pointing out one thing after another, and not uncommonly misses some important feature ; asked what the picture means, he may be entirely at a loss and either gives up altogether or invents some preposterous explanation." [4]

TOTAL APHASIA

Complete absence of language is rare. It is characterised by loss of intellectual, i.e. the more voluntary language ; persistence of emotional, i.e. more automatic, undifferentiated (babbling) utterances, and simple gestures ; the patient can smile, frown, and vary his intonation ; frequent persistence of ' yes ' and ' no,' which, having been constantly used, are highly canalised.[5] The use of these words often signifies the dissolutionary level according to whether they represent emotional utterance only, or correct reply, or the repetition of the ' word.' ' Recurring utterances,' such as swearing and ejaculations like ' Oh, dear,' ' well,' are not infrequent.[6] The patient's behaviour shows infantile traits.

At a lower level of speech disintegration the only observable utterances are inarticulate grunts, screeches, and discordant yells. This is also the level attained by idiots. Some idiots will hum tunes with tolerable accuracy. We agree with Tredgold that "there can be no

---

[1] Gesell, *Infancy and Human Growth*, pp. 128 *et seq*. See also page 37.
[2] semainein ' to signify.' Semantics is a branch of linguistic science which demonstrates the development of meaning, i.e. the relationship between words and the ideas which they indicate.
[3] Head, l.c., i, p. 258.   [4] Ibid.
[5] Jackson, l.c., p. 49.   [6] Ibid., pp. 153–4.

doubt that these often express their feelings, just as do the cries of animals." [1]

HYSTERICAL APHASIA

Psychic and sexual influences, emotional shock, and inferiority feelings, springing from various sources, including speech itself, may lead to a more or less complete inhibition of symbolic expression.

Patients suffering from Hysterical Aphasia dispose of several syllables, or they do not utter at all ; phonation may be more or less completely inhibited (Aphonia). Gesticulation is inconsiderable or very lively. Some patients prefer to communicate by writing, others are averse to it.[2]

It is worthy of note that also psychic disorders of a more or less irreversible nature (psychoses), such as Cyclothymia and Schizophrenia, may manifest in speechlessness depression or negativism.[3]

PROGRESS AND TREATMENT

The stages of recovery of Aphasia follow evolutionary principles.

Severe cases of Aphasia fail to understand what is said to them or what they read to themselves. They are completely speechless, or can only utter the simplest, most highly automatised words like ' yes ' or ' no.' They are in most cases excited by strong emotion. Neither can they repeat sentences or even single words correctly. They cannot write or copy print.

In later stages there appear larger groups of words, such as " walking a little, talking difficult a bit." Hand-in-hand with this goes disturbance of understanding as to spoken or read matter. Writing is possible, but words are badly misspelt, although less so if dictated. Patients understand and execute what they are told, more or less correctly. They may still fail to understand what they read to themselves. Spontaneous speech is slow and difficult, and articulation bad. The latter is helped if they are made to repeat phrases said to them. In regaining the power of speech phrases such as " I don't know, please, good night, just so, to tell you the truth," etc., the patient's name, or address, are correctly given ; thus highly canalised phrases appear first. The patients sometimes cannot pronounce or repeat words or phrases which they recognise.

Aphasic children pass once again, more or less rapidly, through all the stages of infantile speech, such as inarticulate cries, screaming, babbling, primitive sounds, primitive syntax, etc.

If intelligence is not much impaired there arise certain deviations owing to the integration of primitive utterances with more advanced mentality. Thus intonation and gesticulation, babbled sounds, particularly also clicks, are given distinct meanings according to the child's needs. This misintegration impedes to a certain extent the rapidity of the growth of community language.

[1] Tredgold, l.c., p. 156.
[2] Stern, H. (1912). In Gutzmann's *Sprachheilkunde*, Berlin, pp. 616–17.
[3] Brain, W. R. (1933). *Diseases of the Nervous System*, Oxford University Press, p. 84.

As a sequela stammering is not uncommon.

Prognosis.—If the responsible lesion is non-progressive, and if the function of the brain is not too much impaired in general, improvement may be expected. Elderly aphasiacs tend to improve far less than the young. Juvenile patients usually overcome Aphasia rapidly, perhaps because the prevalence of one hemisphere is not yet well established. If, e.g., a brain disease affects the left hemisphere (in a right-handed child), the speech area comes to be established in the opposite (right) hemisphere. Mixed sensory-motor varieties are the most intractable ; sensory types may be ranked next ; simple cases of motor defect offer the best prognosis.[1]

Patients suffering from Sensory Aphasia usually show a more distinct tendency towards spontaneous improvement than those suffering from Motor Aphasia. In the case of children we must be most cautious as to the prognosis for Sensory Aphasia. Motor Aphasia in children offers good prospects for rehabilitation.

The cure of Aphasia, or even improvement of the patient's state, may sometimes take years.

The prognosis of Paragrammatism is not unfavourable. Satisfactory progress is to be doubted in the presence of signs of developmental arrest (see p. 81).

Treatment.—The treatment of Aphasia may only be begun when all the acute symptoms of the underlying disease have disappeared. There is a certain similarity between the rehabilitation of speech in aphasic patients and the way in which infants learn to speak. The technique should therefore follow a behaviouristic line (see Chapters III-IV). The therapeutist should endeavour to train the speaker, and not speech. That is to say, the evolutionary level to which the patient has fallen needs to be considered fully. Dana [2] begins treatment by making the patient repeat exclamatory words. This, is, as the present writer has been able to convince himself for many years, a good start. Being appropriate to an evolutionarily low level, it proves successful so far even in very grave cases of Sensory-motor Aphasia.

Other functions of the brain, such as writing, drawing, reading, and counting, as well as games and manual work in general, represent valuable stimuli for the reintegration of speech. We first make the patient paint all the letters of the alphabet on separate pieces of cardboard. This may also be done in different colours. With the help of these letters we first train the recognising of the symbols by making the patient take a single letter out of a series. The corresponding sound is shown to the patient optically and acoustically, whenever a letter has been selected. Later on we make him form words out of letters. Writing should be done with the hand which corresponds to the non-injured hemisphere (Fröschels).

Lastly we proceed to the copying of small sentences, to writing the names of objects, etc., dictation, writing of letters, etc.

---

[1] Critchley, M. (1936). *Aphasia. British Encyclopædia of Medical Practice*, Butterworth, London, i, p. 706.

[2] Quot. by M. Critchley, *Aphasia*, i, p. 707.

The reading of characters, syllables, words, and sentences (in block letters at first) must go hand-in-hand with the writing exercises.

Drawing exercises ought to be done with the unimpaired hand as well as with the paralysed one so far as this is possible. The patient, to begin with, copies geometrical figures, such as triangles and circles ; then he draws them from memory. At a later stage of the treatment he tries perspective drawing, first from pictures and later from memory.

Counting exercises begin with the counting of little rods, peas, etc. Later we proceed to simple forms of arithmetic. First the patient is helped by doing the exercises with the aid of small objects (little balls, matches, etc.).

Manual training is achieved by all kinds of tinkering and amateur construction.

In playing games, the patient puts little rods, balls, etc., into different shapes and forms ; then he passes on to games such as dominoes, Mah Jong ; later on to games with dice, draughts, Chinese checkers, card and round games (Zumsteeg).

Treatment of Sensory Aphasia depends on whether the patient has merely lost his understanding of speech or whether he is also unable to reproduce what he is told. Patients of the latter group are shown the shapes of mouth necessary for the formation of the different sounds, while we speak the corresponding sound. In this way they learn to connect the acoustic image of a given sound with the motor one. This task is initiated by using pictures of a rather emotional, simple, and primitive character, e.g. animals, the sound of which should be reproduced ; the noises of a saw, a rattle, gurgling, etc. The behaviour of an astonished, frightened, or joyful, person ; laughter, humming, mumbling, grunting, etc., will serve the purpose of bringing forth primitive, slightly articulate utterances.

Here the therapist's powers of imagination, observation, and invention have their full scope.

Step by step onomatopoeic words, interjections, phrases, etc., are practised.

If only the power to understand speech is damaged, and the patient can reproduce what is said to him, he is shown pictures or objects, the name of which is pronounced. This enables him to associate the optic impression with the acoustic image. In the same way written symbols are associated.

Certain motor aphasiacs are highly apractic with respect to the movements of lips, tongue, etc. They must first practise separately certain elementary movements of the speech-producing organs to become conscious of the action of the articulating organs. They are shown how to put the tongue out, how to move it up and down and to the side, how to turn out their lips, etc., how to whistle, blow (with flame of a candle), how to click their tongues, to blow on a mirror, etc. To achieve reproduction of these movements it is sometimes necessary to put the organs of speech into the desired position with the hand or a spatula and then let the patient see the position in a three-part mirror.

The patient learns how to produce the voice by putting his hands on the chest, throat, and under the chin of the therapist, while the latter maintains a long, low-pitched sound (vowels or M). The patient feels the vibrations of the voice and tries to imitate them.

The further integration of the speech-sounds follows the line indicated by phonetics and that used in the re-education of articulate speech in deaf-mute and dyslalic patients (see pp. 94, 160 ff.).

It may be noted, at this juncture, that aphasic patients, who were treated and taught to speak often far away from their native place, regained a speech which was founded on the basis of articulation of their former local dialect. We may therefore conclude that only a certain number of pathways are newly facilitated, until they amalgamate with patterns which have been preserved.[1]

In patients who have lost the faculty of ' designating ' objects, though the recognition of the objects is usually not disturbed, we try to facilitate the connecting of the linguistic symbols with objects and events. We show the patient pictures of objects or the objects themselves, giving the names which he has to repeat. We begin with two pictures, for example, that of a lamp and that of a table. We first present them one after the other and make him repeat what we say. Then we show the same picture in succession to avoid his repeating mechanically ' lamp-table ' and to make him specially concentrate upon the acoustic impression. We then present a series of pictures at the same time, say the name of one of the objects, and make him point out the corresponding picture.

I usually make these patients start a word-book. The pages of this book are divided into two parts by a line drawn vertically in the middle of the page. On one half of the page simple little pictures are pasted or drawn ; the names are written on the other half. This little book enables the patient to train his memory for words at home without the help of others : he must cover the half of the page on which the denominations of the object are written, look at the pictures and try to recall their names on seeing them. It is often advisable to draw only one picture on one page, to assist concentration.

The treatment of paragrammatic patients aims at introducing them to our world. They must learn to realise the relations between objects as we see them and to avail themselves of the means of communicative speech used in their group. This task is extremely laborious and can only be accomplished gradually, for the patient is convinced that the way he realises and verbalises the world is also perfectly clear to us. It is therefore of primary importance that the therapist should adopt a puzzled attitude, so as to make the patient aware of his faulty speech.

The reconstruction of language should be tackled on behaviouristic lines. The patient must be faced with relations between facts to which the therapist reacts by certain utterances. Since most of the words occurring in daily life, and their dictionary meaning, are usually familiar to the patient, the therapist can focus the problem of making the patient understand the relational meaning of words and of grammatical forms.

[1] Stein, L. (1917). " Beobachtungen beim Wiederaufbau der Sprache Aphatischer," *Monatschrift für Ohrenheilkunde,* **51,** pp. 31–8.

Prepositions which convey the meaning of special relation appear comparatively late both in the evolution and in the development of language. In the early history of all languages they probably were nominal or pronominal forms. Through constant usage they were gradually shortened and with the changing phonetic character their original concrete meaning was lost.

The patient should first be presented with the most obvious relations. One of the fundamental conceptions is the sense of position in space. Several objects, such as a box, a drawer, a glass, a match, a marble, are required for instilling the comprehension of relational words into the patient. A wooden box, for example, is put before the patient ; among other parts, particularly its *sides* are pointed to. A marble is then placed beside the box and rolled along one side of it. The question is put : " Where is the marble rolling ? " and is answered : " By the side of (> beside) the box."

A picture of two children is drawn and the idea of *twins* is put before the patient. An apple is then placed in the middle of the two, and the fact that it is *between* them is stressed.

The marble just rolling away is accompanied by the exclamation ' Off ! ' From this interjectional use the other connotations of the preposition ' off ' and that of the word ' of ' [əv] can be deduced naturally by giving concrete examples. For instance, soldiers leaving a fortress are ' the soldiers off (> of) the fortress ' ; strips cut out of paper are ' strips off (> of) paper,' and so on.

This method of approach finds its parallel in the actual historical development of the unstressed form ' of ' [əv] of the preposition ' off.' [ɔf].

In the same manner other prepositions such as in, on, through, etc., are brought to the patient's notice and assembled.

The use of the articles presents great difficulty. Their present meaning is to be derived for the patient from their original demonstrative and numeral meaning. Example : Two marbles, a whole and a broken one, are shown to the child and then hidden. If the child asks for ' ball ' the imperfect one should be given. If he is not satisfied, the therapist must appear puzzled. " Which marble do you want ? " he asks. " This marble," says the child, pointing to the whole one. Familiarity with the phrase and accentuation of the substantive makes the change from *this* marble to *the* marble almost inevitable.

Common ' regular ' forms of nouns, such as the plural, can also be taught by making use of the patient's needs and desires. A child may be given a collection of pencils of different colours. If he asks for them saying ' Pencil,' only one should be handed to him ; when all or some of them are given, the *s* in pencil*s* should be stressed. This example can be varied by using other objects.

The meaning of the auxiliary verb ' to be ' and its forms (is, are, etc.) causes the greatest difficulty. In cases where we intend to express the existence of a thing, paragrammatic patients as a rule merely use the name of the object ; their meaning is rendered more definite by intonation and gesture. It is, however, doubtful whether the highly abstract category of mere existence is conceived by them. Nor can this conception be presupposed for all languages. The language of the

Wintu Indians has suffixes which imply the tense and the person ; they also contain the implications of ' I see,' ' I taste ' (or know through some sense other than sight), ' I infer,' ' I judge,' ' I am told.'　But there is no suffix corresponding to the mere copula (is).　Thus the Wintu can express for example his tasting the goodness of the salmon but he cannot simply state " The salmon is good."　In Indo-European languages the connotation of existence constitutes a comparatively late semantic change of words originally meaning ' to grow,' ' to become,' ' to dwell,' ' to remain ' (see the etymology of ' to be,' ' I was,' etc.).[1] In conformity with this state of development, in dealing with para-grammatic patients the meaning of the auxiliary verbs should be derived from the concrete one.

It is impossible to give a full account of all that is required for the treatment of Paragrammatism.　Much depends on the patient's mental level.　The therapist must avail himself of all the knowledge of comparative philology and psychology in order to guide the patient to the track traced out by the natural development of language and thought.

[1] Wyld, *The Universal English Dictionary*.

CHAPTER IX

MUTISM

Definition.—We have already suggested that behaviour (' to have oneself in hand ') indicates the way in which man responds to the external world, and retains his impressions. The etymology of the word tells us this explicitly. ' To behave ' is derived from the word have, which in its turn has sprung from the same base as Lat. *capere,* ' to seize.' It has afterwards developed the meanings of ' to hold, possess,' ' to retain in the mind,' etc.[1]

The development of normal speech as a mode of behaviour therefore requires normal means of taking possession of the external world, in order to respond adequately. Speech is, as all other actions, acquired and produced by conditioning of pre-formed reflexes. If the means for experiencing the world in all aspects are defective or disturbed, conditioning does not take place, and the development of speech is impeded. The result is *Dumbness.*

We feel constrained to explain the origin of this word, for it shows the stratification of meaning which has been handed on to those using the popular term. The root was probably DHU, ' to fan into flame.' From this two words sprang, viz. ' deaf ' and ' dumb.' The latter carries in itself the meanings of being ' incapable of, slow at, ineffectual in expressing ideas and emotions,' [2] according to the original meaning of ' obfuscated,' and the now common one of being ' unable to utter articulate sounds.' [3] The former, allied to Greek *typhos* (' smoke, darkness, stupor '),[4] had once the meaning of ' dull, stupid,' but is now restricted to that of being " wholly without the sense of hearing." [5]

There is also another word which expresses the same meaning, viz. mute. This word was perhaps originally " imitative of sound made in closing lips," [3] as is shown by the still persisting meaning of the words ' mum ' and ' mutter.' [3] The metaphor is perhaps, as it were, that of closing the door of utterance so as to obstruct the passage for expression.

The term Aphasia is reserved for those kinds of speech-disintegration which are based on the dissolution of well-developed verbal symbolisation. Mutism (Mutitas), on the other hand, should be used only in cases which have not developed speech at all.

Dumbness may be caused by impediments (1) in the receptor organs, (2) in the central pathways, (3) in the effector organs.

DEAF-MUTISM

Aetiology.—Dumbness as a consequence of deafness does not need much explanation. Speech is acquired pre-eminently through acoustic stimulation. If this cannot be activated the speech reflex does not

---

[1] Wyld, *Dict.* [2] Ibid. [3] Ibid.
[4] Skeat, *Etym. Dict.* [5] Wyld, *Dict.*

become integrated. Such persons are called Deaf-and-Dumb (the conjunction ' and ' indicates that in old times it was believed that these human beings were affected by *two independent defects!*). The substantive was Deaf-Dumbness, which for a century has been replaced by the terms now in use, Deaf-mute and Deaf-mutism (French *sourd-muet*).

Deafness, either congenital or acquired in early childhood, before speech is sufficiently canalised (up to about 8 years), naturally results in dumbness. The impairment of hearing may be due to heredity, constitutional or traumatic degeneration of the ear-nerve, infectious diseases (scarlet fever, meningitis, etc.), or chronic middle ear suppuration.

Development.—It is important to note that the first phases in the development of deaf children do not deviate from that of normal children. The new-born cry and scream like other babies, and infants reach the stage of babbling speech. Regarded from the evolutionary angle, the lower patterns of vocalisation are so strongly connected with vegetative ones, and have been so well canalised through the ages, that no external (acoustic) stimulation is needed.

This knowledge must warn the speech therapist to be on his guard when he has to give his opinion of a speechless child. He might in this respect be easily misled by the mother, who does not wish to think that her child could be deaf and therefore interprets babbling utterances as signs of developing speech. As soon as these children have passed through the period of primitive sounds, the lack of the necessary auditory stimulation becomes noticeable: The baby stops babbling, and becomes speechless.

Symptoms.—What remains is inarticulate screaming, accompanied by vivid gesticulation which in course of development serves as symbolic expression and undergoes great differentiation. Deaf-mutes can communicate with each other sufficiently by gesture language.

Treatment.—The modern method of treating the deaf-mute consists in presenting speech visually and tactually. The pupil must be made to feel the vibrations of the larynx walls while the teacher is producing a sound. The shapes of mouth, position of tongue, etc., corresponding to the different speech-sounds, are shown and imitated (speech reading).[1] The complete course of teaching cannot be outlined here as, in the present writer's view, the education and the teaching of speech to the deaf-mute requires such special training that it is wiser to leave it to teachers specially concerned with it.

SPEECH OF THE HARD OF HEARING

If the hearing capacity of a person with canalised articulation is impaired, deviations of utterance may still occur ; their type depends on the nature of the basic ear disease. Diseases of the middle ear more or less prevent the transmission of sound waves by air. Bone conduction is possible, and enables the patient to hear his own voice. But

---

[1] This term should, according to Seth and Guthrie, replace the inadequate term ' lip-reading.'

as he does not hear external noises accompanying the speech of those around him ('masking effect'),[1] he under-estimates the amount of intensity of voice required for intelligible speech. He speaks, therefore, with less intensity than the normal.

Patients suffering from impaired hearing through disease of the inner ear or the auditory nerve are prevented from hearing tones of high frequency conducted through the bone. Being incapable of hearing their own voice clearly, these patients speak much too loudly.

If the loss is less acute, patients may hear something by both air transmission across the middle ear and by bone conduction to the inner ear. " The hearing fails first on the high-frequency range, which includes the formant tones for the fricative consonants, especially the voiceless [s], [f], [ϑ], [ʃ]. These sounds tend to be lost in speech and confused in hearing, and the progressive stages of loss involve the explosive stages of the stop consonants, the voiceless stop consonants, the voiced stop consonants, and finally the vowels and voiced continuant consonants. The general effect on the speech is a slurring of the clearness of the separate speech sounds as well as a lack of control of the durations and separations of the various words. The unstressed syllables and words are weakened or even lost, and so much of the clarity of the thought sequence is obscured." [2]

The capacity of children with defective hearing (congenital or acquired in infancy) to acquire speech varies with the degree of auditory perception (see p. 96).

HEARING-MUTISM

Terms.—Lack of audible communicative means in children is normal up to the age of 12-18 months. A state of speechlessness persisting up to the age of 3 is termed *Retarded Speech Development*. The same conditions persisting after the third year are subsumed in the class of *Hearing-Mutism* (in contra-distinction to deaf-mutism). Equivalent terms are : Congenital Word Deafness, Congenital Auditory Imperception, Audimutitas, Idiopathic Mutism, Mutitas physiologica prolongata (Stern).

Explanation.—The activation of the speech reflex may still be impeded even if the auditory receptor organ is functioning. In Hearing-Mutism the child's hearing is normal ; but the auditory sense-data are not utilised. Thus his ' world ' consists of all sense-data except the acoustic ones. The child will therefore develop responses so far as they can be stimulated by the existing perceptions ; but he will remain mute after the third year in spite of normal general intelligence.

We can explain this state by a simple example : a person looking at something interesting in a shop window does not answer the ' Good morning ' of a friend passing by ; the next day when asked why he didn't respond, he would quite innocently reply : " I'm sorry, but I must confess that I did not hear you." This answer is of course

---

[1] " One tone is said to be a masking tone when it acts to raise the auditory threshold for the second tone." Curry, l.c., § 30, 6.

[2] Ibid., § 32, 5.

wrong, because he was not deaf at the time, that is to say, there was an auditory sensation, but this did not occupy the centre of the psychic field.[1] He could not ' perceive ' what he had heard because the whole of his nerve energy was used for looking at the thing which ' interested ' him ; this is, of course, an exceptional state. In some children this state is permanent ; they hear, but they do not use their faculty of hearing ; their whole nerve energy is used for looking, touching, etc. Thus the usual acoustic phenomena do not act as stimuli, and therefore cannot arouse speech reflexes of a higher order and so cannot smooth the pathway for speech. The result is persisting dumbness. The problem, in view of what was said in the introductory chapters about interest, attention, etc. (see p. 14), is reduced to the question of factors which prevent auditory stimuli from becoming dominant (see below, Aetiology).

Symptoms.—The symptoms of the sensory type of Hearing-Mutism are similar to those in Aphasia. The patients do not attend to speech ; it does not exist for them. In addition they are mute. In some cases utterances are restricted to random inarticulate sounds.

The behaviour of such patients shows lack of concentration ; their attention wanders constantly, they never carry on any game or pursuit for more than a few minutes. In the further course of development they make use of this inferiority, forcing those around them to give in to them by crying and making scenes.

As in Motor Aphasia speechlessness is the conspicuous symptom in the motor type of Hearing-Mutism, while the understanding of spoken words seems at first sight to be unaffected. Closer investigation, however, reveals some lack of understanding. Some children utter a few words in a babbling way.

If thorough examination does not reveal any lack of understanding, the absence of utterance is, as a rule, due to psychic inhibition. A girl of 6, described by Seth and Guthrie, had, according to the mother's statement, " never uttered a single word, although she responded to commands, made known her wants by dumb-show, and appeared quite intelligent. A week after her admission to hospital the staff nurse, entering the ward unexpectedly after a brief absence, found this child talking as well as any child of her age." [2] Apparently the child had been reduced to silence by unsympathetic treatment at home.

Aetiology.—Various factors, such as retarded development of the speech of the parents, hereditary neuropathic traits, adenoids, alcoholism of the parents (Coën), intermarriages, play their part in bringing about Hearing-Mutism. Fröschels found cranial rickets in the majority of cases of Motor Hearing-Mutism ; cases of the sensory type had often suffered from infantile cerebral spasms ; delivery in such cases was often difficult. According to Seemann cerebellar lesions during birth are of decisive influence.

Impairment of sound-perception through diseases of the ear, the auditory nerve, and the sensory centres prevents the activation of the speech loop, for the growing child fails to hear most of the acoustic

[1] Cf. Douglas, l.c., p. 151.　　　　　　[2] Seth and Guthrie, l.c., p. 147.

stimuli. Organic defects of the effector organs of speech, especially
the palate, are obstacles in the motor part of the speech loop.

Hearing-Mutism is often a symptom of general retarded development. Such a backward child does not speak, because he may have
nothing to say !

Last but not least rank unfavourable social conditions (e.g. lack of
playmates), which make communication through audible symbols
pointless.

In *Diagnostic Examination* we must make sure of the patient's
bodily and mental condition. Examination of the nervous system,
and of the cochlear and vestibular functions in particular is essential.
Diagnosis presents difficulties in small children ; it is facilitated in
cases where there is some understanding of speech.

We put simple questions and set little tasks to the child, such as
Where is mother ? Shake hands, etc. In this case we must take care
lest the child read from our lips, and avoid gestures by which our
intention might be detected.

The behaviour of such patients may often hint at the right
diagnosis. Fröschels found that hearing-mute children are sometimes exceedingly restless, thus giving the impression of mania or
idiocy. Deaf-mute children, on the other hand, are mostly good and
amiable.

Differential diagnosis.—Aphasia, Deaf-Mutism, and Feeble-Mindedness have to be taken into consideration in differential diagnosis.

Aphasia can be excluded if the history of the patient reveals that
he had never spoken before. Deaf-Mutism can be left out of consideration if sufficient hearing capacity can be found. This task presents
difficulties, particularly in little children.

For testing the hearing of small speechless children we find the
tuning-fork unsatisfactory, since the child is unable to give us the
necessary accurate information. It is also unnecessary to know
what pure tones the child can or cannot hear, since it is in his
capacity to hear speech that we are most interested. As each
speech sound consists of a series of tones of distinctive frequencies
integrated into a unified pattern comparable to a chord, the child's
response to the notes given by musical pipes gives us sufficient
information, for each pipe produces a fundamental tone and its
harmonics.

An accordion of about three octaves is the best instrument for our
purpose. The examiner begins by sounding a single note or no note
at all. When sounding no note he must make no difference in the
actuation of the accordion. This can be done by use of the wind stop.
His assistant must raise his arm when he hears the note and remain
still when he hears no sound. The child watches this performance for
some time, and is then induced by signs to take the place of the assistant
and give the same response. If he remains still when there is no sound
we conclude that he hears to some extent. If he raises his hand
invariably or indiscriminately we first show him when he should not
have done so, since he may not have understood the purpose. If
after this he persists in raising his arm when there is no sound we

7

conclude that he is deaf. The examiner must also vary his distance from the child.[1]

This procedure can be supplemented by the use of the therapist's own voice.

Testing may sometimes reveal comparatively slight defective hearing which cannot alone be held responsible for the lack of speech. But it prevented many acoustic stimuli from reaching the child's sense, so that the remaining hearing capacity decayed, and made the patient *in practice* deaf. The speech reflex could consequently not be stimulated.

A girl of 12 from the country was reported as being unable to speak or to hear. The child, who was otherwise quite normal, did not produce any sound at all, and did not react to any acoustic stimuli. Repeated examination with a concertina showed the girl to be able to hear all tones from a distance of about 4½ yards. Through hearing exercises (see p. 100) she learnt to speak so quickly and well that she was able to follow ordinary conversation, and to master the work of the first form in nine months.

The father of a boy of 5, who neither spoke nor heard, was deaf-mute ; the mother's hearing was normal, but there were several cases of deaf-mutism in the ancestry. The boy did not react when one called to him. On the other hand, it was impossible to make him imitate the position of the lips when shown sounds. He was most refractory during the examination, and, in addition to outbursts of temper, gave a general impression of imbecility. His mother also showed a letter of an aurist declaring the child to be deaf-mute and recommending him to be placed in an asylum for deaf-mute children. After a few consultations, however, I was able to state beyond doubt that the boy could hear from a distance of 10 feet.

The organic defects in such cases cannot always be removed. But there are a number of psychological factors which are usually of much greater importance than the organic defect. These children, if not actually neglected, rarely enjoy the necessary consideration from those around them. They are often and easily hurt (though this is usually by no means intentional), and they do not receive adequate love and understanding. A further cause of irritation is the derision of other children and the impossibility of joining in the sports and work normal to their age and strength. This explains their wildness and temper. Their normal energy, denied a normal outlet, brings about these unusual outbursts. Any effort or progress which might be made within the limits of their reduced possibilities is promptly checked by the discouragement with which they continually meet. Thus the original state is aggravated, a typical example of neurotic superstructure on an organic defect. This also explains why such children often appear ' backward,' for they have not the appropriate means of training their mental faculties, and they are forced into a

[1] Ewing, A. W. O. (1930), (*Aphasia in Children*, Oxford University Press, pp. 29–36), has developed this ' clinical method ' into a ' laboratory method ' in which an audiometer specially adapted for small children is substituted for the accordion.

position of stubbornness and apathetic inactivity by derision, nagging, and discouragement. If we can convince the parents that the child is mentally sound and likely to improve by adequate treatment, we may be able to restore him to normal behaviour and activity.

To revert to the child of a deaf-mute father and a normally hearing mother. Compelled to adapt himself to the language of signs, because his mother rarely used speech, he was naturally unable to understand the necessity for any other means of making himself understood. As he grew up he discovered that there were certain advantages gained from stressing his inability to hear and making himself understood by signs. He was very much spoilt, especially by the father, and was not held responsible for his actions. Consequently it was difficult in the beginning to make him give up this very profitable attitude. It will be remembered that he would not imitate the movement of the lips when asked to do so, a task which is promptly executed by deaf-mutes. This behaviour might almost be termed simulation. He was altogether completely inactive, and refused to do the smallest duties of little children, such as dressing himself, etc., which shows how well he had assumed the part of an inferior individual.

A healthy 14 year old girl, completely mute, was so wild that it was very difficult to establish contact with her. When she had calmed down she was quite apathetic, and fixed her eyes on the floor, frowning angrily. The sudden changes of attitude which I had observed during her first visit to me made me think of imbecility. The history revealed infantile spasms, suggesting Hearing-Mutism. In the course of treatment the girl was able to learn the sounds, isolated as well as in syllables and words, and the letters of the alphabet within a few months. The further development of her speech showed that it improved in proportion to the dispelling of her feeling of inferiority. She was the youngest of three children. Her two elder sisters were grown up, one of them was married, and she and her husband lived with the parents of the patient, who disliked this sister intensely. This dislike, together with the difficulties of the oncoming of puberty, naturally tended to foster a feeling of inferiority originating in the great difference of age between the sisters. The family doctor had always advised the family to give way to the patient's wishes, and never to demand from her the fulfilment of the tasks and activities of normal children. Thus she had learnt to make her way in life either by passivity or by force, and had never had that most important encouragement which children derive from the feeling of well-directed activity and well-performed actions. Her psychological development and her Hearing-Mutism was thus understandable.[1]

Idiopathic Hearing-Mutism has often been confused with mental defect or regarded as a symptom of general mental retardation. The layman is apt to believe these children to be wholly backward, since their ideas are defective ; but it is the lack of speech which has impeded the development of higher mental patterns.

The distinction between Hearing-Mutism and feeble-mindedness

[1] Stein, L. (1924). "Ueber die psychologische Auffassung von organisch bedingten Funktionsstörungen," *Intern. Zeitschr. f. Individualpsychol.*, **3**, No. 1.

needs close, and sometimes prolonged, observation. Non-verbal intelligence tests are essential.

Prognosis.—The history of many cases of Paragrammatism and of Universal Dyslalia indicates that many such defects may be due to Hearing-Mutism not having been treated in time. We often hear that these children began to speak only at a relatively late stage of their development. The inability to express themselves as well as other children often makes them very backward at school. Out of eighteen children with retarded speech development five showed Paragrammatism, and thirteen Universal Dyslalia. A compilation of thirty-five cases of Hearing-Mutism of the motor type proved my diagnosis to have been right in twenty-eight cases. These twenty-eight children developed normally after treatment, and their progress at school was found to be satisfactory. Thus, provided the diagnosis is correct and home conditions are favourable, the prospects of treatment in Hearing-Mutism are good.

Spontaneous development definitely jeopardises the linguistic expression, the mental efficiency, and the character of such patients.[1]

Treatment.—The treatment of Hearing-Mutism must obviously vary with the relevant etiological factor.

If hearing is impaired, adequate amelioration must first be attempted. The method of approach is outlined in the following section.

Hearing exercises.—Hearing exercises are based on the assumption that the degree of defective hearing is often more severe than the organic lesion would indicate. The central conducting pathways of hearing suffer through lack of use of the organ of hearing, and consequently develop a functional insufficiency of differentiating audition, which may be improved by hearing exercises, though the reduction of hearing which is due to the organic lesion of the auditory organ cannot be so remedied.

Urbantschitsch [2] worked out a scheme of hearing exercises designed to concentrate the patient's attention on the differentiation of various sounds by offering acoustic stimuli adapted to the patient's functional deficiency.

The patient is made to fix his attention on a great variety of sounds of everyday life, such as the noises in the street, the hooting of cars, barking of dogs, the tolling of bells, etc., and to try to distinguish between these sounds. Adults are advised to attend parties, lectures, theatres, and concerts, and so on.

Speech-sounds should be presented predominantly to the weaker ear, the better one being plugged; later on we should speak from different directions. The patient must definitely be prevented from speech reading.

The distance from which we speak to the patient must be such as to enable him to hear only with fullest attention, since the effort to

[1] Stein, L. (1925). " Ueber die Prognose der motorischen Hörstummheit," *Mediz. Klinik*, No. 25.

[2] Urbantschitsch, V. (1901). *Ueber methodische Hörübungen,* Urban & Schwarzenberg, Wien-Berlin.

overcome difficulties increases functional adaptation. Fatigue has, of course, to be avoided. It is much better to do the exercises from a shorter distance in a normal speaking voice and with distinct articulation than to pronounce the words in a loud voice from a greater distance. The latter may be done only if the patient is very hard of hearing indeed. In general, loud sounds produce a disagreeable, sometimes even a painful effect, and may therefore be considered noxious.

The rehabilitation of the recognition of the speech-sounds starts with vowels. We first choose those which are rarely or not at all confused ; this varies with different patients. We might think that [o] and [e], [u] and [i] sound so different as to be easily distinguished, but this is not the case. The power to recognise the different sounds depends on the faculty to hear the harmonics and formants contained in them.

To help the patient's attempts to perceive the quality of a given speech-sound, it is often helpful to draw it out. The patient must repeat what he has heard to prove that he has not only heard but also really recognised the sound. In case of mistakes we repeat first the mistake and then the correct sound to make it easier for him to perceive the difference of the sounds. Needless to say, we must draw his attention to the way in which we correct his mistakes.

We begin the training of syllable hearing by contrasting syllables containing acoustically unrelated sounds, and proceed later to more closely related sounds. Experiment only can decide on the order of practising the different sounds. Next reiterated syllables such as [papa, tete, sisi], and sequences of meaningless syllables, e.g. [bate, pate, pade, bode, bude], are presented so as to make it impossible for the patient to guess sound qualities from meaning. With repetition the syllables follow each other more rapidly.

Then follow exercises of meaningless syllables. Later on normal words have to be mixed with meaningless syllables. In due course stress and intonation must be considered. The combination [pó-ket] (pocket) is easier to understand than [po-két], therefore both must be practised, e.g. pack, packer, packet, [pe-ko], package, packer, [pe-ki], [po-ki], pocket, etc.

The nature of the disease, viz. whether it is a defect of the inner or of the middle ear, must be taken into account when deciding on the arrangement of the exercises, the chosen sounds, and the pitch.

Sentences form the next exercises. They are varied by the interpolation of sentences with meaningless syllables or slightly different words, e.g. the lamp burns, the lamp ' bur,' the lump burns, the lamp turns, and so forth. This prevents guessing on the part of the patient and thus helps to promote his ability to differentiate.

Apart from all these exercises the reading of short passages to the patient often has a favourable effect, especially with children. If the patient makes a mistake, we must repeat what we said to him (several times if necessary) so as to give him a change to correct his own mistakes. This proves very beneficial, notably in the case of children ; reading to them does not tire them so much as training syllables and helps them to gain a more extensive vocabulary.

There must be short breaks between the exercises so as to allow the patient to rest and avoid fatigue which may prove dangerous, especially in the early periods of treatment, as it may cause nervous disturbances. It is therefore necessary to restrict the duration of the exercises from five to ten minutes. They must be repeated several times every day and be carried out by different people as the treatment proceeds, so as to accustom the patient to different vocalisation.

The exercises may profitably be accompanied by noises such as water running, piano playing, and later on by conversation carried on in the same room, etc. This secures differentiation of hearing even while disturbing noises are occurring.

Functional and psychological treatment.—If there is sufficient hearing capacity, our aim must be to stimulate and to integrate the speech reflex. The acoustic and optic impressions which the child gets by being spoken to suffice in normal speech development. But children whose Hearing-Mutism is the outcome of their acoustic inattentiveness must be stimulated by speech presented in a more *systematic* way than is usually the case. Physiology shows that the threshold of response is lowered, if stimuli which are in themselves not powerful enough are repeated several times in succession. The treatment of Hearing-Mutism makes use of this principle. As we do not get any response from the child by simply speaking to it, we keep on repeating single words until the child responds in some, even if inarticulate, way. This must certainly not be done by putting the child in front of us and saying the same word to it over and over again. Psychological factors play a great rôle in the treatment, and the child must neither be bored nor made stubborn. To incite his interest we use pictures of simple things. It is best to have the picture of one object only on one sheet of paper. The ordinary picture books are no good for these children, whose attention is easily diverted. If there is more than one thing on a page they will never concentrate. Now we begin to talk about the picture, using its name as often as possible and laying much emphasis on it, e.g. Look at the *dog ;* nice *dog*, isn't it ? I like *dogs*, and so on.

This sort of exercise is to be repeated several times every day. We may take one or two or three objects for demonstration, but on no account a greater number, lest the child get confused. In general mothers learn this technique quickly ; the danger lies in that they believe, in spite of all they are told, that the more they try to cram into the child the better. They do not understand that the very repetition of an exceedingly limited number of words (three at the utmost) represents the stimulus which is to release the vocal response by its cumulative strength. If the mother does not obey the instructions of the therapist to the letter, it is better to employ a trained nurse. On no account must the exercises last longer than a few minutes at a time. If the child gets tired or bored its attention will stray to other things, so that the acoustic impressions we are trying to create cannot act as stimuli at all. Insistence upon strict co-operation in spite of obvious inattention may lead to obstinacy, and so spoil any chance of the treatment taking effect. We cannot expect the child's linguistic responses to be as articulate as the words we use. This should not trouble us ; what we want to produce is some kind of utterance which can serve as a basis for further canalisation and integration. This is an additional reason for being careful about leaving the exercises to any but trained persons or those who have thoroughly understood what we require of them. The mother who practises with the child in this way is naturally ambitious and anxious that he should make as much progress as possible. She will certainly be happy at the first utterance of the child, but will probably at once try to make him produce something intelligible. Quite apart from the fact that the child is really incapable of doing so, and that his feeling of inferiority must needs be increased in that way, he must not feel that we want to make him speak. Oppositional tendencies must on no account be roused or strengthened by drawing the child's attention to the fact that we are trying to make him speak, an attempt which has been made in vain over and over again. Stubborn children often respond satis-factorily when taken by surprise. They naturally expect the same old methods to be used to make them speak. Apart from the real inability to speak, there is in these children a well-conditioned system of nullifying any attempts to deal with their speech. Then the unexpected happens : they are not asked to speak, but are merely shown some nice pictures and told things about them. As their rôle is an absolutely passive one, there is not much chance for them to offer active resistance. In other cases it may prove helpful to surprise them by using obviously wrong expressions, such as, ' Look at the nice dog,' when we present a marble, and so on. This procedure provokes their tendency to oppose and makes profit of it.

Bearing in mind that neurotic maladjustment plays its part in the development of Hearing-Mutism, adequate psychological treatment must go hand-in-hand with the special speech exercises if the latter are to lead to satisfactory results. Apart from the general lines of re-education which must be thoroughly understood by the parents, there are some important details to be remembered. As we want to increase the patient's acoustic attention, we must try to eliminate all that is likely to draw his attention to non-acoustic phenomena. It is advisable to let the child have as few pictures, toys, etc., as possible in the nursery.

Little by little, and in a reasonable and not too obvious manner the parents should appear not to understand the child's gestures any longer, and should react only to the child's utterances.

Once the child shows a definite tendency to respond by more or less ' babbled ' utterances, he may be left to develop his speech under the care of his parents, nurse, or teacher, if these have understood our instructions and are ready to carry them out.

As a rule speech then develops normally, but some children exhibit Universal Dyslalia which must be treated in its turn, not only to produce intelligible speech, but also to prevent other speech defects which might follow in its wake, especially Stammering. The treatment of Universal Dyslalia in these cases may only be begun when the speech impulse has grown comparatively strong; if we begin too soon we might again discourage the child. For adequate measures to attain articulate speech see pp. 160 ff.

CHAPTER X

DICTION

" Sweet Benjamin, since thou art young,
And hast not yet the use of Tongue,
Make it thy slave, while thou art free ;
Imprison it, lest it do thee."
—JOHN HOSKINS.[1]

Having overcome the difficulties which the acquisition of articulate speech presents, the growing speaker is not yet ready to meet all the demands of expression and communication. We have pointed out (see pp. 41 ff.) that at a later stage the sentence units handed on are, as it were, dissected into the parts which are the conventional words. These in their turn are suitably put together anew. Analysis is replaced by synthesis. The rules and methods of arranging words as members of a sentence are laid down in the syntax of a given language. But syntax does not represent the highest level of verbalisation. Words may be correctly arranged, their inflexion and articulation may be perfect, but the sentence does not necessarily convey the speaker's thoughts and feelings adequately ; nay, it may not convey any meaning at all.

Syntax, therefore, serves, as it were, as a tool for a more highly integrated mechanism, viz. Diction. The word is derived from the Lat. *dicere*, ' to speak,' the original meaning of which was ' to show, to point out, to exhibit.' Diction thus mainly refers to the choice of vocabulary in speaking or writing for the purpose of genuine expression. The speaker not only avails himself of words, forms, etc., in their plain workaday use ; " next, and above and beyond all this, they have, so to speak, an exciting force, a power of stimulating and reviving in the mind and memory all the associations that cluster around them. Nearly all words carry with them, in vastly varying degrees of course, this power of evocation, so that even commonplace terms, words, and phrases hackneyed and worn thin by unceasing usage, may suddenly be invested with a strange and beautiful suggestiveness when they are pressed into the service of the highest poetic imagination." [2] In this sense every one is a poet in his efforts " to present the whole conceivable world—the world not merely of sense and fantasy, but of severest intellectual effort, of subtlest psychological understanding, of the highest ardours of mutinous or consenting passion—to present anything which any faculty of ours can achieve or accept, as a moment of mere delighted living, of self-sufficient experience." [3] Man is continuously faced with a multitude of events and his " experiences are always

---

[1] *Poems by Sir Henry Wollon . . . and others.* Ed. by the Rev. John Haunah (1845), Pickering, London, pp. 84–5.
[2] Quayle, T. (1924). *Poetic Diction*, Methuen, London, pp. 200–1.
[3] Abercrombie, L. (1925). *The Idea of Great Poetry*, Martin Secker, London, p. 16.

unique : they occur in some particular person's mind, in some particular sequence of other experiences. Now poetry is the translation of experience into language ; and the translation has not properly been made at all unless, along with the stuff of the experience, goes a rendering of its peculiar moment, instinct with the moods, implications, references, influences which made the moment unique." [1]

[1] Abercrombie, L., l.c., p. 23.

CHAPTER XI

CLUTTERING

The last quotation refers to the fact that once thought has been dissociated from utterance, the body of ideas and opinions has again to be brought into unison with a sequence of linguistic symbols.

If the processes of thinking and of verbalising fail to collaborate adequately, speech becomes disordered. The disturbance is one of relation and proportion, and not one that affects either of the two processes.

Cluttering is a characteristic disturbance of diction. The term is apparently kindred with ' clatter ' ; the original meaning was to rattle, to tattle, to gabble, the noise being imitated by the word. Similar onomatopoetic terms are the German ' poltern ' or ' bruddeln ' and the French ' bredouillement.'

Symptomatology.—What at first strikes one in a clutterer is the excessive rapidity of his speech. It is so rapid that sounds or syllables are left out, words and phrases are slurred, distorted, jerky, appear in wrong places, and are often reiterated. Reading, writing, and telling tales exhibit the same abnormalities ; in severe cases speech is almost unintelligible.

Weiss has laid emphasis on the deviating pattern of intonation and the more or less accentuated monotony of intonation which according to Stockert seem to indicate a gulf between the flow of thought and its verbalisation. Indeed, these patients may be fully alive to a given situation. But what causes the disturbance is the speed with which the thoughts flow. In most cases the clutterer recognises the possible concatenations of ' atomic facts ' ; he recognises the ways in which the objects hang together like the links of a chain (the structure of the atomic facts).[1] He makes pictures of the facts ; but when he comes to project his thoughts as a proposition in speech, he fails. The various levels in the space of atomic facts jostle one another with such terrific speed that it is scarcely possible to put the thought into coherent sounds and sentences. It is the stratification of the thought which the clutterer fails to transform into a temporal succession of linguistic symbols. His impulse to articulate is so strong that there is no time left to find the necessary words. Moreover, the process of articulation itself is disordered because the excessive speed does not allow the exact execution of the articulatory movements and often alters the succession of sounds.

The total behaviour of the clutterer agrees with his speech in so far as all his movements are hurried.

An important characteristic of Cluttering is that the speaker is originally unconscious of it ; he has the illusion that his expressions are just as correctly uttered as those he hears around him. If attention

[1] Wittgenstein, L. (1922). *Tractatus logico-philosophicus*, with translation by Bertrand Russell, Kegan Paul, London, 2,01, 2,03, 2,032, 2,034, 2,1.

is drawn to his speech, he is usually able to speak distinctly ; after a short time, however, he relapses into his disorder.

Aetiology.—The symptoms characteristic of Cluttering suggest various etiological factors. The over-rapid speed and reiteration bring to mind disturbances of speech caused by diseases of the mid-brain (see p. 121). Occasional fits of weeping and outbursts of temper seem to support this assumption. The impairment of the co-ordination between mentation and verbalisation is the distinctive feature of some types of Aphasia.

It seems possible, therefore, that the final integration of highest levels of speech has been checked during the clutterers' development. This is indicated also in their histories.

History.—We often find evidence of Retarded Speech Development, Hearing-Mutism, Dyslalia, Nasalism or delayed speech in their family history ; the latter occurs frequently. These facts seem to suggest a hereditary disposition to retarded maturation. For Differential Diagnosis see p. 127.

Treatment.—Treatment naturally demands consideration of the possible causal factors, which may all be present. Thus on the one hand the thought process has to be regulated and organised, on the other, the modes of utterance and of action in general must be co-ordinated.

The former task can start with the aid of pictures exhibiting more or less complicated events. The patient should be shown a picture and given time to analyse it into the proper sequence of propositions and to construct the corresponding sentences.

Motor co-ordination should be initiated by various rhythmical exercises.[1]

Elsie Fogerty [2] has drawn attention to the many occupational crafts of a rhythmic character. Thus the swing of the scythe, felling trees with the wood-cutter's axe, grinding, hammering, swinging of the weaver's shuttle, can be imitated.

Concentration on speech can be trained by reading, as suggested in the following technique. The text which has to be read aloud by the patient is covered by a piece of cardboard into which a little window is cut, which permits only one syllable to be read at a time. The patient shifts the window from syllable to syllable. In this way he not only has the opportunity of getting used to a slower tempo, but can also use the articulatory rules he has learned, and is prevented from hurrying on to ensuing facts. The dissection of the text into small, incoherent units keeps him busy making out the meaning of the material presented.

Last but not least the patient should be influenced psychologically. It has been proved that he is able to speak properly if he gives his attention to utterance, particularly when circumstances demand clear expression. It is therefore important to make clear to the patient the social value of speech, as one of the most vital links between the members of a community.

[1] Boome, E. J., Baines, H. M. S. and Harries, D. G. (1939). *Abnormal Speech*, Methuen, London, chapter v.
[2] Fogerty, E. (1937). *Rhythm*, Allen & Unwin, London, pp. 101 ff.

CHAPTER XII

STAMMERING

Terms.—Stammering also is a disorder of diction. It is interesting to note that, in spite of the multiformity of its character, even the layman, with few exceptions, is able to comprehend the various types of this disorder under one concept. This has been given several names, which hint at the outstanding feature of the disorder, viz. the fact that the flow of speech suddenly and unexpectedly comes to a standstill. It is as though the unfortunate speaker were compelled to remain fixed to certain utterances or were stuck because some unknown obstacle is in his way.

The terms used in common English parlance and dialects all refer to the behaviour of the patients. Thus *stammering* and *stuttering* carry the connotations 'to walk with heavy, awkward, unsteady steps; to hesitate, to stagger, to stumble, to totter, to falter.' The former is derived from the base STAM extended from STA 'to stand, remain fixed;' it is also related to Old Saxon and Old High German *stum,* 'dumb.'[1] The latter is a frequentative of *stut;* the original meaning was 'to strike against;' the kindred verb 'to stumble' still conveys the meaning 'to trip.'[2]

The following survey of the symptoms shows how the impression denoted by the aforementioned words arises.

Reiteration of syllables, words, or phrases, e.g. 'how how how are you this morning?', 'I don't don't quite know.' This kind of utterance has been compared with 'clonic,' i.e. repeated muscular spasms in certain nervous diseases. The term 'Clonus' has therefore (mistakenly) been adopted to describe reiterative utterances.

Prolonged articulation of sounds, e.g. 'When [w : : : en] will you come?'

Forced, laboured articulation, varying in length, affecting both reiterated and prolonged articulation. Because of its similarity with 'tonic,' i.e. continuous muscular spasms, the term 'Tonus' has been adopted. "Respiration is jerky . . . and expiration may be completely held up for as long as five or six seconds. On auscultation at the bases of the lungs there is frequently a suspension or marked diminution of respiratory murmur."[3] Other patients paroxysmally press nearly all air out of their lungs, and when almost completely exhausted, succeed in uttering one or two words.

Fröschels[4] subjected clonic and tonic articulations to a close investigation, and showed their pathological significance. According to his theory we are to distinguish the following combinations of clonic and tonic articulation :—

---

[1] Wyld, *Dict.*   [2] Skeat, *Concise Etymol. Dict.*

[3] Boome, E. J. and Richardson, M. A. (1931). *The Nature and Treatment of Stammering,* Methuen, London, pp. 41–2.

[4] Fröschels, E. (1925). *Das Stottern (Assoziative Aphasie),* Deuticke, Vienna.

Tonoclonus is a clonus in which each of the repeated syllables is tonic.

Clonotonus arises if tonic utterances are subjected to iteration.

In all clonic and tonoclonic utterances the time needed for their enunciation has to be measured. When compared with the number of normally spoken syllables, they may prove to be of the same tempo, or of a retarded or accelerated pace.

Any part of the speech pattern may be seized with these motor abnormalities. Thus articulatory, phonatory, and respiratory movements may show quasi-spastic peculiarities.

Parts of the body usually not concerned with speech may be put into operation. These grimaces and gesticulations have been termed *co-movements*, being compared, e.g., with movements such as those which accompany the lifting of a heavy burden. Fröschels rightly suggested the term ' concomitant action,' for reasons which will appear in the next chapter.[1]

Sounds, words, phrases, or meaningless syllables which may be inserted into the sentence, without having any reference to the meaning expressed by it are called *Embolophrasias*.[2] They, too, may exhibit a quasi-spastic character.

Numerous investigations (Fröschels, Seemann, Szondi, Stern, Sovák and others) have shown a great variety of signs of constitutional inferiority in stammerers and their families, but chronic general diseases and defects of the peripheral speech organs play no part in the outbreak of stammering.[3] One of my patients, however, had a purely tonic stammer, due to an extremely short frenulum which made the articulation of all dental sounds hardly possible. The disorder with all its anxiety and inferiority symptoms disappeared after the tongue had been freed by cutting the frenulum.

Adenoids, found by various workers in 20 to 50 per cent. of the cases, are still considered to be of some influence. E. J. Boome and M. A. Richardson[4] emphasise that adenoids " have no greater effect upon the actual speech of the stammerer than upon that of the normal speaker. It is not the *physical* factor that makes adenoidal children stammer, but the *psychical*. Enlarged tonsils and adenoids fill up the buccal cavity, causing obstruction and a sense of discomfort ; when they are removed there is a feeling of uneasiness and a lack of confidence. It is the psychical factor which determines the stammer. In the many cases traced directly to the removal of tonsils and adenoids the cause is usually operation shock or anticipatory fear."

Great significance is generally attributed to left-handedness. In view of the divergent and sometimes obscure records, the question

---

[1] I cannot confirm Fröschels' (*Symptomatology des Stotterns*, p. 43) latest finding that tonic articulation is accelerated, i.e. that pressed articulation loosens comparatively quickly in relation to the efforts made, the more the patient has ' practised his stammer.

[2] Greek *emballein*, ' to throw in.'

[3] Seemann, M. (1935). " Ueber somatische Befunde bei Stotterern." VI. Kongr. d. Int. Ges. f. Logopaedie u. Phoniatrie, Deuticke, Leipzig-Wien, pp. 2–21.

[4] *The Nature and Treatment of Stammering*, pp. 24–5.

whether left-handedness is of aetiological import must be treated with extreme reserve,[1] though there are "instances of left-handed children developing a stammer through being forced to use the right hand." [2] According to Boome and Richardson's statistics, "the number of left-handed children among normal speakers would appear to be about double the number found among stammerers."

Numerous investigations of the stammerer's constitution, which are, however, not yet sufficiently complete, emphasise the striking frequency of signs relating to an inferiority of the lower brain centres (strio-pallidum, thalamus, hypothalamus) and the vegetative nervous system.[3]

Classification.—According to the speech-symptoms, different types of stammerers have been distinguished. Almost any of the vast number of data have been used by the classifiers as characteristic attributes of different stammer forms.

The oldest theory, which has not even yet been fully relinquished, made the spasmodic character of the speech-movements a basis of classification (Kussmaul, Gutzmann). On the other hand, psychological schools (Freud, Adler) rejected all classifications, and regarded all stammer symptoms as equivalent manifestations of the patient's neurotic attitude.[4]

We are indebted to Hoepfner and Fröschels for having indicated new fruitful ways of approach. They have not only described the symptoms as precisely as possible, but have also brought them in logical connection with the mentality of the patient, and have established the relation between a given symptom and its time of onset. They have thus come to the opinion that the symptoms of stammering can only be grouped with regard to their special character in conjunction with their temporal sequence. Their investigations have led them to the view that stammering is a specific neurosis, in the development of which the conscious will of the patient plays a conspicuous part.

The following interpretation is based on the results of these two workers, but it deviates in many points as a result of my own investigations and basic ideas, as explained in the introductory chapters.

[1] Seemann, M. (1935), l.c.

[2] Boome and Richardson, l.c., pp. 19–20.

[3] Stein, L. (1937). *Sprach- und Stimmstörungen und ihre Behandlung in der täglichen Praxis*, Weidman, Wien-Leipzig-Bern, pp. 130–2. Stein, L., in Fröschels, E. (1925). *Lehrbuch der Sprachheilkunde*, Deuticke, Leipzig-Wien, ch. 16. Fröschels und Moses (1926). *Ueber Konstitution assoziativaphatischer Kinder*, Wien. med. Woch. Stern, H. (1925). *Zur Pathogenese der Dysarthria spastica*. Stratton, L. D. (1924). "A Factor in Aetiology of a Sub-breathing Stammerer," *Journ. of Comp. Psychol.*, 4. Szondi, L. (1930). *Die Revision der Neurasthenie-frage*, Novak, Budapest. Sovák, M. (1933). "Poměry sympatických reflexů u koktavých," *Čas. Lék. Čes.* Jellinek, A. *Discussion to Seemann*, l.c. Pollak, E. und Schilder, P. (1926). "Zur Lehre von den Sprachantrieben," *Zeitschr. f. d. ges. Neurol. und Psych.*, 104, pp. 480–502. Seemann, M. (1931). *K etiologii koktavosti*, Sborník Zemanův, Praha. Bray, G. W. (1937). *Recent Advances in Allergy*, London. Kennedy, A. M. and Williams, D. A. (1938). *Brit. Med. Journ.*, 2, 1306. Loewenthal, L. J. A. and Wilson, W. A. (1939). Ibid., 2, 110. Gordon I. (1942). "Allergy, Enuresis and Stammering," ibid., 357.

[4] As to the present state of the problem see Boenheim, C. (1939). *Practical Child Psychotherapy*, John Bale, Ltd., London.

DEVELOPMENTAL INTERPRETATION

First Stage.—Numerous inquiries have shown that the onset of developmental stammering or its exacerbation takes place as a rule in periods of rapid growth. This is on the average to be found in the 2nd, 5th, 7th,[1] or 14th years. These are the phases in which the higher forms of speech and of thought differentiate out of the original unit, and new, highly specialised and independent units emerge.

Once they have originated they do not necessarily remain in the proper proportion with each other. The ideal proportion would be : thought (TH) : expression (E) = 100 : 100 ; but this proportion is never reached.

During the growth of intelligence, two types of disproportion may be expected. Type A. TH : E = 100 : 100 − x.
$$\text{Type B.} \quad TH : E = 100 - y : 100.$$

A few examples may illustrate that disproportions of both type A and type B may result in similar deviations of utterance.

Type A.—Supposing an intelligent child of three came into a warm room in which there was an electric heater which he had never seen. He might have the idea of " something to keep the room warm," he might perhaps like its appearance, etc. ; but he may lack the words when wanting to talk about it to his mother. He would perhaps exclaim : " Loo loo look mother, what a nice . . . fireplace." The deviating form of utterance has obviously arisen through the inadequacy of the child's vocabulary, which does not provide him with names for heating devices hitherto not seen.

Another time the child coming home from the nursery school may be asked what he had been doing there. The answer might sound : " The mistress ta ta ta taught me writing." Why ? The child obviously knows the verb he wants to use ; but he knows also other verbs of a similar pattern, e.g. reach, screech. Every one who has learned a foreign language will realise that the child may find himself in a dilemma as to how the verb should sound in the given case. For there are the forms reach, reached ; teach, taught competing. His uttering fluency will therefore be held up until he comes to a decision. Thus a lack of grammar plays the same part as a lack of vocabulary.

The case may also be as follows : When asked the same question, the child may revive a general impression of all that has happened at school. But the ' atomic facts ' (see above p. 107) are not yet transformed into logical propositions and sentences and arranged in an adequate sequence. Thus several ideas may jostle one another, forcing their way toward verbal expression. The form of utterance will thus be the same in spite of adequate means of expression. Deficiency in arranging mental material in an adequate sequence has taken the place of lack of grammar or vocabulary. Richness of imagination may increase the difficulty.

At all events the normal co-operation between the various physiological and psychological substrata concerned with meaningful utter-

---

[1] Boome and Richardson, l.c., pp. 28–31.

ance is impaired. The disproportion between thought and expression [1] must at least give rise to temporary dissolution, manifest in a speech behaviour which corresponds to the next lower level of development. Other factors, such as mental or physical shock,[2] slight concussion, sunstroke, encephalitis, intoxication, post-morbid conditions, rickets, rheumatic infection,[3] etc., operate likewise.

Organic cases support the view that the symptom of reiteration which appears both in evolution and dissolution is operated by the unbalanced relation between the speech area in the frontal lobe and the striatal system.[4]

Climate and the nature and degree of civilisation can play a similar rôle. Stammering " is, for instance, rare in Rumania, Spain, Portugal, and Italy, the lands of soft sounds and of the warm climate which precludes rush and hurry. Again, those countries whose people have fewer repressions and inhibitions, and consequently less mental conflict and nervous strain, will produce proportionally fewer stammerers. In Germany and Poland stammering is very common." [5]

Clonic stammer.—The form (pattern) of utterance representing this level is *reiterative* (see Development of Speech, p. 32). As a stammer symptom it·is termed *Clonus*. Its origin clearly shows that its nature can neither be that of a genuine spasm, nor can will play any part.

We have to stress here that the child is not conscious of *how* he speaks. Reiteration is not a purposely chosen symptom. He is as little aware of it as we are of reiterated syllables when they occasionally occur in our speech under exceptional conditions such as, embarrassment, perplexity, confusion, or dilemma (see Development of Speech, Evolution of Speech, pp. 39 ff., 50 ff.).

The evolutionary outlook not only explains why the speaker repeats at all, but also why just this form of utterance appears and not another one (say a pause). It is not surprising that the intelligence quotient of stammerers is in the majority of cases above the average.

Type B.—The few cases in which a low I. Q. is found (mental backwardness) do but prove the rule. The ratio of disproportion is here inverse : TH : E $=$ 100 $-$ y : 100. Consequently the same dissolution process, namely, the reaching of an earlier stage of speech development with its characteristic reiterations must take place.

In addition we find in these cases other symptoms (very often overlooked) which should arrest our attention and make us careful as to our opinion. These stammerers are frequently most garrulous and verbose ; however, their thoughts are poor indeed, their propositionising exceedingly slow and defective. Careful examination shows that they can hardly settle a situation intelligently. Their bodily movements are quick, irregular, unharmonious, quasi-unchecked and inco-ordinate.

To the inexperienced observer they thus make the impression of being bright through their deceptive swiftness in expression which, however, is in fact mere utterance of little significance.

[1] Aristotle, *Hist. An.*, lib. i, cap. xi.
[2] Boome and Richardson, l.c., p. 25.   [3] Ibid., p. 18.
[4] Pollak, E. and Schilder, P. (1926). " Zur Lehre von den Sprachantrieben," *Zeitschr. f. d. ges. Neurol. u. Psycgiatr.*, 104, pp. 480–502.
[5] Boome and Richardson, p. 27.

Stammer in adults.—It does not surprise us that stammering is in the majority of cases a developmental disorder, since in childhood the top levels of standard language are not yet well canalised, so that they are apt to succumb to dissolution. But patients have been under the observation of some therapists and of the present writer, who had assuredly never stammered in childhood and yet developed a stammer in adult age.

We must expect that only strong factors can bring about a dissolution of well-organised language. Patients are sometimes seen who have over-exerted themselves to such an extent that general inanition prevents them from translating their thoughts into sentences. In other cases close examination and study of the history of the disorder reveals previous more or less serious and widespread organic processes in the brain. Such patients may first suffer from mild Aphasia, or Dysarthria which in turn may cause a stammer ; others may develop a stammer, though there had not been any previous speech disorders. Patients of the latter- kind may have overcome diseases of the brain, manifesting themselves in general signs (e.g. high temperature, tiredness, somnolence, restless sleep, seeing double, fits of crying) to which the patient did not impute particular significance as to speech. Patients therefore, as a rule, do not mention these previous illnesses at all. Only after persistent inquiry will they report ailments such as sunstroke or ' influenza ; ' medical examination may disclose the signs and symptoms of past encephalitis.

It is understandable that these cases also, under the influence of such strong dissolutionary factors, develop a reiterating kind of stammer according to the rule delineated in the case of developmental stammerers.[1]

The rare cases (children and adults) who deviate from this rule will be dealt with below (see p. 119).

Development of clonic stammerers.—Stammerers of type B often reiterate for years unless maturation equalises the disorder, as it does, in a minority of cases. As a rule they never " grow out of it " ; in the end, sometimes after many years, degenerative processes in the nervous system become noticeable (e.g. Imbecility, Parkinson's syndrome).

The type of stammer does not change, as the patients are not aware of their disorder. If their attention is drawn to it they mostly do not worry about it, for their mental capacity does not allow them to realise the social consequences.

There are two possible ways of development of type A : (1) it may be overcome spontaneously ; (2) it may change into a persisting stammer.

In the majority of cases stammering of type A is apt to disappear spontaneously, but it would not do so if any ' assistance ' were given.

The explanation of the disappearance of the reiterations is a simple and brief one. In a case of dissolution where the nervous systems is

---

[1] For the contributions to the elucidation of the disturbances in different areas of the brain, made by Hoepfner, Schilder, Trömner, Brown and others, see L. Stein's reports in " Der Stand der Logopaedie und Phoniatrie " (1929), *Monatschrift für Ohrenheilkunde*, **63**, pp. 1316–26. " Die Behandlung der assoziativen, Aphasie " (1934), ibid., **68**, pp. 920–35.

still fit, evolution is going on at the same time (see Chapter V). Thus as time and growth goes on, the further development of linguistic faculties required for transforming thoughts will be well under way. The more the disproportion between thought and linguistic expression decreases, the less occasion is there for reiterations.

This development must naturally be a steady and smooth one; and this requires both time and abolishment of all circumstances which could obstruct this progress (see Prognosis).

There are cases in which clonic stammering remains unaltered during the whole life and is not complicated psychically. Freund [1] calls this type " rudimentary stammer."

Second Stage, First Phase.—Let us now consider the position as to speaker and listeners. Those around a young stammerer in the initial stage have been watching him for several years and have been seeing that his growth and intellectual progress have been quite satisfactory, nay, in most cases exceedingly good. Also the child's speech has hitherto been developing normally.

When they see that his speech is affected there arises at least surprise. Being ignorant of the very nature of the disorder, those in charge of the child will inevitably follow a mistaken course in dealing with him, regarding this change as a " bad habit." It would consist mostly of remarks meant to be helpful, such as: " Why are you talking like that ? " " Do not talk like that," " If you talk like that I shall not listen to you," " Talk properly," etc.

The stammerer's response may be twofold :

1. Some children " duly note " it and keep on stammering in the same manner without worrying.

2. The majority of children and adults consciously wish to get rid of the disorder.

Neurotic use of the clonus.—The first response occurs if the clonic stammer be built into an already existing neurosis of other origin. An example may make this clear. An exceptionally bright and clever boy of five showed a clonic stammer which had lasted for only a few weeks. After a few introductory words I asked the child straight away : " Tell me frankly, *why* are you stammering ? " The boy was astonished, and answered : " Why do you ask me, *you* ought to know." This was indeed the answer I had expected. I then went on : " If I stammered, I should certainly know ; but as it is *you* who do so, *you* ought to know." The boy became pensive, and after a while said : " Really, I often don't know, but sometimes I do it just to bully mother."

The history revealed that the boy—an only child—had for about two years shown symptoms of aggression against his over-anxious mother (he would, for instance, approach the window-sill as if he were going to climb on it).

We should go too far if we thought that the aggressive tendency created the speech symptom. But it is well known that the neurotic character may take a hold on established symptoms which it has discovered would serve its purpose.

[1] Freund, H. (1932). *Med. Welt*, pp. 1243-5.

The mere fact that the symptom is *perceived* (and perception is directed by interest) [1] then clears the way for the further development of the clinical symptoms. These again follow dissolutionary rules which will be dealt with presently.

In the above case the clonus has been used as a weapon by an aggressive child. This neurotic mechanism will show itself more plainly in the ensuing phases.

Centipede attitude.—In otherwise normal individuals there arises a state of surprise. As the stammerer has not yet been aware of what those around him are actually talking about, he will naturally, after being told repeatedly how bad his speech is, begin to examine his own speech. This can only be done by observation followed by a comparison of his own speech with that heard from those around him. The stammerer (adults not excepted !) will then realise that there is in fact a difference between his own speech and that of those around him. Noticing the reiterations he will naturally endeavour to get rid of them ; but this will induce him to attend to the organs which perform speech. This step the stammerer takes is a very dangerous one, since it leads to a state of mind which I should like to call the "*Centipede Attitude*." I am referring here to Craster's little poem, which reads as follows :—

> " The centipede was happy quite
> Until a toad in fun
> Said, ' Pray which leg goes after which ?
> That worked her mind to such a pitch,
> She lay distracted in a ditch
> Considering how to run." [2]

The psychological and physiological significance of this poem is briefly : As soon as we consciously and deliberately deal with activities which under normal (natural) circumstances are unconscious and automatic, their inhibition is achieved. Think of what happens if you begin to observe every single action of the members of the body while, say, walking, writing, etc.

Hesitation.—The natural consequence will be, besides the reiterations, a certain hesitating [3] (i.e. sticking fast, pausing, tarrying) attitude in speaking. If a stammer is described as hesitating, the term should be used to denote this phenomenon only. Unfortunately almost any other type has been denoted likewise, which causes so much confusion that many otherwise valuable case histories have lost their clinical value.

The stammerer who suddenly finds himself stuck, not realising the manifestation of the "centipede attitude," acquires an unnatural sensation as to his speech organs. In fact it has been observed how stammerers of this type manipulate with their lips or tongue.

These and all the following explanations are derived from patients'

---

[1] See Blanshard's elaborate explanations, l.c.
[2] Craster, E. (1871). "Pinafore Poems," publ. in *John O'London's Treasure Trove*, George Newnes, London, p. 106.
[3] Intensive form of Lat. *haerere*, ' to stick.'

own spontaneous reports. They stressed their sudden surprise at getting stuck, which, after a short period of unconcern, was followed by dislike. They came to feel the ridiculous and comic character of their speech. Children are often made the laughing-stock of their school-mates ; but adults can also in many cases not keep back a smile.

Ridiculousness of stammering.—A brief remark may be inserted here. How is it that so many people may be induced to laugh at stammerers ? Because they unconsciously sense the archaic feature of such speech ; the speaker exhibits all characteristics of a normal individual, excepting his utterance which appears to belong to an earlier period. And this incongruity irresistibly leads to laughter, just as if someone wore modern clothes and a helmet of the sixteenth century.

The stammerer soon comes to know this changed atmosphere around him, which in its turn leads to embarrassment ; and a Chinese saying runs : " Embarrassment leads naturally to anger."

Second stage, second phase.—When the stammerer's attention is drawn to the fact that his speech is ' bad,' the task of speaking seems so formidable as to make it difficult to contend with. The mental response to the emotionally tuned do's and don'ts may be of two different kinds. If the reaction is too violent it leads to complete discouragement, which manifests itself in mutism and other symptoms of depression—gloom, immobility, apathy, etc.

The individual seeks safety in flight, and will then only be capable of emotional expressions used by small babies : crying, thus reaching one of the lowest dissolutionary levels (see Chapter IX, Mutism). But comparatively few children give up in this way ; the majority try hard to overcome the difficulty.

It appears obvious, and has been proved by the statements of many stammerers in the initial stage, that they are puzzled by these ' queer ' reiterations, and are eager to refer it to some cause. The stammerer soon begins to believe that the speech abnormality has something to do with the mouth (speech organs). Many children can be found manip-ulating their ' disobedient ' speech organs. Their attempts to reduce them to obedience are still promoted by the adults' words such as " Pull yourself together," " Be careful," " Make an effort," etc. And the little stammerer follows the advice !

Adults give themselves the same advice. They attribute their odd utterance to some mysterious ' weakness ' which they resolve to get rid of at all costs.

Let us bear in mind that we can never ' invent ' methods but only utilise and improve those mechanisms we find in existence (see De-velopment of Speech). Also we must not overlook the fact that in any dissolution process, evolution is still going on. We have seen that, during the period of normal speech development, the child, for the sake of social advantage, i.e. of being understood and of the fulfilment of his desires, has to fight the iteration tendency. This can only be effected by suppression.

He mistakenly attributes the difficulty to the speech organs them-selves. But " a little learning is a dangerous thing ; " and thus the next conscious conclusion jumped at by the speaker is *that he must make an increased effort* in order to suppress the reiterations or hesitations.

It is obvious that this inference is wrong, since it is due, so to speak, to a disarranged perspective ; for (1) speech is in reality not a toilsome task, (2) the origin of the symptom is to be sought neither in mentation nor especially in the speech organs and their function. It has arisen from their *mutual relation*. C. G. Jung has pointed out that "it depends on quantitative relationships . . . whether the struggle leads to health, to a neurosis, or to compensatory over-functioning. . . ." [1]

Tonus.—The stammerer, in view of the apparent uphill work, will use more energy than the natural compensation would require. The result will be morbid tension (*Tonus*). It is clear that this new symptom cannot be regarded as a genuine spasm, since it is gained by the exercise of will and attention.

Increased attention paid by the speaker to his utterance can be found in Motor Aphasia and paralytic speech disorders where it brings about strained articulation and concomitant movements (see below). On the other hand, delirious conditions (delirium tremens, pneumonia) which impair attention, relieve the tonic articulation. [2]

Slow tonoclonus.—This laboured articulation also seizes the original and still persisting reiterated utterances, thus giving rise to the Tonoclonus. Its tempo is slower than that of the ' pure ' Clonus, as the tonicity hinders the usual rhythmic repetitions.

Disturbances of respiration.—The respiratory disturbances, which have often been regarded as the primary cause of stammering, prove themselves to be consequences of the laboured articulation.

Rôle of the Strio-Pallidum.—We will now consider what the application of force really means. In the effective contraction of the muscles the necessary tension is produced originally by the influence of lower levels of the central nervous system, particularly the spinal cord, the sympathetic nervous system, and their central nuclei, Hypothalamus, Thalamus, and especially the Strio-Pallidum. The conscious efforts of the untrained are made by eliminating the inhibiting influence of the highest cerebral levels, which under normal circumstances plays its part in co-ordination, i.e. the balance between lower and higher strata.

I have been able to show that the tense accompaniments of stammering disappear if the vocal cavities are rendered insensible by administering anesthetics, e.g. Percaine. [3] Two explanations are possible. On the one hand the anesthesia of the sensory nerves themselves prevents the proper use of the effector organs (remember the condition you feel in your tongue and lips after a cocaine injection into the gums !) and thus the application of excessive force ; and on the other hand—according to Seeger's [4] interpretation of my experiments—the

[1] Freud, S. (1937). *The Origin of Psycho-Analysis. A General Selection from the Works of Sigmund Freud*. Ed. by John Rickmann, Hogarth Press, London, p. 38.
[2] Stockert, F. (1935). *Die Psychogenese des Stotterns*. VI. Kongr. d. Int. Ges. f. Logopaedie u. Phoniatrie, Deuticke, Leipzig-Wien; p. 24.
[3] Stein, L. (1937). *Sprach- u. Stimmstörungen*, pp. 151, 157.
[4] Seeger (1935). Discussion to Stockert, *Psychogenese*, l.c.

anesthetic through reabsorption alters the tonus of the vegetative nervous system (see p. 9).

If, now, the lower levels are allowed to act as top levels, forms of action reappear which were observable when, during developmental and evolutionary time, those levels were in fact top levels. We shall meet them when dealing with the further stages of stammer development, and we shall be obliged to recall many infantile gestures.

In view of all we know about the development of speech, Bacon's catchword, " The remedy worse than the disease," may well be applied to what is taking place and promoting further deterioration.

The patient's deliberations are certainly ' logical,' and thus justify the assumption of an ' inner logic ' in the development of the stammer stages.

These absurd conclusions and extravagant actions of stammerers are, to use H. Jackon's words, " the survivals of their fittest states " [1] (see Chapter V, Dissolution). Their manifestations will appear plainly during the following phases.

Before dealing with them, a few words must be said about the fact that in some cases all details obtained from the patient's history and from analysis seem to indicate that stammering had started with tonic symptoms, without having passed through the clonic phase. This fulminating outbreak is entirely in concordance with our scheme of dissolution, representing simply a severer degree of trauma. Grave shocks or diseases may disintegrate so many of the higher evolutionary levels of speech and behaviour as to make the patient lapse to levels corresponding to physiological dumbness.

The patient on the one hand perceives his inability ; on the other hand, he tries to overcome the deficiency. As he misinterprets the origin and nature of the deficiency, he falls into error as outlined.

From now on neurotic mechanisms make themselves clearly noticeable. The speech disorder appears as a welcome means to serve the purposes of the neurotic mind. A girl of 25 began to stammer clonically shortly after a serious operation with subsequent complications apparently of a septic nature. She did not mind it at first, and was expecting a spontaneous improvement. After a short time she became impatient and tried to overcome the stammer by effort, which activated the tonus. In spite of (or because of) advice from elocutionists, she could not get rid of it. The riddle can be solved if it be taken into consideration that two years before the operation, while working in a foreign country, she had fallen in love with a fellow-worker whose world outlook she and her family did not share. The stammer obviously presented to her a good pretext for not returning to him. Numerous parapraxes, such as constant forgetfulness and slips during treatment, gave sufficient evidence for this assumption.

In accordance with what we have already pointed out (p. 118), and in the chapter on development (p. 14), we must assume a strong affinity between tension and its introspective aspect of attention (notice the common etymological base !) on the one hand, and tendencies of flight or of aggression on the other. These factors check

[1] Jackson, l.c., pp. 46–7.

reintegration along the biologically normal pathway, though the patient consciously strives towards the standard. As the normal way is blocked, he is forced to strive after normal language *by a side way ;* looked upon from the biological angle, it means going *down* the evolutionary scale. Further dissolution is going on ; regression [1] leads to lower levels, that is to say, patterns which will naturally expose more primitive outlooks.

We are here anticipating the *hierarchy* of biological and psychological patterns, manifest in clinical symptoms, which will appear in the ensuing phases.

Second Stage, Third Phase.—By adopting the method of force, the stammerer finds himself in a curious dilemma. On the one hand, the outlawed reiterations are now—to the minds and approbation of the people in his environment—practically abolished. They find his speech much ' better.' We can quite see why they do so. Compare [ma ma mam] with [m : : am] and you will certainly prefer the latter from the naïve acoustic point of view, though you will not consider it quite ' normal.' On the other hand, the stammerer himself must obviously dislike this type of utterance for two reasons : (1) he realises that it is still a ' stammer,' (2) it also needs considerable effort, whereas his former stammer type was ' easy.' There then arises a contest between the will to speak and the will to keep silent.[2]

Conception of difficulty.—Thus the type of speech he observes in those around him appears to him a remote ideal. And his conclusion is : *speech is difficult.* This conclusion, drawn from wrong premises, will dominate the stammerer for ever, and will itself serve as a premise for further conclusions which will obviously also be wrong, unless psychological treatment corrects the premises.

Speech anxiety.—At the same time the stammerer's emotions of discomfort gradually turn into definite anxiety. He fears speaking, and may again adopt two modes of approach : (1) he may more or less avoid speech, (2) his conscious idea will be, in most cases, that he is to blame for his failure inasmuch as he did not make sufficient effort.

Turning to the neurological basis, it may tentatively be suggested that the influence of the thalamus and its communications with the corpus mammillare on the one hand, and with the cortex on the other now prevails.[3] They constitute the pathways along which concentration on interpretation and effective ' tuning ' of a given situation operate.

Glottal stop.—Even if we had no reports on the stammerer's feelings of embarrassment and anxiety, we could infer them from a symptom which arises simultaneously with the psychological ones. It is the *glottal stop*, which has already been fully discussed in the description

---

[1] " The flight from the unsatisfying reality into what we call, on account of its biologically injurious nature, disease, but which is never without an individual gain in pleasure for the patient, takes place over the path of regression. . . ." S. Freud, *The Origin of Psycho-analysis*, p. 36.

[2] Schneider, E. (1922). " Ueber das Stottern," *Zeitschr. f. psychoanal.*, Pädagogik.

[3] Cf. Grünthal, E. (1939). " Ueber das Corpus mamillare . . .," *Confinia neurologica*, 2, pp. 64–95.

of the crying period (see p. 28). The glottal stop may, and does originate as an independent symptom of fear (see p. 48). That is to say, it is not, or need not be, primarily attached to the articulation of the word intended. But the stammerer often, not knowing its significance, infers that it is part of the ' difficult ' word.

Rapid tonoclonus.—The tonoclonus grows faster until its speed finally exceeds that of the normal syllable sequence. Fröschels holds that this is due to ' practice.' In my view this symptom, in conjunction with the appearance of the tendency to hurry in speaking and the inability to stop, manifests the increasing power of the strio-pallidar level ; for patients suffering from organic diseases of this system (encephalitis lethargica, pseudo-bulbar palsy) sometimes show a similar peculiarity called Palilalia.[1] This manifests itself in the " repetition of a phrase which the patient reiterates with increasing rapidity." [2] The disorder is rare, and its nature not well understood.

The blind alley.—What the stammerer does not see, is that he has missed the right track at a point of bifurcation indicated by reiteration. The patient has experienced frustration ; he has not been able to meet the requirements of social reality ; interference from those around has inhibited the natural recovery (the three outstanding factors leading to neurosis.[3] As the straight track proves impassable, he now walks along a path which will later on prove to be a *blind alley.*

Seen from the dissolutionary angle, this blind alley not only leads sidewards, but also downwards to lower strata, whose manifestations will be seen presently. The postures on which the speech movements are based (see p. 11) can accordingly increase in intensity to such an extent that, in the end, utterance is entirely frustrated. The impulse to speak is not noticeable, but can be recognised from pneumographic curves which show expiratory impulses. To call this type ' forme fruste,' as Biaggi [4] does, is misleading, since this term would suggest that the disorder has not developed to its full extent. But, in fact, it constitutes an advanced stage and, therefore, a severer degree of the disorder.

Second Stage, Fourth Phase.—His deliberate efforts have brought the stammerer " out of the frying-pan into the fire." He is now quite convinced that speaking is hard work, and is puzzled about how other people can master it. He now follows the rule which we all follow when our motor attempts are not successful : we think we have not made *enough effort.*

Imagine your attitude when you want to lift a table or cupboard which you think is too heavy for you. You will consciously and deliberately use the whole of your energy. But this is more than would correspond to the capacity of your arms. There arises, therefore, an overflow of energy which manifests itself in all sorts of tense movements of organs which have nothing to do with the work.

Co - movements.—These concomitant movements usually show features peculiar to each stammerer, e.g. closing the eyes tightly,

---

[1] Greek palin, ' again ' ; lalein, ' to speak.'　　[2] Brain, l.c., p. 82.
[3] Freud, *Selection*, pp. 70 *et seq.*
[4] Biaggi, R. " Sulla balbuzie frusta," *Arch. ital. di otol.*, 9, p. 293.

wriggling, fidgeting movements of the extremities, stamping the feet on the ground, grimaces, expressing fear, disgust, rage, audible gnashing of teeth, etc. The behaviourist and the evolutionist can easily recognise lower more emotional levels being set free. The psychological histories of the patients are sure to confirm the validity of these clinical symptoms. A stammerer exhibited violent tonic and tonoclonic articulation, and rigidity of the whole body. Concomitant movements represented the typical attitudes of flight and aggression. He clenched his fists, and drew the corner of the mouth sidewards and upwards, thus exposing the teeth. Simultaneously he ducked his head. Analysis revealed distinct sense of frustration and strong rebellion against the father and father-substitutes (dictators).

The canalisation of attitudes of fright or of aggression leads to the general hypertonicity in stammerers, which has been stressed especially by English workers.[1] From what has been said it appears to be the effect of the stammerer's neurotic development, but not the cause of the stammer.

Seen from the dissolutionary and neurological angle, the lower parts of the brain (such as the brain stem, the strio-pallidar system, the hypothalamus, and the thalamus with their interconnections), which are known to be the somatic substrata of emotion, attention, and tonicity (see p. 119) seem to obtain increasing control.[2]

Clicks.—The appearance of clicks (see p. 49) also evidences the activity of lower evolutionary levels. They are used to express emotions of embarrassment, anger, contempt, impatience, fear; meanings which they still convey as interjections in normal speech (see p. 50). Clicks in stammering are often accompanied by grimaces and gesticulations which have the same significance. The fact that clicks and corresponding gesticulations may present themselves simultaneously suggests that the patient has reached a level where the primitive pattern of less differentiated expression is still preserved.

Sound-anxiety.—At this time, sometimes earlier (say in the tonic phase), the stammerer may go astray into a further side-path through a dangerous logic. He has for some time been observing his speech-movements closely, without, of course, knowing their true nature. Still consciously wishing to conquer them, he begins to dissect them in a way that does not conform to the biological and psychological stratification. This aberration draws his attention to units which certainly are artificial, namely, sounds.

Naturally developed speech does not know single sounds, but only sequence of sounds; there are, phonetically, more sounds contained in a syllable or word, than orthography can represent. It is the spelled symbols that the stammerer, in consequence of what he has learned in writing and reading, regards as the bearers of the evil. Thus the original word- or syllable-anxiety develops into sound-anxiety.

For the most part sounds at the beginning of a word or phrase move more and more into the foreground; but those in the middle of

[1] Boome and Richardson, l.c.
[2] Cf. Brown, F. W. (1932). *Amer. Journ. of Orthopsychiatry*, **2**, pp. 363-76.

a word may also appear dangerous. These patients are then not even able to articulate single meaningless sounds easily. Consequently they are sometimes inclined to omit these hard sounds altogether.

Which sounds acquire this meaning of hardness depends on the individual circumstances. As a rule, those frequently used or those charged with strong emotions are endowed with the danger quality.

Analysis of one of my patients brought to light that he had entirely repressed various difficulties with his fiancée, named Ruth. This factor caused hardship in the sound R, inconceivable to himself. In a girl, psychotherapy uncovered that the difficulty in J [dʒ] arose when she one day wavered between two utterances. She was sitting with her lover in the office situated behind her father's shop, in which at the same time the apprentice was working. The maid came down asking her if the apprentice could give her a hand. Her real intention was to agree, realising that it would be an opportunity to be alone with her admirer. On the other hand, her morals prevented her from saying so. In her state of indecision she stammered. The name of the apprentice who was the obstacle was ' Joe ' !

Especially family names cause most patients to use strained articulation for fear of being held up, failing to say their own name, or to greet people properly, and so on.

Clono-tonus.—At this stage when all efforts to speak result in exhaustion, the stammerer must give up and then renew his attempts over and over again. Thus laboured utterances are repeated, i.e. tonic words become clono-tonic.

In a next stage this mechanism turns into a back-swinging, in order to get a fresh impetus. We shall meet the, to the stammerer's mind, improved mechanism in the third stage (see p. 126).

Second Stage, Fifth Phase.—In any process and at any time automatisation goes on. Thus during the development of a stammer all the subsequent actions become canalised and facilitated. This must not be misunderstood. There is not, and cannot be, such a thing as a pure deviation of speech, but only an expressive response of a reacting organism (the speaker) under particular circumstances. What becomes canalised is the unit of psychic and bodily reaction to the sum total of the stimulating psychical and sociological factors. This partly explains why the disorder does not occur constantly. The external and internal conditions vary within smaller or larger periods and the speech reaction with them.

That is why, for example, the stammerer can usually talk properly when he is alone in a room ; but when he expects somebody to come in, he at once relapses into the disorder. Singing or declamation usually causes little or no difficulty for the same reason. Speech is a social action. The stammer deteriorated under the influence of certain social conditions. And it is this complex of phenomena that is canalised. As soon as speech loses the social aspect, i.e. if it is no longer a means of communication (as in the above instances), its inhibited character disappears.

Pike attitude.—The concepts and the kind of perceptual thought thus enforced on the stammerer make him sooner or later unfit for further struggle.. Canalised inhibition of his actions renders him, as it were, a prisoner. Thus a further step downwards is taken, which again reminds us of what we explicitly see in animals. Möbius put a pike " in one end of a tank, and in the other end a troop of minnows, which the pike contemplated hungrily through a glass partition. It cost the pike countless nasal collisions, which almost literally beat the conclusion into his head, to learn that the minnows were beyond reach ; but he did master this in the end. However, he was only a sadder not a wiser pike, for now the partition was removed and the minnows swam all round him in safety Having got it fixed in his head that the minnows were not for him, he could hardly get it out again." [1] This ' pike attitude ' of the stammerer means a complete change of the stammerer's character. He is now no more an individual doing his best to assimilate his deviating speech to that of those around him. He takes his stammer as an inborn, inherited or in some way enforced evil with which he has to get on as best he can. The behaviour and mental attitude of many stammerers towards their disorder seems to show " How use doth breed a habit in a man." [2]

Our speaker still moves among his fellows, but he begins to withdraw, he leaves them alone, he does not embarrass them with his speech, and he is thankful for not being addressed ; but the needs of life occasionally enforce contact with his fellows.

Second Stage, Sixth Phase.—The position has now to be considered again. The series of conclusions drawn from wrong premises has led the stammerer to the very bottom of the blind alley. He still seeks the ' good ' speech he hears and cannot attain. But he cannot find the way out ; he longs for it, particularly since social conditions make him suffer because of his deficient speech the more as he grows older.

The stammerer in the maze.—But—logically—there does not seem to be any measure left which could be taken. Once he is convinced that he is right in inferring that effort is one of the most *necessary* factors for obtaining perfect speech, the stammerer becomes desperate, realising that he cannot afford *more* than the whole of his energy. He finds himself in a *maze*, from which he has not been able to find the way out, and so turns again to scrutinise his speech position. What does he find ?

Eluding manœuvres.—Examining his speech and the circumstances anew, he may make various ' discoveries.' These will, naturally, in each case be tuned and determined by the stammerer's previous experiences. A patient may find that the word ' yes,' for example, has never caused any difficulty. In fact well-canalised short symbols such as ' yes, no, of course, well, thank you, you see, don't you know,' and others are usually not affected, obviously because they had never involved the possibility of a disproportion between the proposition and its verbalisation.

Embolophrasias.—The stammerer, to be sure, does not realise this explanation. Various other sounds, e.g. [ə], syllables [am], and words,

---

[1] Quot. by Blanshard, l.c., i, pp. 244–5.
[2] Shakespeare, " The Two Gentlemen of Verona," Act V, Sc. 4.

phrases, sentences, or their parts, not belonging to the sentence intended, are put wherever there is difficulty ; they are called *Embolophrasias.*

Patients gradually obtain such skill in using embolophrasias as an easy start that only close observation can unmask them as stammerers. When, however, they use senseless and queer embolophrasias they can easily be recognised. An assistant of the physician J. Frank, for example, used to insert the syllable-sequence ' hedera federa ' in between the words of a sentence.[1] Curiously enough these embolophrasias often undergo the changes demonstrated above ; they become reiterated and then tonic.

Other tricks.—Another method frequently used is that of replacing ' hard words ' by those that appear easier. This often necessitates the reconstruction of the whole phrase or sentence. We can easily realise that this technique, though at first giving quite a satisfactory outside result, means an enormous inner strain, for the whole proposition and its verbal expression must also be transformed.[2] This task, in its turn, gives rise to a disproportion between thought and expression with all its consequences, such as clonus, tonus, and so forth. The stammerer thus moves in a vicious circle ; the gulf between thinking and uttering which still persists makes him stammer, and the enforced transformation of propositions again causes a similar disproportion.

Others give themselves airs of meditating, which often proves useful, since it grants a short respite ; but it becomes conspicuous and ridiculous when the stammerer, asked his name, poses as one pondering the question.

Many stammerers do not even shrink from giving obviously wrong or stupid answers, just because apparently easier words can be used ; e.g. 2 plus 2 make 6 ; apples are vegetables, etc. Patients even go so far as to feign ignorance, answering any question by " I don't know," and so on.

This state of affairs has given rise to the opinion commonly held that stammerers are dull, backward, etc. Stammerers in this advanced phase make a virtue of necessity, when they ape the silent, thoughtful, careful, ruminating man. All these tricks aim at hiding the mistakes which the stammerer is convinced he must make. Fröschels therefore termed this stage that of concealment ; Hoepfner calls it the sensory-aphasic form of Associative Aphasia. The stammerer at this stage may be said to have achieved a real Cadmean victory. He has defeated his enemy, speech, inasmuch as he can now keep up appearances ; but the loss which the self suffers is great.

Third Stage.—In the end the patient no longer considers himself a normal person. He no longer believes in his health, which he feels is impaired by the special inability in speaking. Indeed, he does not regard himself as an individual who incidentally stammers, but as a stammerer, and so he resigns himself to his fate.

---

[1] Gutzmann, *Sprachheilkunde*, pp. 420–1, footnote.

[2] Cf. Wendell Johnson, *Because I Stutter*, quot. by Boome and Richardson, l.c., p. 45.

Masked Stammering.—Feelings of inferiority and ill-health, anxiety and strong emotions prevail, whereas motor speech-symptoms are in the background. The power of judgment deviates from the norm, social and moral behaviour deteriorate.[1]

Environmental circumstances may either bring forth useful over-compensations, or may lead to the decay of the personality.

For records illustrating the development of the stammerer's psychological attitude in all its vicissitudes see " The Stammerer's Point of .View," in E. J. Boome's and M. A. Richardson's work.[2]

Clonus again.—Pathological symptoms in overt speech may now have almost completely disappeared. Occasional fast (sometimes very slow) clonus, manifesting itself mostly in words and phrases, exhibits the concept of the ' improved ' mechanism which we saw arising at an earlier stage (see p. 113).

At this juncture the diagnostic value implied in the minute distinction of the various utterances of a reiterated character should be noted. The dissolutionary significance of the stammer symptoms furnishes a fairly reliable means to assess the gravity and the prospects of a given stammer.[3]

In differential diagnosis the discrimination between Developmental Stammering and ' Infective ' Stammering (acquired through social contagion) must first be considered. We have seen that in the developmental type there is a stringent temporal sequence of the symptoms, due to dissolutionary factors and the patient's conscious meditations. But if, for example, a patient shows a pure clonus and unduly excessive concomitant gesticulations, the inconsistence is plain. The existence of these aids to expression presupposes the patient's awareness of great difficulty in sound production. But this is just what does not happen in a pure clonus. The given symptomatological feature of the stammer must therefore have been acquired through inexact observation on the part of the patient. The child may, for instance, have overlooked the hypertense component in the tonoclonus of his model (Fröschels).

Similar considerations apply to the intentional simulation of Stammering. Rothe and Fröschels have pointed to the diagnostic import of the movements of the sides of the nostrils, which often occur in stammerers. This symptom can only be imitated with difficulty, if noticed at all. The malingerer therefore can scarcely be expected to make use of this symptom. Consequently its existence bears witness to genuine stammering, whereas its absence proves nothing.

The nature of the nostril symptom is not known for certain.

---

[1] Hoepfner's third sub-phase or moral-psychopathic form of Associative Aphasia. See Stein, L., *Sprach- und Stimmstörungen,* p. 134.

[2] *The Nature and Treatment of Stammering,* chapter viii. Cf. also Aldous Huxley's *Half-Holiday,* and W. Nuttall's "Memoirs of a Stammerer," *Psyche,* 1937, xvii, pp. 151-84.

[3] The purely psycho-analytic aspect of Stammering has necessarily been touched upon only occasionally and superficially, because the available psychoanalytic case histories have not paid due regard to the relationship between the clinical syndromes of Stammering and unconscious processes.

Hoepfner holds that it is a striatothalamic automatism.[1] Others consider it a result of the breathing disturbance.[2]

Finally, Stammering must be distinguished from Spastic Dysarthria (see p. 169).

The differential diagnosis between Cluttering and Stammering is not always easy in view of the reiterated syllables and occasional checks in the flow of speech, often accompanied by slight tension, which occur both in Cluttering and Stammering. The distinction between the two disorders may be facilitated by the use of the following tabulated survey, based on that compiled by Freund :—

	Stammering	Cluttering
Awareness of the disorder . . .	yes	no
Concentration on the disorder . .	yes	no
Speech in the presence of strangers .	worse	better
Speech when at ease . . .	better	worse
Brief definite answers . . .	difficult	easy
Repetition of at first faulty sentences .	often worse	better
Essay writing, spelling . . .	normal	mostly equally faulty

It must, however, be borne in mind that a present stammer may have developed out of a former clutter. In such cases speech is hasty and monotonous and the symptoms of Stammering are interspersed with frequent cloni and tachylalia. The patients seem to understate the degree of their disorder (D. Weiss).

Prognosis.—Being a functional and psychogenic disorder, stammering may, on the whole, be given a good prognosis. The prospects of recovery depend on the stage of its development, the degree of automatisation, and on etiological and environmental influences.

In the majority of cases a stammer in the first stage tends to disappear spontaneously. Advice is rightly given by many teachers, family doctors, and nurses, who are often consulted in the first instance, that for weeks or months it is of the utmost importance not to interfere in any way. Those who give this advice should realise that it may be necessary to instruct the immediate associates of the stammerer on the best method of avoiding interference (see Treatment, p. 135).

Stammerers in the second or third stages are not likely to ' grow out ' of their disorder. Treatment offers good prospects provided the environmental circumstances do not counteract the efforts of both the stammerer and the therapist.

Reported spontaneous recovery of severer cases is to be judged with great reserve ; close examination often reveals certain symptoms which have been concealed.

Treatment.—Innumerable methods of treatment for stammering have been advocated. We need not dwell on the discussion of the various tricks, instruments, diaphragm exercises, and so forth ; they

[1] Hoepfner, Th. (1929). 3rd Congr. of the Int. Ges. f. Logop. & Phon., Deuticke, Vienna, p. 94.
[2] Newekluff, ibid., p. 95.

can—as methods—justifiably be placed within the category of ' quack remedies.' Boome and Richardson have convincingly illustrated the fate of the unhappy victims resorting to these ' methods.' [1]

The leading principle in the treatment of stammerers should be relaxation. " It is impossible to insist too strongly upon this point ; and it is only necessary to watch the mildest case to see the reason for this insistence. Hypertension is present whenever the act of speaking involves a struggle, and this tension must be overcome and replaced by ease before the patient can feel any confidence in his ability to speak." [2] I feel sure that this need has been clearly seen by all workers. And yet their methods vary greatly, according to the basic views each holds on the principles of nervous mechanisms.

Let us bear in mind that ' relaxation ' is an abstraction, and for this reason does not furnish any guidance for action. This can only be attained by experience or by experiments which refer to such still integral ' relaxed ' activities as allow the natural ' emergence ' of speech. It is this insight which indicates the track that should be followed. I believe, therefore, that the following technique is one of the possible pathways leading to relaxed speech. Its flexibility allows the inclusion of other techniques applied by the schools of speech therapy and of medical psychology. [3]

The protean nature of stammering makes it impossible to go into every detail of treatment. It must suffice to outline the general plan founded on the principles laid down above. [4] The essential is to instil into the patient full comprehension of his particular form of stammering. Consciously he is only too anxious to know all about his insidious foe who plays these underhand tricks upon him. He should therefore be thoroughly enlightened as to the nature of his disorder. The task can suitably be begun by explanations of concepts such as disorder, canalisation, pattern, therapy, and of questions of speech development and its particular deviation. The therapist is referred here to all the details given in the introductory chapters i-v.

Re-creative, bio-psychological treatment.—We have seen that in stammering the speech-pattern (including the corresponding mentality) undergoes dissolution. This may halt at various levels. Therapy has naturally to re-integrate the speech-pattern from the given integral level. Thus treatment is based on the principles indicated in the introductory chapter (pp. 25 ff.), but its technique must conform to the given stage of disintegration. The method of approach should be on lines corresponding to the way in which stammering develops, viz. it should proceed from the connection between the clinical symptoms and the level of dissolution, and thus analyse the particular significance of the symptoms in a pragmatic way. Using the simile of the blind alley, the *natural* course to pursue is to *go back* until the stammerer reaches the right track, whence natural healing can take place. The

---

[1] Boome and Richardson, l.c., p. 78.   [2] Ibid., p. 101.
[3] Other methods based on ' speech gymnastics,' such as those described on pp. 209 ff., can be left out of consideration, since any therapeutic attempt that does not take into account the bio-psychological framing of disintegrated speech as it manifests itself in the stammerer's attitudes is unnatural and must fail.
[4] See Stein, L. *Sprach- und Stimmstörungen*, pp. 159-85.

point of bifurcation is, as a rule, the clonic stage of stammer. He must therefore allow himself to 'stammer' as he did before he tried to *stop* 'stammering.'

Unfortunately, to the mind of the stammerer and the public at large, this means to stammer more and worse. Imagine the difference between, for example [ɪt ɪt iz ɔn ɔn ðə saɪ saɪdbɔ : d] (for " it is on the sideboard ") and ['ɪt iz 'ɔn ðə s̄ ꞉ ꞉ ꞉ aɪdbɔ : d,][1] and you will certainly agree with the patient and his listeners that the second kind of articulation is " less objectionable " and therefore " better." But from the dissolution standpoint the latter type represents a lower stage. Also from the patient's and the psycho-biologist's point of view its degree must be considered more serious and harder to overcome. As we have seen, the patient's endeavours are usually fruitless.

It should be the aim of the speech therapist to use all proper means and devices to induce the patient to retrace his steps to the clonic stage, though in view of all the social impediments, automatisation, etc., this is difficult for both patient and therapist.

At first the patient is asked to imagine that he is a baby whose babbling utterances have not yet got any communicative meaning. As a rule he succeeds in imitating sequences of reiterated syllables. The patient is then reminded of the developmental stage in which the child on the one hand tends to reiterate, and on the other to imitate a standard word, e.g. la la lamp for ' lamp.' He is then asked to start each word which he is about to stammer tonically, with a series of reiterated syllables. He may reiterate until he is able to proceed with the following sounds of the word or phrase. Thus the first move towards reintegration of emotional into significant utterance has been made. Patients generally agree that this mode of utterance does not involve —much to their surprise—any hypertonicity.

Under adequate guidance patients soon get used to transforming speech into reiterated utterances ; but at the same time a strong resistance makes itself felt. Though the patients appreciate the easier flow of speech and the absence of any tension, they are obviously not disposed to adopt this method in conversation because they fear the social consequences. Expecting that they will have to persevere in ' babbling,' they anticipate appearing childish, and thus ridiculous. In such cases to hint at the occasional reiterations in normal speech proves helpful. The stammerer has for long been concentrating on the speech of those around him, being eager to imitate it but incapable of achieving this. He will therefore be only too ready to discover this same defect in his fellows. Having made sure that these reiterations scarcely penetrate the consciousness of the listeners, he will *occasionally* try to introduce deliberate reiterations into his speech in place of the tonus. A few successful trials give considerable encouragement.

But the wedge is pushed farther in by another discovery. Patients spontaneously report that once they had made up their minds to reiterate they were quite surprised to find that the necessity for ' babbling,' i.e. for producing too large a number of reiterations, was

[1] ' = glottal stop. ꞉꞉꞉ = lengthened articulation. ‾ = laboured articulation.

far less than they had presumed. This progress seems to be due to the changed attitude of the speaker.

The time is now ripe for putting the patient's imaginative power into operation. After careful psychological preparation he is advised to picture himself as though going to reiterate. This image brings about the desirable relaxed posture in advance. The patient no longer assails speech but just lets it go.

The neuro-motor aspect can be suitably illustrated by the simile of horse training. The unbroken young horse, still dominated by the flight instinct, pulls the bridle in its attempts to run away. Its posture and movements are highly tense. The skilled trainer achieves an equipoise between the pulling action of the horse and his own restraining force. In the same way the thalamus puts the vital question as to what ought to be done, but the rein (represented by the striatum) is loosened by the exercise of the cortex which, by its power of judgment, adjusts posture and movements to the situation. Thus stammering is mastered by looking upon it from a ' higher ' viewpoint (see p. 19).

To put the principle in psychological terms : by suggesting the retracing of steps, the therapist allows the patient to adopt an earlier type of speech. He may now enjoy infantile speech which, having been repressed for a long period, is now sanctioned by the therapist.[1] Thus a good deal of confidence and self-control is obtained. The technique resembles that of encouragement advocated by Adler and that of graduated tasks put forward by Herzberg.[2]

The remaining impediments are then cleared away by means of mental exercises aiming at destroying the root of the disorder, viz. the too great disproportion between thought and expression, as described below (p. 134).

Leading the patient towards reiterative speech (babbling) requires careful preparation, especially as to all characteristics of behaviour. The therapist should therefore be thoroughly acquainted with all biological, developmental, physiological, and psychological aspects of standard speech, as well as with the technique of psychotherapy.

If the patient finds himself very deep in the blind alley, i.e. the second or third stage, thus too far away from the point of bifurcation, the proposed babbling type of speech presents too much difficulty, for the way back towards iterated speech is blocked by well-organised (canalised) pathological patterns. Especially in cases where attention has been drawn to the artificial units of speech, i.e. ' letters,' or sounds, the therapist has to contend with considerable difficulties. Such patients suffer from excessive ' sound-anxiety ' and morbid attention. Every attempt to integrate sounds into syllables naturally fails, and thus strengthens the stammerers' belief in their inferiority. From the viewpoint of the still intact psychological and linguistic levels they can be regarded as ' sucklings ' (see p. 31). Reintegration must accordingly start from such peculiarities of the prelinguistic period as are not infected by morbid attention.

[1] Stein, L. (1941). " A New Method of Treating Stammer," *Lancet*, p. 813.
[2] Herzberg, A. (1941). " Short Treatment of Neuroses by Graduated Tasks," *Brit. Journ. of Med. Psychol.*, xix, pp. 19-36.

All emotional vocalisations of that period, such as laughing
([hə hə hə . . .]) constituting voice initiated aspiratedly, the murmuring
of satisfaction ([ə : : : : : . .]), humming ([m : : : : : . . . , n : : : . . . .]),
which are all attacked softly, can easily be performed by any stammerer.
These actions once experienced, can, if necessary, be subjected to
further deliberate practice as shown on pp. 210 f.

Likewise the noises originating from sucking movements can easily
be produced. This should be done in a behavioural way trying to
perform actions indicated by words, such as sucking, sipping, smacking,
and the like (see pp. 30 f., 49).

It should be explained to the patient that any given phonetic
structure (syllable, word, etc.) is the outcome of the original integration
of voice with iterated sucking movements (see p. 31).[1] That this
statement always meets with the strongest resistance on the part of
the patient is intelligible from the psychological angle. As the execution of this task means not only going back to an early (infantile)
stage, but also drawing the necessary conclusions as to practice, the
patient shrinks from performing that which he has 'theoretically'

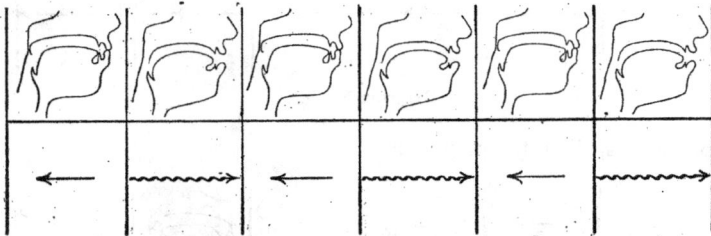

Diagram No. 2.

admitted. Cautious guidance is therefore indispensable and can be
greatly aided by experiments which should also be supported by
parallels from the normal development of speech.

The patient is asked to initiate voice and to prolong it, as, for
instance, in groaning.

Next he is asked to perform rhythmically repeated ' smacks.' The
therapist can profitably avail himself of the opportunity to show the
patient that he can produce such noises with as much effort as he likes
without feeling that he is then stammering.

Once the patient is acquainted with the underlying infantile
patterns of phonation and of articulation we pass on to the integration
of the two. The bars of Diagram No. 2, indicated by vertical lines,
are horizontally divided into an upper and a lower line. The lower
indicates the continuous flow of voice, the upper shows the iterated
insertion of the smacking click. In conformity with the remarks as
to the origin and evolution of babbled utterances (see p. 31 and p. 50),
the patient will experience the interruption of phonation by the clicks,

[1] Cf. Fröschels' method of breath-eating, p. 212.

for phonation, i.e. the expulsion of air, is essentially incompatible with the rarefaction of air implied in clicking. The result will be phenomenally a series of reiterated syllables which as to their mode of production consist of one, though interrupted, stream of voice, and iterated clicks. In phonetic spelling the resulting acoustic effect may be represented thus : [də də də], [d̄] (a ' p ' turned upside down), indicating the click which is the basis of the p. See Diagram No. 2.

In the next exercise the patient is advised to abolish the difficulty of combining phonation with an implosive sound by giving up one property of the click, viz. the rarefaction of air, and replacing it by some mode of expiration. The motor result may either be

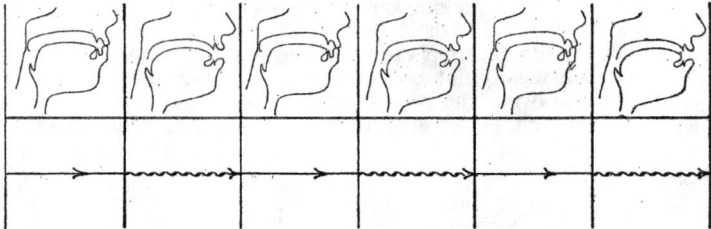

Diagram No. 3.

in phonetic spelling [pə pə pə], or

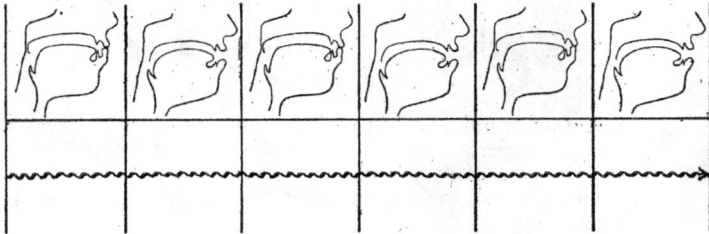

Diagram No. 4.

in phonetic spelling [bə bə bə], according to whether non-vibrating or vibrating air escapes. These exercises should be modified by utilising other ' clicking ' patterns.

It is curious that patients, when asked how they would write what they have just uttered, usually fail to think of a way. When they discover that their deliberate action ' is ' speech, viz. [pə], or [bə], they are quite surprised.

A task of great import has thus been accomplished, as the aim of psychotherapy is to bring about the change of *meaning* (see p. 67).

The experiment, by which the patient has unwittingly produced a syllable which otherwise would have caused great difficulty and

anxiety, has then to be put into a kind of mathematical equation
(see Diagram No. 5).

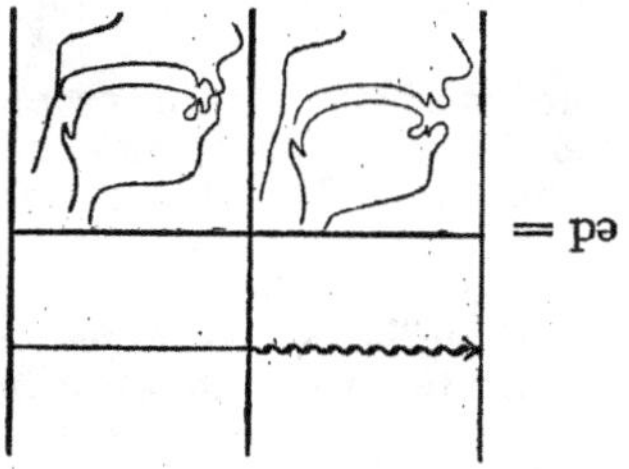

$$= p\mathrm{\partial}$$

Diagram No. 5.

The right-hand side of the diagram shows the 'unknown value' [pə],
that is to say, the 'hard' syllable ; the left-hand side gives the solution
of the riddle. It shows that the syllable, as an acoustic phenomenon,
can easily be produced if two patterns which the patient has admittedly
mastered are integrated. The one is the unit of aspirated voice represented by ――――――――――. The other is a sequence of clicks.

The achievement of [bə] is represented in the equation illustrated in
Diagram No. 6.

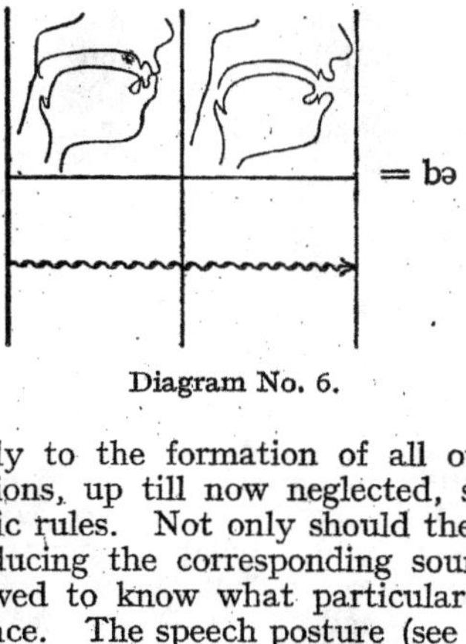

$$= b\mathrm{\partial}$$

Diagram No. 6.

These rules apply to the formation of all other syllables. The
specific vowel positions, up till now neglected, should be explained
according to phonetic rules. Not only should the shape of mouth be
shown without producing the corresponding sound, but the patient
must never be allowed to know what particular speech-sound he is
expected to pronounce. The speech posture (see pp. 11 ff.) has been
made comprehensible by drawing attention to behavioural patterns.
Activities of the speech organs should be mimed, which operate, for
example, if silence be imposed (s, sh), if admiration (m), vexation (ı),
contempt (d), indifference (mb), surprise ([a :], [o :]), fright ([u :]),
and so forth, be expressed. At this stage we need not hesitate to add
exercises which help to overcome the natural atactic clumsiness (see
pp. 209 ff.).

The tormenting question as to how two sounds are to be joined together now proves superfluous. A glance at the diagram convinces the patient that it is the *unit* already mastered ————————— or ——————— which, if given a certain resonance, ' carries ' the ' syllable.'

The conscious psychological effect of this procedure upon the patient is very good, since it enables him, as it were, to turn the tables upon speech. He has hitherto adopted a compulsorily aggressive attitude towards his way of uttering, constantly being ready to fight his foe by the use of force. Though he consciously regrets and blames this over-anxious self-observation, he knows no way of getting away from it. Now he may concentrate on speech without any struggle, for he has availed himself of the *natural* pattern. *He* thus defeats the stammer by its own dangerous weapon, self-observation.

This technique contradicts the opinion that treatment should be guided by the principle of entirely diverting the patient's attention from speech. In my experience I have had no success with that type of treatment, except in small children in the clonic stage.

Needless to say, what we mean must be expressed in a way adapted to the patient's intellectual type, a necessity which is unfortunately often under-estimated. The therapist should take pains in narrowing down the ambiguity of terms. Since most words, however, have several connotations, it is necessary, and also helpful, to lay stress upon those which are apt to help the patient in picturing the right pattern of action. Advice must not be over-persuasive, for the patient is much too discouraged and distrustful, though both these peculiarities are usually concealed. The matter has to be put before him in a way that allows him to draw the natural conclusions. The decision whether or not a given step should be made must be left to the patient. The procedure must therefore be very cautious and gradual, so as to make sure that the patient will not fail. To free him from the misconceptions connected with common words, such as sound, syllable, sentence, etc., these should be carefully and plainly analysed. The whole process of speech integration which is observable in the child should, under the guidance of the therapist, be recapitulated by the patient, always having regard to the corresponding behavioural patterns.

Once the correct aspect and execution of syllables is safeguarded, the further procedure follows the line marked out by developmental considerations (see Babbling Stage, p. 40) and by the technique already outlined (see p. 128). Syllables now appear as a continuous flow of air with " peaks of distinctiveness " and lack the dangerous arbitrary division into sound-units.[1] The patient can now, as it were, play with these syllables in a babbling manner.

Finally, when the outward symptoms have almost disappeared, we must set about abolishing the root of the disorder, viz. the gulf between thought and expression. This opportunity is given when there are pure cloni, or slightest tonus, indicating the disproportion already mentioned and perhaps some apprehension. At this point the patient himself would report considerable improvement, but would complain

---

[1] As to the phonetic mechanism see Curry, l.c., chapter v.

—as one patient put it—of having got into "that nasty habit of iterating."

Exercises in transforming thoughts, facts, perceptions, ideas, etc., into a sequence of logical propositions and sentences can be made through the medium of pictures showing more or less intricate occurrences.

It need not be emphasised that during the whole of the speech treatment the therapist should avail himself of every opportunity for readjusting the patient's personality. For further information on this problem we must refer to the textbooks on psychotherapy.

The lack of relaxation in developed stammerers is, as we hope has been made clear, a behavioural symptom, that is to say, it is the patient's response to environmental stimuli. A relaxed attitude can, therefore, be achieved if the method of approach be based on the idea of building from a level the pattern of which is naturally relaxed. Only when this reintegration is going on can the patient be assisted by relaxation practice. For this see Boome, Baines, and Harries, *Abnormal Speech;* Boome and Richardson, *The Nature and Treatment of Stammering;* Boome and Richardson, *Relaxation on Everyday Life.*

Treatment in children.—Considering the amount of concentrated work required for the differentiation or reintegration of the speech *process,* parents and friends of the stammerer should refrain from ' helping ' exhorting, or advising him. Children especially should be allowed enough time to re-develop standard speech. " If parents understood the amount of concentrated work required, they would be less inclined to force the child and would allow him to develop this new talent at his own pace. It is a great temptation to show off the child to friends and relations, to prove his superiority to all other children by making him go through his linguistic paces, but it is a temptation that should be resisted. . . . The critical adult who insists upon repetition of difficult sounds with ' Say it again, dear,' may very easily make the child speech-conscious and be the means of fixing a faulty speech-sound or of inducing hesitation that may grow into a stammer.[1] Such advice given by doctors should be regarded as malpractice.[2]

Thus in little stammerers, who usually show clonus or hesitation, active treatment is neither necessary nor desirable. Their speech-patterns are not yet well canalised, so that their re-integration can be left to be effected by the natural progress.

It goes without saying that all organic conditions that might impede our therapeutic efforts need medical attention, with which this book is, however, not concerned. Let me just quote one instance. Boome and Richardson find — with Cameron — that most of the ' difficult ' children benefit greatly by extra sugar ; " not only should they have a larger quantity in tea and pudding, but we recommend barley sugar in addition, and with excellent results in nearly every case." [3]

---

[1] Boome, Baines, and Harries, *Abnormal Speech,* chapter iv.
[2] Stein, L. (1922). *Ein therapeutischer Kunstfehler,* Wien-klin-Woch, No. 20.
[3] Boome and Richardson, *The Nature and Treatment of Stammering,* p. 34.

As far as possible children should keep in the open air. When indoors they should preferably be occupied with handicraft. They should not be given too many toys, nor are books and party games recommended. In short, everything in the child's surroundings should be adapted in such a way as to give him time and opportunity to harmonise the disproportion between thinking and verbalising.

CHAPTER XIII

DISORDERS OF ARTICULATE SPEECH

Articulation.—In discussing the development of normal speech and also its retardation (Hearing-Mutism), we have seen that the production of ' speech-sounds ' is, at first, an integration of sounds which originate ' at random,' being noises accompanying vegetative responses of the organs of respiration and digestion.

A further integration is established in *Articulate Speech.*

We must necessarily dwell a while upon terminology before entering on the clarification of the physiological and pathological phenomena.

The terms ' articulation ' and ' to articulate ' suggest a stratification of meaning which must not be forgotten when approaching its deviations. The source of these words is the Indo-German root AR, ' to fit,' ' to join,' whence its use in talking of the junction between two bones, or parts of a plant ; finally, it has become a term for the motor function whereby words, having been formulated, are converted into sounds.[1] It denotes " the part played by the super-laryngeal organs in modifying the sound-waves produced at the larynx." [2] So far as sounds are arranged in units through specific adjustments of the speech mechanism,[3] regardless of their content,[4] they are articulated.

The adjective ' articulate ' means (1) ' united by a joint, composed of jointed segments.' It has adopted the stricter meaning of (2) ' *distinctly* (i.e. possessing differentiating characteristics, clearly perceptible or discernible by the senses or the mind), jointed or marked.'

Used of sound, its meaning has undergone a further extension ; it expresses the feature of being divided into distinct and also *significant* parts ; thus, speaking intelligibly.[5]

There is also a word expressing the lack of the properties mentioned above. Thus ' inarticulate ' means, in anatomy, ' not joined,' and used of speech, ' indistinct, persons not capable of speaking distinctly or of expressing their ideas and feelings.' [6]

One can agree with Stopa in that an inarticulate sound cannot be used in normal speech, because it does not accomplish the psychological principle of a speech-sound, viz. to be a discernible symbol of thought.[7] But by looking more closely we discover that the underlying process he assumes, viz. ' irregular, inco-ordinate movements,' does not exist.

All movements or actions, so far as they exist in a given individual, are already co-ordinated in some way, i.e. they spring from the common action of various organs which work together in a certain order.

Their irregularity means merely that they deviate from a conventional pattern put up by individuals, whose articulations, however,

---

[1] *Shorter Oxford Dictionary.*   [2] Curry, l.c., § 5, 1.
[3] Sievers, E. (1901). *Phonetik. Grundriss d. Germanischen Philologie.* Ed. H. Paul, Karl J. Truebner, Strassburg, i, p. 287.
[4] Kussmaul, l.c., p. 46.   [5] *Shorter Oxford Dictionary.*
[6] Wyld, *Dict.*   [7] Stopa, R. *Die Schnalzlaute,* p. 327.

cannot be said to be fully standardised. So this term is an expression of relationship, and the present chapter has therefore to deal (1) with the organs performing co-ordination of speech movements (articulation), (2) with the results of the function so far as they mean something to both speaker and listener (articulate speech).

Ultimately many parts of the body, such as the extremities, the muscles of the face, even of the back, can be used as means of expression by more or less primitive peoples.

We will confine our interest to those movements which result in auditorily perceptible phenomena. These actions are performed primarily by the organs of breathing and digestion—mouth, throat, nose, chest.

CHAPTER XIV

DYSLALIA

Types.—We begin with types of utterance which are on the one hand regarded as speech, i.e. a method of expressing and communicating mental states, and yet on the other hand, deviate in ' articulateness.'

Such utterances are included in the class of Dyslalia (*dys*, ' badly, with difficulty ; ' *laleo*, ' I speak '). In conformity with the use of the Greek prefix *para*, ' beside,' in the formation of the term Paragrammatism, we may also accept the term ' Paralalia ' for "the production of distinctly different sounds from those desired, or the constant substitution of one sound for another." [1]

The gradations of deviation have been variously named. Universal Dyslalia means a disturbance of articulate speech which affects almost all sounds, thus rendering speech more or less unintelligible. Partial Dyslalia manifests itself in the disorder of one sound or one phonetic group, so that the communicative character of speech remains fairly untouched. Severe degrees of Universal Dyslalia are called Idioglossia (Greek, *idios*, ' own,' *glossa*, ' tongue '). In Hottentotism, speech is restricted to a stream of voice modified into few distinct vowels and interspersed with occasional dental consonants (Fournier).

UNIVERSAL DYSLALIA

Symptoms.—Universal Dyslalia is a very frequent speech disorder of childhood, and is sometimes retained for a very long time. It is also—though less frequently—met with in adults. Its degree is variable ; there are children whom only those who are quite used to their way of speaking can understand, whereas others speak comparatively distinctly, so that in spite of the anomalies in their speech they are fairly generally understood.

We may in many cases find a patient being quite talkative, using the usual intonation and stress, but it may take a certain strain to understand what the patient's utterances *mean ;* and this because their *phonetic* character is different, so that it seems as if we were hearing a more or less strange, unknown language. There is a certain resemblance with what we saw in Sensory Aphasia.

Yet it can soon be found out (1) that the patient's understanding of speech is entirely intact, as far as we can judge from his responses, verbal and acting ; (2) that he means to use our words ; but though his utterances are distorted, he does not notice it, or, if he does so, he still retains them.

It is in many cases impossible to deny that there is a similarity of form and meaning between the child's utterance and that used around him. Sometimes, however, the phonetic feature deviates so much

---

[1] Robbins-Stinchfield, *Dictionary of Terms Dealing with Disorders of Speech,* p. 18, quot. by Stinchfield, *Speech Disorders,* p. 53.

from the usual that only by close investigation can the correlation be found.

In some cases we notice so severe a lack of adaptation that we may think of this speech as ' gibberish.'

Let us take a few examples at random. An English-speaking child said,

(1) " Iss 'oo doin' det me a 'itoo fis' ? " instead of, " Are you going to get me a little fish ? " [1]

An Austrian child produced the following utterances :—

(2) [dotatea] for ' grosser Verkehr ' (big traffic) ; (3) [tiʃe] for ' Kirche ' (church) ; (4) [tetl] for ' Sessel ' (chair). Another patient said, e.g., (5) [huʃe] for ' Küche ' (kitchen), but pronounced (6) [ter] for ' Scheere ' [ʃe : re] (scissors). The latter changed after a few months (without treatment) into (7) [ter].[2] In the speech of a girl (8) the fricatives [ç] (as in Germ. *ich*), [j] (as in Engl. *young*), and [x] (as in Scot. *loch*), were changed into [ʃ] and [ʒ] ; the plosives [k] and [g] became [t] and [d]. It was striking that this process had taken place also before the back vowels [o] and [u]. The riddle was solved through X-ray pictures taken during articulation. They showed that the blade of the tongue was abnormally raised against the front palate (as in [e] and [i], during [o] and [u]. The audible effect, however, was not distinct enough to be perceived. One patient replaced (9) [n], [j] and [r] by [l], but used to say also [r] instead of [l], e.g. [laize] becomes [rais] , [flaiʃ] becomes [ʃrais]. In a similar case (10) ' Spatz ' [ʃpats] (sparrow) was pronounced [pas], but [Susi] (Susan) changed into [tuti].

It is striking that the vowel-sounds in Dyslalia are very little affected so far as the acoustic impression they convey is concerned. Closer investigation shows that this is due to the fact that the auditory deviation is below the threshold of acoustic discrimination for those hearing the dyslalic child.

Idioglossia.—An understanding of idioglossia should now present little difficulty. A patient of W. S. Colman's,[3] quoted by Tredgold,[4] serves as a good example. This boy of 6 reproduced the Lord's Prayer as follows : " Oue tabde ne nah e nedde, anno de di na ; i dede ta, i due de di ou eeth a te e edde. Te ut te da oue dade de, e didde ap tetedde, a ne adiu to tetedde adase us, ne notte tetate, mime, utte een, to i aite-vene, pore e dande, to edde e edde. Ame." " At first sight it appears to be an extreme form of ' lalling ; ' but it is evident that it is some-thing more than a mere persistence of baby language. . . . It consists in such an extensive substitution of sounds for the correct ones that the child speaks a language peculiar to himself; hence the name ; but he generally uses the same sound for the same word." [5]

S. Stinchfield [6] describes the peculiarities in some twins with whom

[1] Stinchfield, *Speech Disorders*, p. 54.
[2] ' above a consonant is a ' modifier ' indicating palatalisation, i.e. the simultaneous anticipation of the articulation of the following sound resulting in the [t] being pronounced with the blade of the tongue raised against the hard palate.
[3] Colman, W. S. (1895). *Lancet,* **1**, p. 1419.
[4] Tredgold, l.c., p. 147.   [5] Ibid., pp. 146-7.
[6] Stinchfield, l.c., pp. 52-3.

she has worked. They were found to be dropping or "mutilating initial, middle, and final consonants, and sometimes to be modifying the root vowel. In some instances they gave the vowels in the correct sequence and quite clearly." Most consonants were replaced by labial ones.

The description shows that Idioglossia represents, phonetically, the same process on which Universal Dyslalia is based, only enormously magnified. It is the child's individual language, but it is not invented, as one might perhaps think. Furthermore, we may infer that the patient's " view of the world " is so different from ours that further adaptation of speech is not necessary. This fits in well with the fact that it can be found in mental defectives,[1] to which it is, however, not confined. Idioglossia can be found in neurotic children of any type.

Twins.—I have seen many cases of Universal Dyslalia in brothers and sisters of almost the same age, and in twins. It was striking that the linguistic characteristics of their Dyslalia showed only trifling resemblances. The feature of a child's group feelings up to about 4 or 5 years (see section on Standard Speech, p. 44) is apt to explain this divergence of articulation and also the relatively insignificant rôle of imitation in Dyslalia.

Adults.—Dyslalia is by its nature (see below) pre-eminently a disorder peculiar to childhood. Once language has been adapted to social needs, it is not likely to go downhill, especially if canalised throughout the years. Only very strong forces would have the power of disintegrating it. Thus we can find Universal Dyslalia in mental diseases, e.g. Paranoia (a psychosis characterised by fixed and systematised delusions), or Dementia paralytica (General Paralysis, chronic inflammation of the brain of syphilitic origin). In the course of dissolution of the cortex both psychoses naturally again reach a stage where those levels which are the substratum of a childlike attitude become dominant.

When psychotic patients of this kind have got so far downhill they show articulatory deviations which are surprisingly similar to those found in childhood. Here are a few examples : tanjiff instead of Germ. Schlangengift (poison of snakes) ; fripipp instead of Germ. Friedrich (Frederick) ; jutbitter instead of Germ. Gutsbesitzer (owner of estate) ; autetiehn instead of Germ. ausgestiegen (got out, alighted).[2]

Various types of Aphasia also show a similar disintegration of articulate speech. Head's patient No. 13 (Syntactical Aphasia after injury of the left temporal lobe by a shell fragment) [3] furnished the following examples (I retain Head's transcription). The words ' speak, foot, C.C.S.,' being rendered as ' speat, pook, she she es,' fit well with our assertion, that Dyslalia does not consist in a lack of articulatory power ($k = t$, $t = k$, $s = \int$). ' Nozzer, ās, Jan-wy,' for ' another, asked, January,' show the elision of unstressed sounds which is an important factor in language development.

[1] Tredgold, l.c., pp. 146–7.
[2] Liebmann, A. (1903). *Die Sprache der Geisteskranken*, Marhold, Halle.
[3] Head, l.c., ii, p. 199.

Aetiology and nature. — We are now in a position to tackle the question of the causes and nature of Dyslalia.

Schultze [1] believed that the child tries to make his articulation of sound easier by shifting it forwards towards the lips. Kussmaul [2] believed it to be due to a mistake in education or to lack of training. Wundt [3] ascribed it to "the imperfect acoustic and optic perception of sounds and sound-movements as well as to the influence of one sound upon its neighbour, which is greatly increased with children."

Fröschels [4] gives a number of reasons for Universal Dyslalia, such as central disturbances of ' chord hearing ' and other hearing disturbances, clumsiness, weakness or deformation of the peripheral organs of speech, diseases of the motoric nervous system, and lastly, imbecility. He also mentions inattentive children who sometimes articulate correctly, sometimes incorrectly.

On close examination these arguments do not always hold water, since expressions, such as ' lack of training,' ' shifting to the front of the mouth,' ' imperfect perception,' ' inattentiveness,' etc., obviously lack clear reference to known facts.

There is always the underlying idea of there being some ' difficulty ' in articulating, which the particular patient, for some reason or other, cannot overcome. This, however, seems somewhat improbable, since most of the Universally Dyslalic patients show no ' defect ' to justify the assumption of an inability to articulate properly ; so it would seem that there are other tendencies at work here which have nothing fundamentally to do with the child's faculty of articulation.

The character of Dyslalia suggests a comparison with the development and evolution of language in general, which might lead up to the explanation of the disorder. We have seen utterance developing from vegetative noises into meaningful expression. When these expressive sounds are responded to by those around the child, they become integrated into means of communication. The acquisition of sentences used by adults makes steady progress. Later on the sentence patterns which have been handed on are analysed and free use is then made of sounds. In other words, the power of ' articulating ' grows into that of using ' articulate speech.'

We have also seen that the utterances are, in all individuals and at all times, subjected to continuous phonetic changes.

At a certain level the chain from the perception of the external facts to their verbalisation, both in respect of movement and sound, and to the acting and speaking response of those around the speaking child, constitutes one unit. This is in constant process of differentiation, thus generating new independent but co-ordinated parts of the unit. Their further development will depend on the need for adaptation.

It happens at times that these units satisfy the requirements of the individual (child or adult), though the phonetic features of his utterances deviate.

[1] Schultze, F. (1880). " Die Sprache des Kindes," *Darwinistische Schriften*, No. 10, Ernst Günther, Leipzig.
[2] Kussmaul, l.c., p. 240.
[3] Wundt, W. (1911). *Die Sprache*, Engelmann, Leipzig, pp. 315 ff.
[4] Fröschels, E. *Lehrbuch der Sprachheilkunde*, p. 192.

The unit of utterance and the unit of mentality must be subjected to separate investigation.

For the elucidation of the phonetic structure of Dyslalia we must follow the path taken by philology when it sought to clarify the relation between languages a hundred years ago. Etymology, for instance, was regarded as one of the most foolish [1] sciences because the etymologists used to explain the origin of certain words through comparison with words of similar meaning or pattern in other languages ; thus they established a relation between words of several languages which, in fact, were not at all kindred. They failed because they did not know the rules which govern the evolution of languages. These rules and laws now being established, etymology and comparative philology are no longer considered foolish, and have obtained remarkable results.

In the case of Dyslalia we have to compare the speech-sounds of the dyslalic patient with those of the ' mother-tongue,' and we must find out the way in which the sounds of the pattern are changed in the disorder. An example from historic language development may indicate the method of approach. The Latin word for dog, for instance, was *canis* [ᴋanis] ; nobody would doubt that the French word *chien* [ʃiē] originated from the Latin word, but why does it now sound quite different ? The sound [k] is replaced in the French word by [ʃ], represented by the two letters ' ch ; ' the spelling shows us that a few hundred years ago the French may have pronounced a sound similar to the Scotch [x] (e.g. in ' loch ') and gradually this fricative sound changed into [ʃ].

The change of [x] or [ç] into [tʃ] and subsequently into [ʃ] is due to ' palatalisation ' ; i.e. a sound-change which any consonant may undergo if it absorbs the tongue articulation of a palatal vowel following it. In our example it is the [i] of the diphthong [ie]. There is no doubt that this diphthong corresponds to the Latin [A] ; it shows us that the original articulation of the old [a] was gradually brought forward, the tongue which was originally elevated at the back now being elevated in front. The phonetic description of the vowels shows that particularly [e] and [i] are pronounced with the elevation of the front of the tongue. This diphthong [ie] then influenced the articulation of the [x] so that the articulation of the [x] was also brought forward. We know that the frictional sound produced by an elevation of the front of the tongue is [ʃ].[2]

When applying this method of approach to Dyslalia, one important fact should be stressed. While, for instance [t], replaces [ʃ] in one word, e.g. [tere] for [ʃere], Germ. Schere, ' scissors,' [ʃ] may nevertheless be pronounced as a substitute for another sound in another word, e.g. [huʃe] for Germ. Küche, ' kitchen.' The importance of this fact will be evident when we remember that earlier authors attributed Universal Dyslalia to some kind of general speech disability.

To illustrate the correspondence between historical and dyslalic

---

[1] " L'étymologie est une science où les voyelles ne font rien, et les consonnes fort peu de chose " (Voltaire), quot. M. Müller, l.c., ii, p. 262.

[2] Meyer-Lübke, W. (1913). *Historische Grammatik der französischen Sprache,* Winter, Heidelberg, pp. 28, 133, 266–7.

sound-changes, I quote at random some parallels from the history of languages. The development of Lat. CANIS to French *chien*, [ʃiẽ], 'dog' (certainly through an intermediate stage [çien]); Old Slavonic [duchïa] to [duʃa], 'soul,' corresponds to the examples Nos. 3, 5, 8 (see p. 140). Nos. 2 and 3 exemplifying the sound-changes of the velar plosives [k] and [g] into the dental plosives [t] and [d], follow the line of development in Greek dialects, e.g. the equivalent form of Attic *tis* in Thessalian is *kis*.[1] Indo-Germ. *g* before *e* or *i* appears as *d*, e.g. the base *golbh*, ' that which is swelled,' has given rise to both Greek *delphys*, ' womb,'[2] and to Sanskrit *gharbat*, ' womb.'

The underlying process is Palatalisation. This is a phonological tendency in which the articulation of the tip of the tongue against the front palate in sounds such as t, d, n, s, l, r, is complicated by an elevation of the tongue blade. There arises an intimate amalgamation of these sounds with [i] or [j] (French ' consonnes mouillés '). If velar sounds, such as [k], [g], and [x], are influenced in this way they become dental consonants, that is to say, [k] changes into [t], [g] into [d], [x] into [s] or [ʃ].[3]

These examples contradict the assumption that the dyslalic patient simplifies articulation because he cannot master it. In fact the abnormality consists in a more complex articulatory pattern. It originates from the mutual influence of neighbouring sounds. Example No. 1, ' itoo,' [itu], (see p. 140) recalls the sound-change of the French plural *chevals* [ʃəvals] into *chevaux* [ʃvo :], ' horses,' or Lat. *alba*, *alter*, into *aube*, *autre*. The [l] was apparently articulated whilst the back of the tongue was simultaneously raised against the soft palate into the [u] position.[4] This process has also taken place in the standard pronunciation of Engl. ' people.'[5]

Example No. 8 shows the noteworthy fact that a phonetic tendency does not simply affect some sounds at random. There is always a certain conformity between the sounds of a group, so that it is generally a whole group of speech-sounds which is changed. If in a given language the tip of the tongue lies back during the articulation of, say, [t], we may expect [d] and [n] not to be articulated against the front teeth. These facts indicate what is meant by ' articulation basis ' of a given speech or language ; and it is this which is changed in Dyslalia. The examples Nos. 6 and 7 (p. 140) illustrate how far such tendencies may reach.

The comparison of dyslalic sound-changes with historical shifting of sounds shows a noteworthy similarity. Dyslalia hardly ever shows any shifting of consonants in a direction opposite to that observed in the historic development of language. Both dyslalic and historical sound-changes are ruled by similar primitive inherent tendencies. The changes of sounds in dyslalic speech are not always what we should

[1] Giles, P., l.c., p. 113.
[2] Hence *adelphos*, ' brother ' (cf. Philadelphia).
[3] Mikkola, R. (1913). *Urslavische Grammatik*, Winter, Heidelberg, i, pp. 32 *et seq.*
[4] Meyer-Lübke, W. (1913), l.c., p. 137.
[5] Jones, D. (1937). *The Pronunciation of English*, Cambridge University Press, p. 22.

expect according to the language group of the patient. Nor can we predict what particular feature a national language will adopt in its further development. It is, however, not the change of single speech-sounds, but rather the underlying general principles of sound-change which is of import. Mechanisms such as assimilation, palatalisation, elision of unstressed syllables, etc., are indeed found both in the normal development of language and in Dyslalia.

Thus the fact that Dyslalia, not being a disorder affecting single *sounds* but one affecting the whole of the fundamental articulatory 'conduct' (like in the development of normal languages), justifies the conclusion that there are very old tendencies at work here which, though common to all people, have, for some reason or other, not had the same effect on the development of their respective languages.

Dyslalia seems thus to correspond with dialect or, from a historic point of view, with an epoch or even several epochs in the development of languages.

There arises now the paradox that Dyslalia, viewed from the angle of evolution of language, represents *progress* in speech rather than a phenomenon of decay, as it was once thought to be.

The older philologists, such as Bopp,[1] Humboldt,[2] Grimm,[3] Schleicher,[4] when they saw sounds, inflexions, etc., fading away, were induced to compare human speech with leaf, blossom, and fruit, gaining first a state of perfection and beauty, and then declining and dying. But Grimm already saw that, on the other hand, " human language is retrogressive only apparently and in particular points, but looked upon as a whole it is progressive and its intrinsic force is continually increasing." [5] Jespersen then evolved the latter opinion to outstanding heights.[6]

The sound-changes observed in the historical development of languages, in dialects, and idioms, as well as those constituting Dyslalia are, in the first instance, to be considered mere variations, which we should refrain from valuing. The tendency towards sound-change undoubtedly plays an important part in the evolution of normal languages. Many deviations regarded as abnormal in regard to their too rapid development and their excessive difference from the group speech appear normal changes from the philologist's point of view. Left to develop by themselves these deviations, as in some African tribes, may bring about an entirely new language from one generation to the next (see also p. 141). Rousselot described a sound-change within a group of people whose language was little influenced from the outside. Palatalised [l] changed into [j], which the older generation must have felt to be a mistake, though the younger accepted it without question. Lucian, in a pleasant dialogue, described the Sigma (s) being the plaintiff against the Tau (t) which had expelled it step by step from the words of its inheritance. " Some earlier occasional

[1] Bopp, F. (1816). *Das Conjugationssystem der Sanskritsprache*, Frankfurt.
[2] Humboldt, W. v. (1836). *Verschiedenheit des menschlichen Sprachbaues.*
[3] Grimm, J. (1822). *Deutsche Grammatik*, 2nd ed., Göttingen.
[4] Schleicher, A. (1876). *Compendium der vergleichenden Grammatik*, Weimar.
[5] Quot. by Jespersen, l.c., p. 62.   [6] Ibid., pp. 319 *et seq.*

attempts (as when he took *tettarakonta* for *tessarakonta, temeron* for *semeron*, with little pilferings of that sort) I had explained as a trick and peculiarity of pronunciation." [1]

From the viewpoint of the *raison d'être* of language, such a change is regarded either as a defect or as a normal new formation. Thus the parallel between the tendencies at work in the development of dyslalic speech and that of normal language seems to be established.

What then distinguishes the phonetic pattern of Dyslalia from that of normal language ? It is obviously not the sound table in itself which characterises Dyslalia. In view of what was said about the quantitative criteria in biological, historical, and individual development (see p. 46), it is the terrific speed of transition that strikes the observer. The fact that dyslalic sound-changes take their course with a rapidity exceeding that found in the development of individual, or even historical speech responses (cf. example No. 6, p. 140) calls up the idea of morbidity.

The development of Universal Dyslalia might thus be compared with the growth of tumours. Here, too, we can see the augmentation of cells taking place through the same influences and factors that we observe in normal growth ; but in some way these forces seem to be unbridled, unchecked. A certain degree of inhibition seems to be necessary for maturation. As the growth of the unit of cells is unchecked, the cells themselves cannot become mature ; they always manifest a juvenile aspect. Dyslalia exhibits a similar feature regarded as infantile.

This brings us to the mental part of the speech unit which, as it were, plays the part of the checking cells in our simile. Investigations made by myself [2] and my former collaborators, Edith Goldberger de Buda [3] and Karoline Dworak, have shown a typical a-social or infantile attitude of these patients. They are as a rule easily frightened, isolated, attached to one person, pampered ; they do not want to grow up or to gain the membership of a community beyond that of the mother. A few characteristic utterances may illustrate their outlook.

A boy of 4 always turned to his mother when his speech could not be understood, with the pitiful appeal : " *You* understand me, Mummy, don't you ? " The characteristic neurotic symptom of a schoolgirl of 6 was that she always appeared not to remember her age, though she was intelligent and had often been told it.

These patients seem to live in a world of their own, to which their progressively changing speech corresponds. They do not realise that they should become members of an ever-enlarging group.

The community seeks to enforce upon the individual certain rules of conduct, although the rules are not usually codified. " So far as the code goes, the members of a group are expected to behave alike." [4]

---

[1] *Dike phoneenton* (1905). Translated by H. G. Fowler and F. G. Fowler, Clarendon Press, i, pp. 26–30.

[2] Stein, L. (1925). " Das Universelle Stammeln im Lichte der Entwicklunggeschichte," *Zeitschr. f. d. ges. Neurol. u. Psych.*, **95**, pp. 100–7. *Sprach- und Stimmstörungen*, pp. 66–73.

[3] Goldberger, E. (1933). *Mon. f. Ohrenheilk*, **67**, p. 73.

[4] Woodworth, l.c., p. 123.

This limitation requires a functional adaptation of the child's mind. On the other hand, " the child's rôle is to be little and dependent, but, no less, to grow and become more and more independent."[1] The way in which the child solves this dilemma depends on the skill of those around him in helping him to compensate his natural feeling of inferiority (which itself is not the cause of neurosis) and to find the best way to raise his position in society.

Speech, to be sure, is such an important social link that the child has to adopt the group modes of behaviour in this respect, or else the *raison d'être* of speech to a great extent disappears. There emerges a struggle between naturally developing functional tendencies and rules imposed by the social group.

If the restraining yoke of social feeling is imposed on natural articulatory tendencies, speech gradually assimilates itself to the standard, that is to say, it is supposed to become ' perfect ' and ' definite.' (Bear in mind that ' perfect ' originally meant ' thoroughly made ' and ' definite ' meant ' finished ! ').

The child, in his very first attempts to get in harmony with his environment,. experiences a real defeat. The more complete this defeat the nearer the child's speech approaches to that which is standard [2] (see p. 44).

If natural tendencies prevail, the child goes his individualistic way, showing then a neurotic behaviour. We may expect it to impress its character also on speech. Thus articulateness is diminished. The individual really wants to utter his thoughts and also expects them to be intelligible. This kind of speech can be followed like any other foreign language, if it is familiar to the listener. But owing to certain deviations of articulation and grammar, this speech is not intelligible to all members of the social group in which the speaker has grown up.

In standard speech, what was once forced is now conventionalised. This conventionalised speech is that which answers to the rules and authoritative or recognised examples of correctness and perfection, which are imposed by the social group. It is evident that these characteristics are mere ideal qualities, imagined as perfect or fully developed.[3]

The linguist recognises that there cannot be any speech standard. Language and speech change day by day ; each speaker has his own patois, altering at each moment. The deviations, of course, are and must be very slight, so that they cannot always be differentiated. Mostly the dialect of the ruling classes becomes the standard speech. During childhood the ruling class is represented by the parents, nurse, etc., of the child. They are, however, not always the perfect examples that the definition assumes ; but even if they represent or are standards, these can never be reached (or equalled), since this means either (1) perfection, or (2) some definite degree. (1) is impossible, since nature

[1] Woodworth, l.c., p. 123.

[2] Stein, L. (1940). " On Disorders of Articulate Speech," *Brit. Med. Journ.*, 1, pp. 902 ff.

[3] See *Oxford Dictionary*, s.v. norm, normal, standard, type, ideal, perfect.

does not know any finality, and is always changing and developing ; (2) presumes a forced and thus unnatural stop.

In the days of Curtius (70 odd years ago) the natural evolutionary tendency which is opposed to the conservative tendency characteristic of adults represented a paradox. According to him we are tempted to reduce the normal phonetic laws to a striving after comfort and ease, qualities that are almost abnormal. The conservative tendency should, on the one hand, preserve the sounds from decay, and on the other, interfere with legitimate tendencies leading to decay. Marty [1] has, also, pointed out that any ' logical ' consideration of speech must be rejected if it regards as abnormalities, even as speech defects, all linguistic appearances not in accordance with certain patterns.

It is obvious that we must abandon this method of valuing deviations and disorders in favour of an evolutionary consideration of the psychic and philological aspect of speech. This point of view helps to explain the paradox that an advanced stage of articulate speech is at the same time a disorder. When speech is handed on to children, or adults of another tongue, natural and social speech tendencies must counterbalance each other. In Dyslalia the harmony of the two functions of language, namely, as an instrument of thought and a means of communication, is disturbed. The former looks rather advanced, the latter is more or less ineffective. In consequence of the psychic peculiarities described above (p. 146), speech strives forward unchecked, hence, too rapidly, while its social function is vanishing. Expressed in physiological and anatomical terms : higher levels of the brain cannot acquire, or have lost, their influence on the activities of lower ones. Dyslalia, therefore, regarded from the psychological, analytic, and physiological angle, certainly possesses an infantile or more primitive character. This is shown by the fact that Dyslalia does not only occur in children, which we have used as examples. Here it is caused by unfavourable psychological environmental influences or by deficient maturation. But it has, so far as I can see, been overlooked that the same vehemently progressive sound-changes can be found in adults who, through dissolutionary factors of any kind, have fallen back on the next earlier level or pattern of evolution (see p. 141). This is also supported by the fact that some symptoms of Dyslalia—elision and substitution of sounds—reappear if a subject is, through hypnosis, put into an earlier age.[2]

Characterisation.—The essential characteristics of Dyslalia are :

The faculty of shaping the cavities of resonance in such a way as to produce any sound is preserved ; the individual is thus able to articulate distinct sounds.

The power of perceiving *articulate* speech, i.e. utterances which are divided into distinct and meaningful constituents, is intact.

What is impaired is the reproduction of articulate speech. The

---

[1] *Über das Verhältnis von Grammatik und Logik. Symbolae Pragenses,* pp. 102 f.

[2] Winkler, F. (1929). " Zur Psychologie und Psychotherapie des Stammelns." III. Kongr. d. Int. Ges. f. Logopaedie u. Phoniatrie, Deuticke, Leipzig-Wien, p. 79.

articulatory patterns show disproportionately progressive changes because primitive articulatory tendencies are unchecked, that is to say, lower levels of behaviour have become dominant.

It is obvious that the disturbance is one of relationship with the meaningful environment.

I submit that Dyslalia should be classified as a disorder of *articulate speech*, whereas Dysarthria is a disorder of *articulation*.

Differential diagnosis.—The causes of the disorder may be functional or organic ; thus, from the aetiological point of view we can distinguish functional and organic types of Dyslalia (see p. 65). But according to our definitions of functional and organic diseases (see p. 64) and to the doctrine of dissolution, we need not attach too much significance to that discrimination in delimiting Dyslalia.

In Dysarthria the activities of the organs concerned (e.g. lips, tongue, palate) are so restricted as to prevent the primitive functions of eating, breathing, swallowing, chewing, and so on, as well as speaking, in the adult. In the child this impairment naturally impedes the specialisation of vegetative functions into speech. The term Dysarthria sensu strictu has hitherto been restricted to the disordered production of speech-sounds caused by either organic or functional disturbances within the central nervous system. According to my findings, I see no reason why the term could not be applied to disorders of sound production caused by defects of the peripheral speech organs (e.g. cleft palate speech).

PARTIAL DYSLALIA

Types.—So far we have seen that dissolution in Universal Dyslalia is uniform, that is to say, the whole system of articulation is under the same conditions or evil influence.[1] It has also been stated that the sound-changes concerned are not really affections of the sounds themselves, but of their articulation basis (see p. 144).

Hand-in-hand with the further specialisation of articulate utterance certain sounds come, according to their acoustic or motor properties, to form classes such as those of the sibilants, fricatives, plosives, or that of sounds characterised by high frequency formants (see pp. 31 and 50). All sounds belonging to one group more or less obey the same rules of sound-change.

It is in this sense that the term Partial Dyslalia should be understood. In Partial Dyslalia disorders are included which affect larger or smaller groups of sounds.

As far as the disturbance affects sounds as single units, the diagnostic terms have been derived from the Greek names of the corresponding symbols by the addition of the suffix ' -ism.' Thus, e.g., disorders of the sounds [k], [g], [l] are named Kappacism, Gammacism, Lambdacism respectively. If the character of the affected sound has completely disappeared, e.g. if [k] is replaced by [t], it has been the custom to indicate this in the diagnostic term by the prefix ' para ' (*para*, ' beside '), Parakappacism, and so on.

[1] Cf. Jackson, l.c., ii, p. 47.

Multiple Interdentalism.—Multiple Interdentalism (Fröschels) [1] may prove a suitable introduction to this subject. This disorder is, as it were, a transition from Universal Dyslalia to Partial Dyslalia.' It affects more or less all sounds articulated by the *tip of the tongue,* such as [s], [t], [d], [n], [l], [ʃ] ; [ϑ] and [δ] are naturally also affected, unless we admit that their proper articulation is interdental, a misconception often found in German books.

" The letter TH represents two standard English sounds. The one, whose phonetic symbol is ϑ, is a breathed dental fricative, articulated by the tip of the tongue against the upper teeth, the main part of the tongue being more or less flat. The symbol δ stands for the voiced form of ϑ." [2]

In Multiple Interdentalism all or some of the aforementioned speech-sounds are articulated interdentally, that is to say, the necessary shape of mouth is altered by putting the tip of the tongue between the front teeth.

Evolutionary Explanation.—Multiple Interdentalism as such has only recently been clearly recognised, because acoustically the interdental articulation of [t, d, l, n] is scarcely noticeable. Only the interdental pronunciation of the sibilants [s, z, ʃ, ʒ] strikes the ear.

In Multiple Interdentalism a uniform tendency to protrude the tip of the tongue in all tongue-tip sounds is obvious. Now the view that all sounds are the outcome of the integration of vegetative motor tendencies brings to mind the fact that the protrusion of the tongue is a common behaviour of babies. Analytical and developmental considerations seem to suggest that it is associated with sucking movements. The tongue may thus ultimately represent the nipple, and manifest a primitive libidinal tendency. The protrusion of the tongue is frequent in mental defectives. It can also often be observed in children, and in adults, where it betrays emotional attitudes, such as perplexity, surprise, and so on.

It is therefore little to be wondered at the frequent occurrence of Multiple Interdentalism in early childhood. In the course of development it usually disappears through adaptation. If it does not, it is considered ' childlike,' and therefore ' sweet ; ' and it is significant that especially female patients with this disorder are found ' attractive.' This is all the more striking as all other speech disorders are generally believed to be symptoms of some mental inferiority. The question, ' Why is Multiple Interdentalism not regarded as contemptible ? ' is therefore justified. It is undoubtedly its emotional (erotic) meaning which influences the opinion of the listener by reminding him of all he holds dear, i.e. children and the fair sex.

Trude Newekluff, having regard to the view which I had propounded on dyslalic disorders, subjected Multiple Interdentalism to a psychological and statistical examination. She found that interdental speech occurs in children up to the fourth year, that is to say,

[1] Fröschels, E. (1924). " Zur Aetiologie einiger Sigmatismen," *Festschift für Hugo Pipping.* (1926). "Beobachtungen an Sigmatismen," *Zeitschr. f. Hals-Nasen- u. Ohrenheilk,* VI, No. 4.
[2] Jones, D., l.c., p. 29.

while the tongue serves the child's infantile desires (sucking). It can therefore be regarded as a physiological phenomenon in the child's speech development.

If the child later on adapts himself to the social surroundings, he corrects the deviating auditory impression of the interdental [s] ; but the original tendency to speaking interdentally betrays itself very often in the interdental articulation of other dental sounds. The resulting state of speech was termed ' Sigmatismus sine sigmatismo ' by T. Newekluff. It should more appropriately be called ' Interdentalism without sigmatism,' as the [s] is normal, while the acoustic feature of [t], [d], [n], and [l], in spite of their interdental articulation, does not deviate perceptibly.

Premature ceasing of physiological interdentalism is due to disturbances in the child's oral-erotic attitude.

Similar psychological characteristics as those outlined in cases of Universal Dyslalia, such as accentuated infantility, particularly in younger or only children who are spoiled or sickly (cardiac defect), were found by Newekluff in Multiple Interdentalism.

Many parents consider Interdentalism ' pretty ' and therefore cultivate it in their children.[1]

From the evolutionary angle it is interesting to note that interdental speech can often be observed in erotic states or in tender and amorous moods.[2]

Multiple Interdentalism is thus not a ' merely functional ' disorder, but is based on primitive mental attitudes. The patients themselves are unconsciously aware of its infantile or erotic significance. In this context it is perhaps interesting to mention that Multiple Interdentalism is the only speech defect which is commoner in girls, according to Stinchfield's survey.[3] It is important to bear this in mind when treatment is contemplated (see pp. 153, 162).

Sigmatism.—Among the consonants articulated by the tip of the tongue the sibilants [s], [z], [ʃ], [ʒ], [θ], and [ð], and their combinations with other consonants, deserve special consideration, inasmuch as their pattern, both from the motor and the acoustic viewpoints, is rather complex. It is therefore all the more apt to be disintegrated.

Description of the normal dental fricatives.—In [s] the tip of the tongue forms a narrow passage between itself and the front teeth, the lower teeth being behind the upper ones. The tip of the tongue can either be elevated behind the upper incisors or lowered behind the lower incisors. What is, however, essential is the formation of a groove in the median line of the tongue, its lateral parts being raised and touching the molars. The air passes along this groove and so produces a hissing sound.

If voice is used with this friction between the tip of the tongue and the teeth, [z], as in Engl. ' zeal,' is sounded.

[1] Gumpertz, F. (1929). *Discussion to* Newekluff. See below.
[2] Newekluff, T. (1929). " Ueber die Häufigkeit der multiplen Interdentalitaet." III. Kongr. d. Int. Ges. f. Logopaedie u. Phoniatrie, Deuticke, Leipzig-Wien, pp. 90–3.
[3] Stinchfield, l.c., p. 76.

In the spelling of various languages the characters 'x,' 'c,' and 'z' do not represent single sounds, but groups of consonants, such as in Engl. X-rays [ɛks ɹeiz] ; Germ. zehn [tse : n], 'ten' ; Czech, co [tsɔ], 'what' ; Ital. zelo [dzɛ : lo], 'zeal.'

[ʃ], e.g. in Engl. shoe, is a breathed dental fricative, articulated by the tip of the tongue against the upper gums, the front of the tongue being considerably raised towards the hard palate. Some articulate the sound with the blade, keeping the tongue tip against the lower teeth. The voiced form of [ʃ] is [ʒ], as in Engl. measure [meʒə].[1]

The sounds heard in English church, judge, are combinations of t or d with [ʃ] or [ʒ] respectively.

[ɵ], as in Engl. think, thorn, is a breathed dental fricative, articulated by the tip of the tongue against the upper teeth, the main part of the tongue being more or less flat. Its voiced form is [ð], as in Engl. though, than.[2]

The hissing sounds represent resonances containing very high overtones and formants. The range of formants in S extends from d flat[4] to e[5], in SH [ʃ] from f[3] to e flat[4], the range of the latter thus being considerably lower.

It should be mentioned that the range of formants in F and CH (as in Scotch 'loch ') lies almost within the same limits as that of S (d flat[4] to d flat[5], e flat[4] to d flat[5])[3] (see p. 156).

The corresponding voiced fricatives [z, ʒ, v, ð, ɹ] show a similar pattern with the addition of the fundamental and the first few harmonics.[4]

Types of Sigmatism.—Deviations from the delineated articulations cause differences of resonance which are comprised in the class of Sigmatisms (Sigma is the Greek letter expressing the sound [s]). The diagnostic classification of the types of Sigmatism has been made in accordance with the acoustic and/or motor character of the deviations. It will, however, prove necessary to classify Sigmatisms also with regard to behavioural patterns. This, in its turn, will be of some help in treatment.

Interdental Sigmatism.—The symptomatology of Multiple Interdentalism shows that it is not a disturbance affecting only the hissing sounds, but a manifestation of a general tendency to protrude the tongue. All sounds produced by the articulation of the tip of the tongue against the front teeth are therefore affected. The conclusion is that, psychologically, Multiple Interdentality represents the integration of infantile and primitive erotic responses into speech-sounds.

A similar explanation evidently applies to Interdental Sigmatism. (Lisping sensu strictu.) This is a disorder which resembles Multiple Interdentalism in so far as the tongue-tip articulates between the front teeth ; but it differs from it in that this interdental articulation is restricted to the hissing sounds [s], [z], [ʃ], and [ʒ]. Folklore seems to indicate that the roots of this tendency and its integration with utterance are to be sought on the same level. An English proverb

---

[1] Jones, D., l.c., p. 30.   [2] Ibid., p. 29.
[3] Stumpf, H. (1926). *Die Sprachlaute*, Berlin.   [4] Curry, l.c., p. 59.

runs : " A lisping lass is good to kiss." This seems to indicate that lisping has a deep erotic significance. I have received confirmation of this from many sources.[1]

It is not clear, however, why adaptation to the norm has taken place in all sounds except the sibilants ; but I suggest tentatively that, if the individual still finds any necessity at all to exhibit his psychic tendencies, it can be done only through the hissing sounds. For the other sounds do not show any acoustic deviation if uttered interdentally. Thus Multiple Interdentalism may gradually become restricted to Interdental Sigmatism, which in some cases persists only as a relic of the former condition. It must not, however, be overlooked that organic reasons may also play their part in the genesis of Interdental Sigmatism. The tip of the tongue must find a firm point against which to articulate. If during the period of sound adaptation the front teeth are missing, the protrusion of the tongue is naturally facilitated. This is also shown by a similar occurrence in a recognised language. The Otyi-hereros' pronunciation is lisping, owing to " the custom of the Va-herero of having their upper front teeth filed off, and four lower teeth knocked out. It is perhaps due to this that the Otyi-herero has two sounds similar to those of the hard and soft ' th ' and ' dh ' (i.e. [θ] and [ð] ; note by the present writer) in English." [2]

The appearance in adults of disorders of the S sounds is due to similar factors. In certain cases after extraction of the front teeth and the fitting of an artificial set, [s] and [ʃ] come to be ' lisped.' The tip of the tongue, however, does not protrude and the S is articulated like the genuine English TH. The reason is obvious. The articulation of the S requires a highly refined kinesthetic feeling. If the position of the new set of teeth is only slightly different, the whole mechanism breaks down. Patients report that they feel as if their tongue were no longer quite at home in their mouth.

I have seen foreigners with Interdental Sigmatism who, when imitating the English [ð] produced an excellent [z] (not interdental). These sound-changes z > ð and ð > z show that a patient suffering from even a well-canalised Interdental Sigmatism is capable of producing the right S, but he does so only in words in which he hears the interdental z [ð], the articulation of which is familiar to him.

Lateral (Lambdoid) Sigmatism.—What we hear in Lateral Sigmatism (Lambdoid Sigmatism) is a hissing sound and an l-sound simultaneously. The tip of the tongue articulates against the upper teeth or gums, and so produces a friction, but the necessary elevation of both of the lateral edges of the tongue is missing. The main part of the tongue obstructs the air passage in the middle of the mouth. The expired air, therefore, escapes on either or both sides of the mouth, thus creating the impression of [l].

In many cases the lateral articulation is accompanied by drawing one corner of the mouth sideways. Very often the same lip action

[1] The wife of Bath (Chaucer's *Canterbury Tales*) was buck-toothed and—had five husbands ! I am indebted to Dr. D. S. Murray for this parallel.
[2] Sir G. Grey's Library, i, p. 167. Quoted by Max Müller, *Lectures*, ii, p. 178.

can be observed, apart from speech, as a kind of tic.[1] The biological and psychological roots of such automatic actions are, as a rule, to be found on low levels.

As to the significance of drawing back the angle of the mouth and thus showing the canine tooth, I refer to Darwin. He pointed out that " the action is the same as that of a snarling dog ; and a dog when pretending to fight often draws up the lip on one side alone, namely, that facing his antagonist." [2]

It would thus appear that this symptom is preponderantly an aggressive one. The psychological examination of patients with Lateral Sigmatism justifies the assumption that their specific Dyslalia may be the expression of such a repressed aggressive tendency.

A girl of 23, when seeking treatment, gave this reason : " I attack everyone with my tongue." Further investigation showed that she was very aggressive in all respects, such as towards her parents, and towards religion. She was not good at making friends. Her attitude while at school was, " I hated the world and everybody."

I therefore submit that Lateral Sigmatism preserves primitive patterns of articulation. This assumption is not only supported by the aforementioned behaviouristic and evolutionary facts, but also by linguistic considerations. Primitive languages still preserve lateral clicks, and it is not improbable that they are the roots of the lateral S (see Evolution of Language, p. 49). Even in normal adults one can sometimes detect a lateral (inspiratory or expiratory) S as the expression of a feeling of danger, combined with embarrassment and pain.

Nasal Sigmatism is characterised by the conjunction of a hissing sound with a nasal one. The tip of the tongue may take up the normal position required for the sibilants, or it may be somewhat drawn back. In some cases the necessary friction is produced by a narrowing of the air passage between the main part of the tongue and the palate.

The soft palate remains lowered so that the air escapes through the nose as well, sometimes giving rise to a snoring sound (Silbiger).[3]

Nothing is known for certain about the genesis of the Nasal Sigmatism. Many years ago I made an observation [4] which I have been able to repeat on several occasions. If one has to give an answer hurriedly, while, say, eating a hot morsel, or while anything prevents the articulation of the tip of the tongue (e.g. dental treatment), the fricative pattern of [s] becomes more or less impaired. Curiously enough, the resulting sound is always nasalised, the soft palate being inactive. Fröschels [5] made similar observations in lisping patients while they were using his wax plate (see p. 160). In slovenly speech, when the tip of the tongue is scarcely articulating, there appears a nasal h [ɦ] instead of [s] or [ʒ]; one often hears[ɦæŋkju] instead

---

[1] A tic is a convulsive twitching of the facial muscles.

[2] Darwin, C. (1890). *The Expression of the Emotions in Man and Animals*, 2nd ed., John Murray, London, p. 261.

[3] In Fröschels, E. (1931). *Lehrbuch der Sprachheilkunde*, Deuticke, Vienna, p. 321.

[4] " Proc. of the Oesterr. Ges. f. experim. Phonetik," *Wien. med. Woch.*, 1918, No. 34.

[5] Discussion, ibid.

of [ʒæŋkju]. Thus there seems to exist a primitive connection between the articulation of the tip of the tongue and the elevation of the soft palate.

One might thus seek for the origin of this disorder in a neurotic suppression of the articulation of the tongue-tip. I have evidence of a similar causation in a kindred type of Sigmatism, viz. Guttural Sigmatism.

Guttural (Velar) Sigmatism is a very rare type, of which I have found no description in the textbooks. It does not, so far as I can see, occur in developmental Dyslalia, but mostly in traumatic cases. The sound [x] which appears in the place of [s] is not due to sound change, but to sound substitution.

One of my patients, a 30-year-old Irishwoman, stated that she had suffered from this speech disturbance since early childhood. She said she did not mind it at all, but came only because of her dentist's opinion that it was very bad. All articulations, including those of [ʃ] and [ʒ], were normal! Only the [s] and [z] were replaced by [x] and [ɣ]. Her behaviour was strikingly motionless and taciturn ; the play of the facial muscles was stiff. Blowing into a key (see Therapy) produced an excellent result immediately without hesitation or random trials. The patient was cured after a few interviews.

The bare fact that the patient was able to find the correct articulation instantaneously must give rise to the suspicion that the normal S pattern had actually developed but was repressed and replaced by an acoustically kindred sound. The assumption was justified later on, when the patient's elder sister stated that the patient had been articulating all sounds, including [s] and [z], normally until her 10th year of age. At that age she had an accident which caused painful wounds of the lips and palate and the loss of several incisor teeth. She also suffered from shock. The fact that the patient herself had completely forgotten this comparatively recent accident, together with her inhibited attitude, clearly reveals repression.

In *Laryngeal Sigmatism* a sound produced by friction of air between the ventricular bands replaces [s], while the tongue is inactive. The disorder, described by Sokolovsky,[1] is rare. I can only remember having observed it in cases of cleft palate. Here it may owe its origin to the fact that the patient does not find it in any way possible to produce a fricative sound in the mouth. It seems to conform with the substitution of the glottal stop for dental or velar stops.

Labiodental Sigmatism, described by Nadoleczny,[2] arises if the lower lip is placed under the upper teeth, as in the articulation of [f], while the tongue is in the position peculiar to [s]. The acoustic result is a very sharp whistling noise.

Lacking exact investigations, it seems to me that this constitutes an unsuccessful attempt to convert an impure S into a normal one, by directing the stream of air downwards with the help of the lips.

[1] Sokolovsky, H. (1921). " Eine noch nicht beschriebene Form des Sigmatismus," *Mon. f. Ohrenheilk.*, **55**, p. 1640.

[2] Nadoleczny, M. (1926). *Kurzes Lehrbuch der Sprach- und Stimmheilkunde*, p. 67.

In *Strident Sigmatism* a very sharp [s] is produced, the middle groove of the tongue being too deep and narrow.

Addental Sigmatism (Fröschels' *Sigma Multiloculare*).—This disorder arises if the tongue is pressed too much against the teeth. The necessary groove in the middle of the tongue cannot be formed, so that the air has to pass over a great part of the tongue surface. The resulting sound is similar to [ʃ].

In some cases the tip of the tongue comes so near to the front teeth that the air passage is completely obstructed. No friction is therefore possible, and the [s] appears replaced by the explosive sound [t].

Examinations carried out by Fröschels and Fremel,[1] and by the present writer,[2] showed that this abnormal reproduction of the [s] is often due to a bilateral lesion of the inner ear acquired in early childhood. The degeneration of the sensory cells or the fibres of the auditory nerve impairs particularly the perception of very high tones, but may allow the growing child to acquire speech. Thus the child cannot hear the whole sound complex of [s], as the necessary formants (see p. 152) are not perceived.

Addental Sigmatism, therefore, often constitutes a most important sign of a lesion of the inner ear, since those around the patient and the patient himself may fail to notice his defective hearing.

Palatal Sigmatism.—In some cases the articulation of the tip of the tongue is combined with a simultaneous lifting of the blade of the tongue against the palate. The acoustic result is a sound which exhibits the characteristics of both [s] and [ç].

Sigmatismus palatalis is certainly kindred to similar tendencies in Universal Dyslalia (see p. 144). As it can often be found in the sound table of dyslalic patients, it seems that, if isolated, it represents the last remnant of a former Universal Dyslalia, in which palatalisation tendency had played its part. X-ray examination showed that other dental sounds, such as [d], [t], [l], and [n] were also—though not audibly—affected in the same way.[3]

Aetiology.—The types of Sigmatism thus seem to originate from different evolutionary levels. Interdental and Lateral Sigmatism appear to be integrations of low behavioural patterns. The nasal, guttural and laryngeal types probably owe their origin to a traumatic destruction of the motor part of the sound pattern, whereas the addental form is based on an incomplete acoustic pattern. The Palatal Sigmatism is the last remnant of the shifted basis of articulation in Universal Dyslalia.

Most forms of Sigmatism show a psychological attitude which fits well into the developmental structure of the sounds.

Diagnosis.—The examination of the Sigmatisms is generally made by a rubber tube, one end of which is put into the therapist's ear while the other is passed along the row of the patient's front teeth during

---

[1] Fremel, F. and Fröschels, E. (1914). " Gehör und Sprache," *Arch. f. exp. u. klin. Phon.*

[2] Stein, L. (1929). " Sigmatismus und Innenohraffektion," *Monatschr. f. Ohrenheilk,* **63,** p. 414.

[3] Stein, L. (1927). " Ueber das Wesen des Sigmatismus," *Mediz. Klinik,* No. 13.

articulation. The observer can thus distinctly feel and hear where the air escapes.

The experienced speech therapist will in many cases be able to diagnose the type of Sigmatism by audition and by vision.

KAPPACISM AND GAMMACISM

Symptoms.—The essential motor factor in the pattern of the stop consonants is the momentary blocking of the air passage, which is then forced open by the air. The block can be made at any point in the mouth. In [p] and [b] the lips are closed. If the obstacle is offered by the contact of the tongue with the palate, a series of stops is produced, the resonance of which varies from the distinct [k] or [g] sounds (velar plosives) to [t] or [d] (dental stops).

In Kappacism and Gammacism the velar stops [k] and [g] are changed, usually into the respective dental stops [t] and [d]. Sometimes the glottal stop substitutes them. If the sound table of the patient's language contains the sounds [x] and [ç], they are often replaced by [s] or [ʃ] like sounds.

Investigations made by Gumpertz and by the present writer have shown that the above description is not quite accurate, inasmuch as many intermediate varieties of lingual stops occur, which cannot always be perceived by the unaided ear.

The exact position of the tongue has been ascertained by Palatography. The tongue is smeared with some dye (e.g. methylene blue), which thus colours the palate (or a plate inserted there) where the tongue articulates with it during the production of a sound.

The palatogram shows that in Kappacism and Gammacism all the above-mentioned articulatory deviations may occur ; the tongue may even be in the t- and k-positions simultaneously.

These peculiarities recall, on the one hand, the characteristics of the sucking movements and of the clicks (see p. 31) ; on the other, they remind us of the shifting of the basis of articulation, as in Dyslalia Universalis, inasmuch as the K- or T-character of the disordered articulation often depends on the surrounding sounds.

Evolutionary aspect.—The stops [p, b, t, d, k, g] are generally among the earliest acquired by the child. The historical phonology of most of the language families more or less confirms that the stops were the characteristic sounds of ancient and primitive speech.[1]

For the last three to four thousand years the general tendency in all language families has been to shift the articulation from the back of the mouth to the front—from the uvular and velar positions to the palatal and alveolar.[2] The growing child in the babbling period has not much difficulty in producing stops ; but the tendency to abandon the back articulation as in [k] and [g] plays its part in the acquisition of standard speech.

In some primitive languages the wavering, undecided articulation is still noticeable, so that—as in Kappacism—for an observer not

---

[1] Chatterji, Suniti Kumar, l.c., pp. 332–4.   [2] Ibid., p. 334.

acquainted with, say, the languages of the Sandwich Islands, it is impossible to tell whether he hears a guttural or a dental stop.

It would thus appear that in regard to the evolutionary explanation of Kappacism, the same rule applies which we have delineated for Universal Dyslalia.

Also the sound change of [k] and [g] into the glottal stop has its parallel in the normal evolution of languages (it is quite familiar to us in modern Cockney). Primitive languages, such as Tahitian, Hawaian, Samoan, lack guttural sounds. In these dialects the [k] is indicated—in M. Müller's words—' by a hiatus or catching of the breath,' which seems to signify the glottal stop.[1]

RHOTACISM

The Diverse Types of R.—When we speak of sound-changes affecting the R, we are, though mostly unconsciously, thinking of the *letter* R. The history of languages has shown that this symbol stands for a number of speech-sounds which differ in manner and place of production, and in sound.

The sounds spelled R vary greatly according to language or dialect. In Germanic, Romance, and Slavonic languages standard R is normally produced by the tip of the tongue against the front teeth, gums, or front palate (dental, alveolar, palatal R), except for a few dialects where it is formed by the uvula, e.g. French. In both cases the articulating organs (tongue-tip or uvula) are either caused to vibrate : trilled or rolled [r] and [R], or to produce fricative sounds : [ɹ], [ʁ] or even [χ]. In Germanic languages uvular [ʁ] and [R] are certainly later substitutes for dental r.[2]

The fully rolled r is common in Northern English. A semi-rolled r [ɾ], which consists of one single tap of the tongue, is commonly used in Standard English between two vowels, as in ' period, arrive,' or after th [θ, ð], as in ' three.'[3]

The sound regularly used in Standard English is a voiced dental fricative, articulated by the tip of the tongue against the upper gums, the front part of the tongue being rather hollowed. In some dialects the latter shape is more distinct, the tip of the tongue being turned back towards the hard palate, inverted r [ɻ].[4]

Symptoms.—In Rhotacism any one of the above variants may take the place of the standard r of a given language. Apart from the afore-mentioned sounds, [l], [ŋ], [x], [ɣ], [j], or [w] may substitute the r. It may be doubted whether the sound-change should be regarded as a disorder or merely as an idiomatic variation of the language community to which the patient subscribes. In some cases the disorder follows the model of those found in historic phonology. Particularly the substitution of [l] for [r] occurs in all languages and at all times. Cf. Engl. *plum*, Lat. pruna ; Engl. *silk*, Lat. *sericum ;* this word " is supposed to have passed into Slav via some languages which have

---

[1] Müller, M., *Lectures*, ii, pp. 180-4.   [2] Sievers, l.c., p. 297.
[3] Jones, Daniel, l.c., pp. 24-5.   [4] Ibid., pp. 30-1.

confused -r- and -l-."[1] This confusion has also been observed in Japanese, and in some African and Polynesian languages.

Fröschels submitted that the inability to differentiate between [r] and [l] is a symptom of regression. He sees evidence for it in the fact that this inability is found in Japanese ; but it is by no means evident that Japanese is on a lower evolutionary level than European languages.

A solitary variety of a rolled alveolar consonant is the Czech [ř]. It is produced by vibrations of the tongue-tip which is approximated to the dental ridge. The stream of air is less interrupted than in [r] and is only temporarily damped. The ear therefore perceives the [r] and the [ʃ] almost simultaneously.

Czech patients may fail in producing the [ř], because the articulation of the alveolar [r] is defective, that of the [ʃ] being normal. [ř] is replaced by the uvular [R] + [ʃ] or [ʒ]. In many cases [ʃ] and [ʒ] substitute ř. Here also the pathological process takes the course indicated by the evolution of language. The comparative history of Slav languages shows a tendency of [r] before palatal vowels ([i], [e]) or diphthongs to change into palatalised (mouillé) [ŕ], as in Russian, then into [ř], as in Czech, and finally into [ʃ] [ʒ], as in Polish. Silbiger [2] based his elucidation on the parallelism between dyslalic and historical sound-changes, which I had detected and which had given me the clue for the explanation of Universal Dyslalia.[3]

MINOR TYPES

Finally, some other types of Partial Dyslalia may be briefly outlined, being of minor importance.

In Lambdacism the [l] is replaced by [r], [j], [n]. In Betacism [v] replaces [b]. [g] and [k] sometimes take the place of [d] and [t] (Deltacism). [f] is in rare cases articulated by the upper lip against the lower front teeth.

Treatment of Dyslalia.—We have seen that under normal conditions the child himself succeeds in adapting his speech-sounds at a time when the patterns are still ' plastic.' If this time, through the circumstances described above (see p. 146), is missed, the deviating speech-patterns become so well canalised that the patient himself is no longer able to alter them even if he wishes to. In the case of Dyslalia originating in adults it has been made clear that a level representing primitive phonetic tendencies has become dominant. This permits those tendencies to be at work unchecked and to bring about phonetic products which had previously been repressed.

The therapist's task must be to re-create the whole of the speech-pattern out of the material available, i.e. by using functions corresponding to a lower level which must then be integrated. Treatment must consequently take into account not only the sensory, motor, and

[1] Weekly, E. *Etymological Dictionary of Modern English,* John Murray, London.

[2] Silbiger, B. (1929). " Zur Pathologie des tschechischen r," III. Kongr. d. Int. Ges. f. Logopaedie u. Phoniatrie, Deuticke, Leipzig-Wien, pp. 112–19.

[3] Stein, L. (1925). *Das Universelle Stammeln.*

kinaesthetic units of the speech-pattern, but also the psychological attitude of the speaker. The respective techniques apply to cases of Partial and Universal Dyslalia.

Treatment of Sigmatisms.—Although Sigmatism seems to be the most widespread speech defect, it must not be inferred that the S sound presents any greater difficulty in its formation than any other sound, which is obvious when we consider how quickly the correct formation is generally learned under treatment.

All Sigmatisms, with the sole exception of Nasal Sigmatism, may be treated in the same way. In the case of Multiple Interdentalism, how-ever, an attempt must obviously be made to correct the articulation of the other dental sounds (t, d, n, l) too.

The easiest and simplest way of making the patient produce a correct S consists in evoking in the patient's conscious mind the primi-tive behavioural pattern connected with it. The therapist would, for example, ask : " What would you do if you wanted people to stop making a noise ? " In most cases the patient will, as soon as he realises what is required, produce the proper hissing sound.

If this method proves unsuccessful, a kind of whistling into a hole may bring about the desired result. The first step is to make the patient leave his tongue flat in his mouth, close his jaws, open his lips horizontally, and blow gently in this position. Then we give him a little glass tube, lemonade straw, or an ordinary hollow key, which he must put a little below the rim of the lower incisors right in the middle. With lips opened horizontally he must try to whistle into the tube. This attempt forces the tongue to form the channel necessary for the correct articulation of [s]. This whistling exercise should be practised until well canalised. The next step consists in advising the patient to perform the same exercise ; during his prolonged whistling the key or tube is gradually drawn away from the teeth. Thus the whistle disappears, whilst the still persisting groove of the tongue is giving rise to the [s].

Should the patient not be able to learn the [s] in this way, another method (Fröschels [1]) may be tried. A wax plate [2] is softened in hot water and a small triangular piece is cut out of the area corresponding to the front teeth. The plate is placed between the teeth and the patient is then told to bite into it, after which the plate is hardened in cold water. The impressions of the teeth keep the plate in position in the patient's mouth when he puts it in for his exercises. It forces the tongue into the correct position for [s], since the tongue must necessarily lie flat in the mouth ; it cannot get beyond the teeth ; it cannot press against the teeth, because the triangular opening of the plate is so small as to allow the escape of air only if the tongue does not obstruct it by its elevation. Frequent exercises with this plate accustom the tongue to the correct position.

Gutzmann [3] suggests pressing down the middle part of the tongue with a probe to produce the groove necessary for the formation of [s].

---

[1] Fröschels, E. (1913). *Lehrbuch der Sprachheilkunde*, Vienna, p. 205.
[2] As used by dentists for taking impressions.
[3] Gutzmann, H. (1912). *Sprachheilkunde*, Berlin, pp. 502–6.

This method often produces the opposite of the desired position of the tongue. Instead of forming a groove, the tongue rises reflexly against the probe. I have found it more effective to press upwards below the chin in the median line ; the tongue joins in the resistance offered to this pressure and thus produces the longitudinal groove. Patients uninclined to action must be urged to resist the pressure.[1]

If the tip of the tongue is not close enough to the teeth, although its position is otherwise correct, the sound [t] should be articulated before blowing so as to make the tongue remain close enough to the incisors when blowing takes place (Branco van Dantzig).

In Nasal Sigmatism it is the elevation of the velum which must be brought about, the position of the tongue being mostly correct. Gutzmann [2] advises closing the patient's nose and making him blow through the closed teeth. Fröschels makes the patient say [f] for a time and pulls away the lip from the teeth during articulation. The air escapes through the teeth and the endeavour to procure a similar fricative sound causes the tip of the tongue to move forward, thus producing S.

In case of a combination of Lateral with Nasal Sigmatism, the position of the tongue must also be corrected.

If the patient is hard of hearing, special training of hearing (Urbantschitsch) must be tried. Success in these cases largely depends on whether the patient is an acoustic or a motor type, in which latter case the prognosis is better since he can utilise proprioceptive sensations for control.

Once the patient has learned to say [s], we can proceed to teach him to produce [z]. The articulation is the same, the only difference being that it is voiced, not breathed. We revert to making him say [f] and then ask him to hum a tune while retaining the same shape of mouth. The result is [v]. By repeating this procedure with the newly achieved [s], [z] is produced.

Patients achieve the correct articulation of [ʃ] easily when trying to imitate the noise of a steam engine, while the lips are well rounded. In some cases it is necessary to push back the tip of the tongue with a probe, the end of which is bent into a loop, while the patient is trying to articulate [s].

By combining phonation with the articulation of [ʃ], as indicated above, the patient attains to [ʒ].

By practising [s], [z], [ʃ], and [ʒ], while listening carefully to the sounds produced, the patient learns to associate the correct articulation with the corresponding sensory impressions. But this does in no way mean that he is able to utilise the newly acquired articulatory ability in words, since the meaning of the words is so strongly associated with the faulty articulation as to make the patient unfailingly slip into the latter. Mention of anything that might give rise to the old associations should, therefore, be avoided, especially in young children. To achieve syllables beginning with [s] or [ʃ] the patient is advised to start the

---

[1] Stein, L. (1928). "Zur Technik der Sigmatismenbehandlung," *Wien. med. Woch.*, No. 29.

[2] Gutzmann, l.c., p. 509.

11

'whistle' and to continue expiration while initiating an aspirated vowel : [s ha, s he, s hi, s ho, s hu] ; [ʃ ha, ʃ he, ʃ hi, ʃ ho, ʃ hu], and so on. At a next stage the patient should enunciate these combinations in a more careless, lazy, and inaccurate way, which leads to the disappearance of the aspirated attack, thus resulting in [sa, se, si, so, su] ; [ʃa, ʃe, ʃi, ʃo, ʃu] respectively.

The production of syllables with initial [z] or [ʒ] presents no difficulty. The patient needs only to continue phonation while proceeding to shape the mouth for the subsequent vowel. Syllables ending in [s], [ʃ], [z], or [ʒ] are equally easy to achieve.

On such syllables the enunciation of monosyllables in rhyme with each other, such as 'moss, loss, toss,' and so on, can be based. Automatisation takes place quickly, and encourages the patient to further activity. This kind of practice is aided by the innate tendency to reiterate.

Arrangements of two words, the first ending in [s], [z], [ʃ], or [ʒ], the second beginning with a vowel, such as 'Miss Ann' [misaen], 'as I' [aezai], facilitate the production of intervocalic sibilants. Such arrangements of words may be practised along with meaningless syllables such as [asa], [ese] ; [aza], [eze] ; [aʃa], [eʃe], [aʒa], [eʒe], and so on.

The practice of meaningless syllables of the pattern sibilant-consonant-vowel, occurring in words like 'fox, frogs, hats, odds, church, George, jam,' etc., follows.

The treatment of young children must necessarily differ from that of older children or adults. Use should be made of the tendencies to reiteration and onomatopoeia. Dramatic gestures and play should accompany the exercises. The description of pictures facilitates the transition to spontaneous speech. Little poems are helpful.

Older children and adults should read aloud passages in which the sibilants have been underlined so as to attract attention and to bring about the necessary association between the motor, auditory, and visual percepts.

Needless to say, the right understanding of the patient, be he child or adult, and infinite patience are most important, as any such patient needs psychological readjustment. To make him self-controlled and independent are aims included in the treatment.

Functional treatment is obviously necessary, since otherwise the patient cannot find the right articulation, for he has never possessed it, and as the abnormal movements are well canalised he cannot easily get rid of them. But in many cases it does not suffice.

Experience has taught me that, especially in female patients, functional treatment does not present considerable difficulties at the commencement. The patients are, after a few weeks, able to pronounce the hissing sounds properly and to use normal sounds in reading and telling stories, but when it comes to conversation they often fail, and this failure persists much longer than in the average case. They cannot concentrate sufficiently.

Now concentration, interest, and similar concepts refer to motivation ; and indeed in many cases analysis reveals that the patients unconsciously want to keep the ' sweet ' pronunciation since they have the feeling that the correct articulation would deprive them of a considerable part of their sex appeal.

Neurotic Sigmatism. Treatment.—The same difficulties arise in treating Sigmatism of purely neurotic origin. The right articulation has very often been repressed for many years, and the wrong one has for the same time been canalised. The rehabilitation thus seems to be in many cases extremely easy as the patients find—by the means already shown—the right articulation without particular difficulty.

As soon as reading, sometimes as soon as syllables are tackled, the patient begins to assure the therapist how very much he wishes to get rid of the ' awful ' lisp, how hard he tries, etc. On the other hand, he uses all sorts of subterfuges, pretexts, and mental reservations, such as " I am too old," which, so to speak, baffle the therapist altogether.

Psychotherapy is therefore indicated ; but this proposal is generally rejected by the patient, the defect being not ' worth while.' The therapist should therefore be extremely careful as to his prognosis, and also cautious in his therapeutic attempts.

Treatment of Kappacism.—In Kappacism and Gammacism the ability to produce lingual plosives such as [t] and [d] is preserved. The speech therapist will profitably avail himself of this tendency. The first task to be accomplished is to make the tongue touch the palate at the correct spot, i.e. to set back the place of articulation along the palate. While the patient says the series [tə tə tə . . .] or [ta ta ta . . .], [də də də . . .] or [da da da . . .] and the like, the therapist slides a spatula gradually backwards along the surface of the palate. The tongue trying to touch the teeth to form [t] or [d] endeavours to escape the spatula, and rears its hinder part in the direction of the back of the palate thus producing [k] ([g]). We must never press the spatula against the tongue, else either the movement stops completely or [h] or [ʔ] are produced.

After a short treatment with the spatula its introduction into the mouth or, a little later, the mere sight of it suffices to produce the association and thus the desired result.

[k] and [g] are never practised as isolated sounds but always in syllables, first with random syllables and later on in words.

Hearing exercises help the patient to distinguish [t] and [d] from [k] and [g], and prevent him from substituting [k] and [g] for [t] and [d] where the latter are correct. A little boy whose mother tried to make him say *kiss* instead of *tiss*, etc., asked, " Mummy, can I have my kea and koast ? "

Treatment of Lambdacism.—In the treatment of Lambdacism Gutzmann [1] recommends making use of the fact that the positions for [n] and [l] are alike except that the tongue lies with its whole rim against the edge of the palate when producing [n], and that there are oval gaps between the side rims of the tongue and the teeth, through which the air escapes laterally when [l] is produced.

One way to produce these oval gaps is to pull the tongue down with a tape put across its back. The patient should close his nose with

---

[1] *Sprachheilkunde*, pp. 513–14.

thumb and forefinger, open his mouth, and so produce [l]. Although
the position of the tongue is achieved mechanically, the correct co-
ordination will result without this help after some training.

As a rule, it is sufficient to make the patient open his mouth and
put the tip of the tongue against the upper incisors or the alveolar
ridge. Thus he produces [l] actively. His efforts may be supported
visually, or by adjusting the position of the tongue with a tongue
depressor.

The treatment described above naturally applies also to the
severest form of Universal Dyslalia, Idioglossia. " Any exercises that
will help in the development of the speech faculty should be given.
Sense training apparatus and pictures are most helpful to give the child
a feeling of the right use of words. It is important to stimulate his
interest in his surroundings in order to counteract the sense of isolation
which his speech gives him. This isolation may be deliberate, induced
by a desire to live in a world of his own. Sometimes Idioglossia
occurs in the younger of two children, especially if the elder is of a
dominating nature ; the older child understanding the language of the
younger, speaks for him. A sense of independence must be instilled
and the child made to speak for himself." [1]

Psychotherapy.—The bio-psychological basis of dyslalic disorders
shows us why we must often fail to cure a dyslalic person if we confine
ourselves to the use of those means which are usually efficient in the
production of normal articulation. The patient may acquire a new way
of articulating, but will not use it. He is in many cases an introverted
character who does not seek any social contact. Our aim must therefore be not only to enable the patient to acquire the new articulation,
but at the same time to educate or re-educate his personality, so as to
bring about the adequate social feeling.

As to the psychotherapeutic methods of approach we must refer
to the textbooks, as this subject exceeds the compass of this book.
A few remarks may, however, be of use.

If we attempt to teach the child correct articulation by exercises
only, and do not help him give up his a-social attitude, he will
not derive any lasting benefit from our treatment. Let us assume
that the child is not so obstinate as to make the mechanical treatment
impossible, and that he is cured of his Dyslalia. He can speak intelligibly, but has not given up one iota of his neurotic attitude. These
tendencies are sure to find another way of defending his position :
having given up one symptom of his defence, he will speedily produce
another. This symptom may be of a completely different nature, but
it will still prevent the child from developing his full powers of usefulness and from becoming a happy member of the community.

On the other hand, the importance of functional treatment must
not be under-estimated. It is almost impossible that children whose
speech has been dyslalic for a considerable time should learn to speak
properly without mechanical help. The correct co-ordinative control
has not yet been acquired or stabilised, whereas the dysfunction is

[1] Boome, E. J., Baines, H. M. S. and Harries, D. G. *Abnormal Speech*,
pp. 33-4.

fixed. We must bear in mind that a comparatively quick progress towards normal speech means a great encouragement and, consequently, aids in the psychological readjustment. If a child who gives up his neurotic attitude and tries to adapt himself to social life is continually discouraged by his inability to speak normally, he will speedily lose what little courage he may have gained by psychological treatment, and again relapse into his former attitude.

An example may illustrate the effective collaboration of treatment by exercises and psychological re-education. E.K. was a little boy of 5. He was pale and thin, suffering from rickets and from seborrhoeic eczema. His hearing was normal. He could definitely be called an intelligent child. His parents were strikingly tall and healthy people. The father was very kind and easy-going, the mother rather too energetic and severe. She ruled the house, and had naturally "taken a lot of trouble educating the boy." Almost all consonants were disordered, especially [r], [k], [g], [j], [ʃ], [l]. The little boy came in trembling, ready to cry. He had apparently been made very miserable already by being constantly told to speak properly. The mother reported that she had taken endless trouble to correct his speech, but that he "didn't try hard." The boy, who was very timid and frightened (he winced when the therapist inadvertently lifted his hand, although he was not even speaking to him), had always been very isolated. He was quarrelsome in contact with other children, and always wanted to have his own way. He was constantly admonished because of picking his nose, whereupon he did it all the more. Excessive masturbation occurred in former years, which he gave up on being very much admonished by his mother ; he also wetted his bed till he was three years old. He was an extremely poor eater, got up from table after having had a few mouthfuls, and never asked for anything to eat. He formerly made a great fuss about going to bed. Now he went quietly, but refused to sleep alone in a room. He had been much jeered at because of his speech, and had often been spanked.

During the first consultation the correction of [k] was begun, with the help of a tongue depressor. He was 'good' but offered passive resistance by dodging the tongue depressor with his tongue. After several attempts [k] was sporadically articulated correctly. During the pauses in the treatment he repeatedly asked, "Aren't we soon done ?" He was quite willing to do what he was asked, although he did not like it, and was very much afraid. The next consultation had the same result. His mother said that she had shown the child repeatedly how to speak correctly, whereupon she was strictly told to leave him alone. After a few consultations he was able to articulate [k] easily and confidently if helped by the tongue depressor. Hand-in-hand with this treatment there was constant encouragement ; he was told that he did these things very well, etc. At this time it sufficed to rest the tongue depressor on his tongue to make him produce the correct [k]. The mother was then shown how to use it, which she learned to do correctly ; but although she was able to make him say a correct [k] with the aid of the tongue depressor when she was at the therapist's, she did not succeed at home. After a week, however, the boy had gained so much confidence that his mother could succeed at home. The mere sight of the tongue depressor made him produce a correct [k]. The better he could articulate, the less he asked if one had done with him. In the end he did not ask about that at all. He got more self-assured in general, was happy when articulating properly, and began to look quite different. He seemed to grow when he was praised, and did not seem afraid any more. His general behaviour changed considerably for the better, his fear, tyranny, etc., disappeared.

We cannot doubt that the weak and sickly boy, who suffered from rickets, and was therefore nervous and irritable, as most of these children are, had been very much spoilt by his parents, who were naturally concerned about his health. This was bound to have a noxious influence upon the child. The tyranny of the mother was an aggravating factor. She tried to educate the boy by force. Her claims upon his faculties and obedience increased as he was growing up, so that we can easily understand that his best way through these accumulated difficulties lay in being a helpless little child as long as possible. The great contrast between the extraordinarily tall and strong and healthy parents and the unusually small and sickly child certainly played an important part in this development. Children usually feel small and inferior before adults, as Alfred Adler clearly pointed out. This natural feeling of inferiority is usually compensated for and fully overcome by means of adequate education. In the case of our patient, however, the additional fear might have arisen from the conviction that he would never become as strong and big as his parents. It does, therefore, not surprise us that he simply gave up trying to ' grow up.' His feelings of inferiority were not compensated by normal and healthy activity, but gave rise to a strong craving for power : hence his active tyranny in the company of children and his hidden tyranny at home by being passive and helpless. He also punished his mother effectively by being an open failure. It is characteristic that she could not at first succeed with the exercises at home. With his growing courage and self-confidence, in combination with the ability to articulate correctly, he no longer had need to keep up his neurotic attitude. The mother had, of course, been made to understand the psychological foundation of the case and to act accordingly. The change of the home situation, the constant encouragement and help by the therapist, and the quickly growing conviction that he could speak like other human beings, made him change completely and grow into a normal child, a thing which neither psychological treatment alone nor an isolated mechanical treatment by exercises would have been able to achieve.

CHAPTER XV

DYSARTHRIA

There can be no doubt that articulate speech is located ultimately in the cortex of the brain. From this region those higher processes are controlled which maintain the phonetic structures in such a state as to remain significant in their fixed arrangements. The lower levels of the nervous system play their part in stimulating the production of such noises as can be used in meaningful speech. If the effector organs and their stimulating neurones are affected, that is to say, if the physiological side of the pattern becomes in some way disturbed, particularly through organic diseases, we must expect disintegration of sounds. Disorders coming about in the latter way are named Dysarthria. If sound production is entirely impossible, we speak of Anarthria. (*Arthros* is the corresponding Greek word for *articulus*, 'joint'.)

It is well known that alcohol in larger doses acts as a poison which has a special affinity with the lipoids of the cells of the cortex. An intoxicated person, therefore, serves as a good example of the effect of dissolution. The top layers of the cortex are out of action; consequently lower levels become dominant, so that the first function to suffer is cortical control. It is therefore not surprising that correct articulation is also impaired. Jespersen has pointed out that under the influence of alcohol "the tongue is not under control and is incapable of accurately forming the closure necessary for [t], which therefore becomes [r], and the thin rill necessary for [s], which therefore comes to resemble [ʃ]; there is also a general tendency to run sounds and syllables together." [1]

Dysarthric disturbances are produced if the nerves which carry impulses to the speech muscles, or from the organs of the special senses, are damaged through injury, inflammation, or degeneration. The nerves concerned are: the N. phrenicus, which innervates the diaphragm and, if affected, causes difficulty of respiration (dyspnoea). The facial nerve, which is essential for the movements of the lips; paralysis of this nerve impairs the pronunciation of the labial sounds, especially B, P, M, and the vowels which require collaboration of the lips (rounding, stretching sideways).

The hypoglossal nerve innervates the tongue. Unilateral paralysis does not cause considerable Dysarthria. The disturbance is hardly noticeable, but the patients complain about subjective difficulty. Bilateral paralysis manifests itself in flabbiness of all sounds articulated by the tongue, especially the hissing sounds, which require a special shape of the tongue (see Sigmatism, p. 151).

The vagus nerve innervates the muscles of the soft palate and of the larynx (recurrent nerve). Its paralysis therefore brings about Hyperrhinophonia and/or Dysphonia (see pp. 173, 193 ff.).

[1] Jespersen, l.c., p. 279.

Finally dysarthric speech disorders come about if the effector organs of speech are themselves defective. To this group belong speech disorders caused by defects of the palate (cleft palate), the lips (hare lip), the gums, the tongue, etc. These disorders will be dealt with under separate headings (see pp. 172 ff.).

Symptoms.—All diseases causing more or less permanent structural changes of the cortex and its interconnections may produce similar disturbances, e.g. injuries, vascular lesions (cerebral palsy), acute and chronic inflammations and abscesses, tumours, degenerative processes of the cortical and subcortical pathways.

Dysarthria due to lesions of the upper motor neuron manifests itself in principle in that the patient's voluntary control over emotional expression is impaired (pseudo-bulbar palsy). The articulatory muscles are weak, or rigid. According to which nerves are affected, certain consonants, especially labials and dentals, are severely disordered, apparently through loss of the power of appreciating posture and passive movements, which is manifest also in other parts of the body, e.g. the digits.[1] As the nerves concerned activate also the movements of eating, chewing, swallowing, etc., Dysarthria is usually associated with dysphagia.[2]

Speech is on the whole somewhat jerky and inco-ordinate, uttered with much labour, with an overflow of energy, often accompanied by concomitant movements of other parts of the body.

It is not the aim of this book to give full accounts of all forms of Dysarthria occurring in organic diseases of the nervous system. Therefore only some of the more characteristic examples can be mentioned.

Diseases affecting those parts of the nervous system which control co-ordinated movement, such as the cerebellum and its connections in the brain stem, resulting in a state termed ataxia, naturally give rise to Atactic Dysarthria.

Speech is drawling and monotonous. Syllables are separated from each other by unnatural intervals—scanned or syllabic speech.[3] Words may be slurred, or jerked out explosively. Voice is improperly modulated, expressionless, and frequently too loud. Speaking requires a considerable voluntary effort and may be accompanied by excessive co-movements of the facial muscles.[4]

Diseases of the spinal bulb also may result in Atactic Dysarthria. In Tabes dorsalis, where especially the posterior nerve-roots, i.e. their sensory fibres controlling motor activity, are affected, we may find excessive movements of the lips, the tongue, the jaw, and the vocal chords; speech-sounds are distorted, lacking rhythm and fluency. Speech is accompanied by grimaces and various co-movements.[5]

Such Atactic Dysarthria of a graver kind is found also in Hereditary Ataxia (Friedreich's disease). Speech is, on the whole, slow (bradylalia), syllables are uttered explosively and scanned, vowels are sometimes broadened, consonants slurred, sometimes nasal. Intonation is more or less impaired.[6]

---

[1] Cf. Head's case, No. 13, l.c., ii, p. 207.   [2] Brain, l.c., p. 81.
[3] Ibid., p. 82.   [4] Brain and Strauss, l.c., p. 166.
[5] Stern, in Gutzmann's *Sprachheilkunde*, p. 582.   [6] Ibid., p. 583.

Diseases producing especially tonic rigidity of the muscles, Spastic Spinal Paralysis, Congenital Spastic Paraparesis (Little's disease), Myotonia Congenita (Thomsen's disease), naturally show difficulty in swallowing and in the articulation of the lips and the tongue. Speech is thus slow and difficult to understand.

Diseases detrimental to the motor nerves and their nuclei (Amyotrophic Lateral Sclerosis, Anterior Poliomyelitis, Progressive Muscular Atrophy, Bulbar Paralysis, Multiple Sclerosis) cause indistinct, nasal, clumsy, slow speech ; swallowing is similarly affected. Aphonia is frequent. In severe stages speech degenerates into an unintelligible mumbling.

Diseases of the brain stem, such as Hepato-lenticular Degeneration (Wilson's disease) [1] and the Parkinsonian Syndrome, show Dysarthria and dysphagia as prominent symptoms.

In the Parkinsonian Syndrome " weakness of the lips, soft palate and tongue leads to slurring of consonants." Voice is monotonous, weak and sometimes of a whining tone. " Mastication is slow, and the swallowing of solids proves difficult in severe cases, probably owing to weakness and hypertonia of the soft palate and tongue." [2]

Extremely characteristic of this disorder is the considerable time which elapses between the patient's resolution to speak and his first utterance. He needs 22-28 seconds on the average [3] in order to pronounce the sentence intended, which is then expelled with increasing speed.

Diagnosis.—The severity of the speech disorder is naturally dependent on the damage to the neurological substratum, which cannot be described here at length.

Diagnosis is not difficult, especially if other symptoms resulting from the underlying lesion co-exist, e.g. paralysis of one limb (monoplegia) or of corresponding limbs on both sides (diplegia), or of the whole of one side of the body (hemiplegia), etc.

Differential diagnosis.—To the diagnostician or consulting speech therapist the diagnosis of grave cases does not give much trouble. But it is the mild cases which he must always bear in mind, since they can easily be mistaken for disorders of quite a different kind. Spastic utterances may, especially at first sight, be taken for Stammering. The spastic movements, the flow of impulses into organs other than those concerned with speech, may induce the speech therapist to confound Dysarthria with the above-mentioned psychogenic disorder which is characterised by similar symptoms. The symptoms are all the more misleading if other symptoms which would confirm the diagnosis of Dysarthria are lacking, or when the slightest amnestic Aphasia feigns some hesitancy or incoherency of speech and thought.

The necessity for extreme caution in every case of spasmodic utterance has been discussed in the chapter on Stammering (see p. 127).

Treatment.—The treatment of dysarthric speech disturbances depends on their nature and causes. " In unilateral cases a great

---

[1] Brain and Strauss, l.c., p. 177.   [2] Ibid., p. 185.
[3] Stern, in Gutzmann's *Sprachheilkunde*, p. 627.

improvement follows re-education, but in bilateral cases recovery is seldom complete." [1] In some cases central Dysarthria can be greatly improved by associating the patient's ideas of speech-sounds with such sounds as are encountered in emotional behaviour (e.g. shuddering, feeling cold, surprised, relieved, angry, and so forth). It should be noted that if in progressive cases treatment is sought, it should be given for psychological reasons only.

rain and Strauss, l.c., p. 168.

CHAPTER XVI

DISORDERS OF NASAL RESONANCE

Nature of nasality.—Normal voice owes part of its carrying power to ' nasality,' i.e. a sound quality dependent on " certain component tones, mainly in the frequency region 300 to 600 cycles." The origin and reinforcement of these tones is commonly attributed to the nasal cavity. It must, however, be stressed that Fröschels' and other workers' recent investigations [1] have shown that the nose is by no means always responsible for nasality.

In certain bass voices the nasopharynx remains open, but speech does not give the impression of being nasal.[2] On the other hand, the so-called ' nasal twang ' of New England (American) speech is caused by a *pharyngeal constriction.*

I have observed patients with fistulous ulcers of the pharynx who produced voice of a definite nasal quality, although the closure of the nasopharynx was not impaired.

The rôle the nose plays depends on its size, shape, the nature of its walls and their lining, and on its communication with the buccal and pharyngeal cavities. The first three factors, viz. size, shape, and walls of the nose, are under normal circumstances unchangeable. The fourth factor is highly variable, as it depends largely on the muscular action of the velum or soft palate, and the posterior wall of the pharynx. They work together as a valve by which the sound-waves can be given or refused direct access to the nose.

Swallowing, retching, vomiting, and the articulation of the oral sounds make the closure of the nose valve necessary. This is achieved by an elevation of the soft palate towards the posterior wall of the pharynx while the latter approaches the former, forming a kind of transversal fold known as ' Passavant's Cushion,' which is probably formed by the raising and folding of the pharynx wall.[3]

The nasopharynx and nose can be regarded as a side chamber off the main air passage. " Wherever, along the tube from the larynx to the outer air, there is a side chamber whose only opening is into the main tube, there is a chamber capable of acting as a cul-de-sac resonator and of producing a quality of tone usually referred to as nasal ; and wherever this side chamber has an accessory opening through it to the outer air, it may still function as a cul-de-sac resonator if the accessory opening is smaller than the aperture connecting the side chamber with the main tube." [4, 5]

[1] Curry, l.c., pp. 98, 116.
[2] Russell, G. O. *Speech and Voice*, p. 18. Quot. by Curry, l.c., p. 98.
[3] Stein, L. (1930). " Zur Frage des Passavant'schen Wulstes," *Wien. Med. Woch.*, Nr. 35.
[4] West, R., Kennedy, L., Carr, A. (1937). *The Rehabilitation of Speech*, Harper & Brothers, New York–London, p. 78.
[5] Russell, G. O. (1931). *Speech and Voice*, Macmillan Company, New York, p. 18.

Since not only the nose but also the pharynx is capable of producing 'nasality' of the voice, the classification of the disorders of nasal resonance could better be based on the acoustic than on the anatomical or physiological aspect.

Types.—Bearing in mind that a certain amount of nasal resonance is always present in normal voice, we can discriminate between various grades of such resonance. Abnormal 'nasality' may thus be either excessive or diminished ; in some cases both qualities may be found simultaneously.

Deviation of nasality can thus be subdivided into three types : (1) Hyperrhinophonia (Hyperrhinolalia), i.e. excessive nasality. (2) Hyporhinophonia, i.e. diminished nasality. (3) Mixed Rhinophonia, in which the above qualities are blended.

HYPERRHINOPHONIA

Aetiology.—Hyperrhinophonia may be due either to organic defects of the palate or to impaired velum function, which in turn is of either organic or psychological origin.

Organic Hyperrhinophonia.—Its causes are mainly defects in the hard or soft palate (congenital cleft palate ; defects of the palate caused by syphilis, tuberculosis, or tumours). In cases of submucous palatal cleft the defect of the hard palate may sometimes be seen through the mucous membrane. As the palate does not always show signs of this cleft, unnecessary operations in the nose are sometimes performed, in the belief that the cause can only lie in the nose. In all suspicious cases digital palpation of the palate should therefore be applied.

Stalactiform adenoids reaching down into the pharynx may also produce Hyperrhinophonia. The velum cannot reach the back wall of the pharynx, but at the same time the air escapes into the nose at the sides of the pedunculations. Adenoids, if not excessively large, do not reduce the use of the velum and thus do not cause Hyperrhinophonia. They may act as a stimulus for increased activity of the soft palate which has to act against a hypernormal resistance.[1]

In the case of large adenoids the velum is hardly ever raised. In the long run, and with increased growth of the adenoids, the inactivity of the velum becomes habitual ; it gets shorter in consequence of the adaptation of its muscular fibres to the obstacle. When the adenoids are removed, the velum, though movable and contractable, may then be too short to reach the back wall of the pharynx.

A reduction of the length of the velum, as a result of imperfect development, is spoken of as Velum Insufficiency (Lermoyez). It occurs in combination with sub-mucous palatal clefts, or may also be an isolated defect. The velum is reduced to a proportional length of 1 : 4 (normal proportion of length between velum and palate being 1 : 2). This reduction prevents the contact between the velum and

[1] Stein, L. (1921). " Ueber Rhinolalia aperta," *Beitr. z. Anat., Physiol., Pathol., u. Therap. d. Ohres, d. Nase u. d. Halses,* ed. by Passow and Schaefer, **16**, pp. 167–88.

the wall of the pharynx. Hypertrophic tonsils may also cause hyper-rhinophonia by putting a mechanical obstacle in the way of the movement of the velum or by impairing its innervation through pressure on the nerve (L. Réthi).[1] The innervation of the soft palate may also be affected by general diseases, such as scarlet fever, parotitis, and diphtheria ; syphilis, encephalitis, bulbar paralysis, pseudo-bulbar paralysis, multiple sclerosis, and infantile paralysis often play their part. Paralysis of the soft palate may also spring from botulism, and may last for years.[2]

The flaccidity of the muscles of the pharynx due to Myasthenia gravis causes Hyperrhinophonia accompanied by dysphagia.

Functional Hyperrhinophonia may be the result of imitation, as in the Oxford drawl, American twang, or 'aristocratic' nasalism in Austria. Habitual dysfunction of the velum often occurs after diphtheria, tonsillitis, or adenotomy. The compulsory cessation of the velum function during the illness, and self-imitation later on, result in the paresis of the velum accompanied by Hyperrhinophonia.

Gutzmann[3] discusses habitual paralysis of the velum as a habit analogous to habitual paralysis of the vocal chords. This holds good only for the initial stage of habitual velar dysfunction. The patient may for a certain time voluntarily refrain from raising the velum, since the movement increases the pain in the throat. In the long run the velum atrophies by inactivity as would any other organ of the human body. In the end the patient is really unable to lift the velum though its innervation may be intact.

Diphtheria as the cause of Hyperrhinophonia by reason of paralysis of the soft palate is sometimes overlooked. This is due to the fact that in most cases the evil influence of the diphtheria poison on the nervous system manifests itself only about a month after the outbreak of the disease, i.e. at a time when the throat symptoms have passed away without other noticeable effects. In many cases nothing is reported with regard to this disease. On insistent questioning, those around the patient recall an illness which they call a chill, a sore throat, or otherwise describe as something insignificant. Mostly they had not considered it necessary to consult a physician as the general state, pains, and temperature were not alarming.

Since in Hyperrhinophonia the articulatory functions themselves are impaired, Hyperrhinophonia represents a relatively low level of dissolution, and may accordingly be regarded as a type of central or peripheral Dysarthria. Other functions ruled from this level, such as swallowing, may also be impaired, as for instance in bulbar paralysis.

In certain cases of pseudo-bulbar paralysis caused by epidemic encephalitis or bilateral softening of the inner capsule, the soft palate cannot be lifted for intentional speech, but functions well in swallowing,

[1] Réthi, L. (1893). *Die Motilitaetsneurosen des weichen Gaumens*, Hölder Wien, p. 34.
[2] Vernieuwe, J. (1920). *Bulletin de l'Académie Royale de Médicine de Belgique*.
[3] Gutzmann, H. (1913). " Untersuchungen über dar Wesen der Nasalitat," *Arch. f. Laryngol. u. Rhinology*, **27**, p. 65.

which is incited by a lower stratum of the brain.[1] Impeded maturation, mental deficiency, and encephalitis often make the patient stay at or lapse to this evolutionary level of speech.

HYPORHINOPHONIA

Aetiology.—Hyporhinophonia is as a rule organic. Nasal resonance may be more or less diminished by various factors which obstruct the air passage in the nasopharynx and the nose, such as compact adenoids (Stalactiform adenoids cause Hyperrhinophonia), nasal or pharyngeal growths, chronic hypertrophic or hyperplastic inflammation of the mucous membrane, adhesions between the velum and the pharyngeal wall, etc.

Functional Hyporhinophonia occurs rarely ; it is caused by violent contraction of the velum and other muscles of the pharynx and the mouth. It is often due to imperfect perception of speech owing to deficient hearing. Nasal vowels and consonants show a strong accentuation of harmonics in the lower region.[2] The perception of these tones is impaired in diseases of the middle ear, so that the acoustic pattern of the nasal sounds, and of the vowels, is deficient.

MIXED RHINOPHONIA

Aetiology.—Mixed Rhinophonia can—though not too often—be observed, if on the one hand the air passage into the nose is free (owing to cleft palate or insufficiency of the soft palate), and if, on the other hand, the nose cavities are obstructed through growths (tumours, adenoids, hypertrophic turbinals, and the like).

Some of the oral sounds acquire hyperrhinophonic character ; especially stops and fricatives are accompanied by snoring clicks. The nasal sounds are hollow, as in Hyporhinophonia.[3]

Diagnosis of Rhinophonia.—In Hyperrhinophonia all consonants and vowels are more or less nasalised. The impossibility of closing off the nose cavity by elevating the soft palate does not allow the patient to produce sounds of an explosive character. The stops [b, d, g] therefore sound similar to [m, n, ŋ] ; [p, t, k] turn into breathed nasal sounds [m, n, ŋ]: sometimes they are replaced by the glottal stop.

In cleft palate speech articulation is so much changed that it is sometimes hardly possible to understand the patient. Hypernasality of the vowels increases from [a] to [o], [e], [u], [i]. In place of the stop consonants the glottal stop is often used. Some patients can articulate the velar stops [k] and [g] by pressing the root of the tongue against the posterior wall of the pharynx. The articulation of the sibilants is usually disordered (Sigmatism).

In Hyporhinophonia [m], [n], and [ŋ] change into [b], [d], and [g]. The vowels bring to mind the notes of blocked wind instruments.

[1] Spiegel, E. A. and Sommer, I. (1931). *Ophthalmo-und Oto-Neurologie,* Springer, Wien-Berlin, p. 312.
[2] Curry, R., l.c., pp. 58–60.
[3] Gutzmann, H. (192). *Sprachheilkunde,* p. 538.

The discrimination between excessive and diminished nasality is facilitated by using a simple rubber tube. One of its ends is put into the patient's nose, the other into the therapist's ear ; this enables the latter to listen to the resonance while the patient pronounces vowels and consonants. At the same time the external ear distinctly feels the vibrations of air. In normal speech no vibrations or escaping air are felt during articulation, except during the nasal sounds [m], [n], [ŋ]. In Hyperrhinophonia the ear senses vibrations during the articulation of all speech-sounds, whereas in Hyporhinophonia the ear does not perceive any vibrations.

If greater exactitude is required, the air escaping through the tube may be conducted to an apparatus for graphic recording.

In Gutzmann's A-I-tests the vowels [a] and [i] are pronounced in turn while the nose is alternately closed and left open. In cases of normal speech the resonance remains unchanged, whereas in cases of Hyperrhinophonia the sounds are considerably dulled when the nose is closed because of the stronger vibrations of the volume of air retained in the nose. A finger laid against the patient's nose can feel those vibrations. A cold mirror held before the hyperrhinophonic patient's nose will be frosted by the air passing through the nose (Czermak).

Differential diagnosis.—On first hearing Hyperrhinophonia may be confused with Nasal Sigmatism. Examination with the rubber tube, or even with the unaided ear, will soon reveal that in Nasal Sigmatism nasality is present only in the sibilants, whereas Hyperrhinophonia affects *all* sounds indiscriminately.

Hyperrhinophonia in cases where the soft palate functions satisfactorily in swallowing must not be assumed to be functional without thorough neurological examination (see p. 173).

Post-diphtheritic Hyperrhinophonia will not be confused with habitual Hyperrhinophonia, if the presence of other pareses, e.g. of the muscles of the eye, is ascertained.

Prognosis.—The prospects of cure in Hyperrhinophonia depend on the nature of the underlying disease. Congenital clefts should be subjected to either surgical or orthodontic treatment as early as possible. Syphilitic and tuberculous lesions are naturally dealt with by the specialists concerned.

Prognosis of Hyperrhinophonia as the result of Diphtheria depends on the potency of the toxin. If only the innervation of the pharyngeal muscles is affected, normal function of the soft palate, and thus normal resonance may be restored within a few weeks. In cases where the muscles of the eye, the neck, the legs, and the heart have been affected, several months are required for recovery.

It must not be overlooked that Hyperrhinophonia without defects of the palate or its innervation may easily become habitual following a disease of the throat or, if grafted on a neurotic disposition, grow into a neurotic disorder.

Treatment of Hyperrhinophonia.—In cases of organic defect, surgical or orthodontical treatment must be given. Palatal holes or clefts must be closed surgically where there is a chance of providing adequate palato-pharyngeal control. Submucous palatal clefts often require surgical treatment, plates being insufficient. Collaboration of the surgeon and the speech therapist is essential in all cases operated upon after speech has developed.

Adequate training must be given to enable the patient to learn the correct articulations for which the conditions have been prepared by the operation. Older children or adults affected with cleft palate should undergo functional treatment (see below, p. 177) before the surgeon operates, so as to facilitate the efforts of the patient to raise the newly formed velum.

Obturators need, owing to the improved methods of palate surgery, rarely be used. Only if the patient refuses to be operated on, or if the chance of producing a satisfactory velum is slender, should the therapist have recourse to this aid. The obturator is a rubber plug which the therapist must shape so as to restrict the passage of air through the nose in speaking without too much impeding quiet respiration. In the course of treatment the patient should learn to contract the pharyngeal muscles in an effort to touch the plug and to close off the naso-pharyngeal cavity thereby. If the air passage can be narrowed down to a width of at least 2-3 mm., fairly normal speech is attained.

If the soft palate is insufficient, adenoids must not be removed unless there are other indications, such as chronic catarrh of the respiratory organs, or repeated diseases of the middle ear, for in cases of velar insufficiency the adenoids may prove a most desirable substitute in effecting palato-pharyngeal closure. In such cases speech may considerably deteriorate after adenotomy, and thus jeopardise the patient's chances in life.

If after adenotomy habitual Hyperrhinophonia persists, functional treatment should be applied. Passive and active exercises aim at strengthening and adjusting the muscles of the soft palate and of the oro-pharynx. Gutzmann [1] recommends raising and massage of the soft palate with a palate-lifter, consisting of a curved nickel wire bearing a piece of gutta-percha on its smaller foot. Fröschels improved this method by means of his 'palato-masseur' which allows a combination of massage and faradisation. I have, following Fröschels' and Gutzmann's ideas, constructed a very simple instrument. It consists of two parts, a small metal jaw to which the electric wire is connected, springing from a handle of insulating material, and a narrow metal bar of about 4 inches in length having a curved spoon-shaped end which is to come in contact with the soft palate. This bar is fixed in the metal jaw by means of a screw so that it can be detached for sterilisation.

For treatment a mild faradic current is switched on and the handle is gently and rhythmically tilted up and down so that the spoon end touches the soft palate and elevates it each time the patient voices a vowel. The patient can operate this instrument himself without considerably hindering the movements of his lower jaw and tongue during the articulation of vowels.

It has been suggested that the retching reflex should be stimulated

[1] *Vorlesungen*, p. 172.

as a means of making the velum rise. To this end the base of the tongue or the pharyngeal wall are touched.

Another way to lift the velum is to close the patient's nose with the fingers and make him say syllables like [ab : : a], stressing the [b] and blowing out his cheeks.

Passive elevation of the soft palate does not help in cases of considerable deterioration of the musculature.

The enunciation of vowels, if energetically carried out, is itself a stimulus to greater activity of the velum and the pharyngeal muscles. It is very helpful if patients are made to thrust their arms down energetically during phonation (Fröschels, Stein). This creates an overflow of energy which spreads to all muscles active at the moment. In this way the velum gets additional lifting impulses which accentuate its action, and the muscular substratum of Passavant's cushion is developed, ensuring a better closure of the naso-pharyngeal cavity. It seems that this exercise is of considerable influence in shaping the pharyngeal cavity so as to decrease nasality.

Treatment is greatly helped by breathing and blowing exercises that involve closure or narrowing of the naso-pharynx (see p. 209 and below). Children will be eager to join in games involving breath control, such as the following suggested by J. van Thal and by Seth and Guthrie.[1] Blowing a whistle or trumpet. Ringing a small bell by blowing at it. Blowing through a funnel at scraps of paper, wool, or feathers, and blowing them at a goal. Blowing a ping-pong ball across a table. Blowing beads out of a spoon into an egg-cup. Blowing paper or celluloid boats floating on water. Blowing a sheet of paper placed against the wall so as to retain it in position when the hand is taken away. Blowing out matches and candles. Blowing bubbles or blowing water from one bottle into another. Blowing over two small cardboard platforms held in front of the nose and mouth. A small object, such as a doll, is placed on each card, and the 'game' consists in trying to blow off the doll in front of the mouth without disturbing the other doll.

Joan van Thal describes a device for 'denasalising' speech. Take a wide-necked bottle with a cork pierced in two places to admit two glass tubes. Mind the tubes fit the bottle snugly so as to be airtight. Put a length of rubber tubing fitted with a mouthpiece on one of the glass tubes. Fill the bottle with water up to the neck. When you insert the cork the water will rise some way above it in the glass tubes. Hold the mouthpiece between your lips and blow. Before you blew the water was at the same level in both tubes, but now it rises in the tube opposite to the one you blew down. Make a fountain spurt up. Blow slowly and steadily and see how long you can make the water stay on the same level.

Elsie Fogerty has devised a 'denasaliser' for vowel and voice practice. This is a wry-necked glass vessel which has to be filled with water. The rest of this simple apparatus consists of a funnel shaped to fit well over the lips without impeding their movement but

---

[1] Van Thal, J. H. (1934). *Cleft Palate Speech*, Allen & Unwin, London. Seth and Guthrie, l.c., p. 170.

not covering the nose ; a rubber tube is fitted over the narrow end of the funnel and inserted in the water. When one speaks in nasal tones the water remains static, but a well-produced vowel sound will cause bubbles to rise, and so provide a visual aid to voice training.

Articulation in general, especially that of the tongue, must be carefully considered. In the case of a hyperrhinophonic boy whose adenoids had been removed because of chronic middle ear suppuration, there was insufficiency of the velum. No result was obtained by thrusting the arms downward during phonation. Strangely enough, he quickly learned to produce a correct [s], while the vowels remained nasalised. As a correct [s] cannot be produced with sagging velum (a condition for nasalised vowels), we must assume that the disturbance was functional. Behind the X-ray screen the velum was seen to sag when vowels were produced, and to touch the pharyngeal wall when [s] was produced. This case suggests the probability that there are certain close and intrinsic co-ordinations between the movements of the velum and the articulation of the tip of the tongue.

This patient had apparently never learned to lift the velum when speaking. When we taught him the [s] he did not seem to grasp that it was a speaking process, his attention being completely focused on blowing into a narrow hole : he was whistling, not speaking. His kinaesthetic perception, however, was not efficient enough to enable him to make use of the same co-ordinations when producing vowels. Our patient, in fact, had always produced vowels by lifting the back part of the tongue. Hyperrhinophonia was much diminished when he learned to employ the tongue-tip in the enunciation of vowels. This case instances an experience of long standing, viz. that singing pupils as well as people with speech defects are unable to make general use of the correct co-ordination which they possess in producing certain sounds. Another patient operated on for cleft palate still produced nasalised vowels and nasal sibilants, although she had learned to articulate stop consonants quite well. When she had partly overcome the difficulty in pronouncing a non-nasal [s] the vowels, too, improved. The vowels of another, only slightly rhinophonic, patient exhibited increased nasality when the tip of the tongue was pressed downward during their articulation.

Injections of paraffin wax into the musculature[1] of the region of Passavant's cushion make the posterior pharyngeal wall project permanently and so facilitate the velum action in articulation against the pharynx wall.[2] This method has proved helpful in cases of insufficiency or paresis of the velum, especially after injury or operation. I have also obtained satisfactory results from this method in cases of Hyperrhinophonia and Dysphagia based on Myasthenia.

Treatment of Hyporhinophonia.—Organic cases naturally require the removal of adenoids or growths. Before adenotomy it must always be ascertained whether or not the velum is insufficient. If so, the removal

---

[1] Injection into the mucous membrane is useless and dangerous, as the deposit may easily slip into the mediastinum.

[2] Neumann, F. (1913). *Mon. f. Ohrenheilk.*, No. 2. Fröschels, E. (1916). " Ueber die Behandlung von Gaumenlähmungen," *Mon. f. Ohrenheilk.*, pp. 91–5.

of the adenoids produces Hyperrhinophonia, a much more unpleasant speech defect than Hyporhinophonia. In this case the excessive resonance caused by the insufficiency of the velum is somewhat reduced by the adenoids which, by filling the naso-pharynx and blocking the posterior nares, prevents the passage of the air into the nose.

Functional Hyporhinolalia demands exercises to remove the hypertension which is present with all sounds, especially the nasals. Drawn-out nasal sounds must be articulated while the patient feels the vibrations of the nasal wall with his finger.   There are patients in whom over-contraction of the velum occurs as soon as they open their mouths ; these must learn to breathe through their noses with the help of a rubber plug placed between the teeth.[1]   The relaxation of the muscles must be encouraged in the same way as in the case of functional disturbances of the voice (see p. 211).

When the correct use of the velum for the nasal sounds [m], [n], and [ŋ] has been achieved, the patient should learn to combine them with vowels and with the other consonants, e.g. [amba, embe ; amda, ende], etc.

The nasal sounds are to be drawn out when practising in order to canalise the newly achieved articulation.

Treatment of Mixed Rhinophonia.—Great caution is necessary for this. Non-malignant growths of all kinds should only be removed gradually, for the removal, though reducing the hyporhinophonic component, may increase the objectionable hyperrhinophonic component.

[1] Fröschels, E.   *Lehrbuch,* p. 229.

VOICE

Evolutionary point of view.—Looking back upon the pecularities of the voice of the baby, especially during the first stages, we discover that certain properties of human sound differentiate very early and manifest certain shades of emotion. Such properties are : pitch, timbre, inflexion, rhythm, intonation, and so forth.

The basic features of phonation are highly automatic, and show a great aptitude for expressing the ever-changing variety of emotional states. In later stages of development the above qualities become standardised, and together with articulateness constitute what is commonly understood as a person's, or a nation's 'accent.' The final integration of phonation is song.

In established speech, voice on the one hand and articulation on the other are interdependent units, each of which follows its peculiar rules.

What are we to understand by 'normal' human voice ? 'Norm' means a pattern, type, model ; a recognised standard. The word is derived from the Greek word gnōrimos, 'well known' (from the base *gno-*, 'to know').[1]

Thus normal is said of anything that agrees with the norm.

Standard is a style, mode, type, accepted and recognised by convention, within a community, at a given time.[2]

In view of the definition we can, indeed, find various types of voice which are said to be normal. We speak of the normal voice of the child, the man in the street, the salesman, the clerk, the singer, the actor, the preacher, the teacher, the 'child of nature,' and so on. Thus normality is a social term. The members of a given group accept a given type of voice if it serves the purpose of those producing it as well as of those hearing it.

But here, as in all other activities of human beings, we can see old biological tendencies at work which in course of evolution have had to be checked so as to bring about a more harmonious result. That is to say, the factors involved in phonation must be 'fitted together' in such a way that each of them adapts itself to each of the others, in order to reach efficiency with the minimum of energy. Only in this way can a new, lasting unit emerge, which is capable of further development. The resulting function naturally conveys certain emotional feelings and brings about aesthetic impressions in the listener. In this case it is accepted as 'normal.'

Physical acoustics.—We now turn to the consideration of those properties of sound with which the community agrees.

Voice is produced by the larynx, the 'voice box,' which may for the present purpose—certainly not for any other, such as the biological

---

[1] Wyld, *Engl. Dict.*   [2] Ibid.

(see p. 48)—be regarded as a musical instrument. Take an instrument, such as the oboe, clarinet, or the reed pipes of an organ. They consist chiefly of two parts, viz. the reed, and the resonating tube. When air is blown into the instrument, the reed is thrown into vibrations. If these occur at more or less regular intervals, they are perceived as 'sound.' If irregular in frequency, the audible result is called 'noise.' The fundamental process by which vibrations in a wind instrument are effected can be observed in the mouth organ. Each of its small boxes contains a metal reed in a slot. Blowing causes compression of the air in the box up to a point at which the reed in the slot lifts and thus allows the air to escape. After this the pressure in the box will decrease, and the reed will, by reason of its elasticity, return to its rest position. The constantly and regularly alternating increase and decrease in air pressure constitutes vibration. The movements of each vibrating particle may be drawn in a system of co-ordinates in which the vertical direction indicates the distance

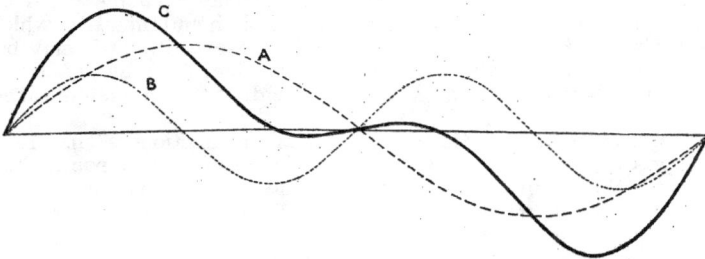

Diagram No. 7.

from the zero point, whilst the horizontal line marks the time when the particle reaches a given distance (see the curves in Diagram No. 7).

In sound waves the maximum distance from the horizontal zero line which the curve reaches, i.e. its amplitude, indicates the degree of loudness which our ear experiences in a given sound.

The pitch of a tone depends on the number of vibrations per second, which is also shown by the length of the waves. The number of vibrations is based on the tension, size, and density of the sounding body.

Almost all sounds are compound tones. If, say, a violin string is set in motion by plucking, it swings as a whole (see Diagram No. 7, curve A), and this would be perceived as a pure tone. But it will also vibrate in its parts. Curve B (see Diagram No. 7) represents a similar pure tone of amplitude $\frac{2}{3}$, and wave-length $\frac{1}{2}$, i.e. of twice the frequency of the first sound. The resultant actual vibration constitutes the algebraic sum of the two; in musical terms, it represents the unit consisting of the fundamental tone and its octave, i.e. the first harmonic (see Diagram No. 7, curve C).

If other sounds are present also, of various wave-lengths and amplitudes, the resultant curve will be more complex in shape. However complex and irregular it may be, if it repeats its shape periodically, it can be analysed into a series of curves, i.e. its sound can be said to be made up of a number of pure tones.

The curve in the last diagram takes quite another form, in which the composing curves are hardly recognisable ; but the conditions in nature are much more complicated, many more partial tones (overtones) being produced. The pitch and intensity of the component tones make up in the main the quality or timbre of a given sound. In view of the superposition of each individual curve demonstrating an overtone, the quality of a sound is illustrated by its curve.

It is obvious that the pitch of the overtones is dependent on that of the fundamental tone. If a gramophone record is turned at an increased or diminished speed, the pitch of both the fundamental tone and the upper partials changes accordingly. The peculiar timbre of the speech-sounds also deviates in this experiment. The phenomenon is due to the fact that every speech-sound is characterised by a group of harmonics within a fixed range of pitch and intensity, which is superimposed on the fundamental tone, whatever its pitch may be. Since the quality of the speech-sounds is completed by the latter harmonics, they are said to ' form ' the sound, and are therefore called ' formants.'

Sound waves radiate through the air in all directions. They may appropriately be compared with the ripples formed on a pond when a stone is thrown in. The sound waves initiated by a vibrating reed, say, of a clarinet, must pass through a tube of a certain length, diameter, shape, and composed of a certain material.

Sound waves may be reflected on striking walls in the same way as are the ripples on reaching the edges of the pond. If the walls are curved, the reflected waves may be brought to a focal point, and this increases their intensity.

The surrounding walls can also be set into sympathetic vibration by sound waves of a periodicity akin to their own. A vibrating tuning-fork placed near a similar one will set it into vibration. A wooden resounding body sounds much louder than the tuning-fork which produces the sound. There will be the opposite effect, however, if the material of the walls is of very low elasticity, so that they cannot be induced to resound.

In a clarinet we have to take into consideration both the production of sound by the reed and the amplification of certain partials by the resounding tube. These two factors interact in such a way that any change of the effective length of the tube influences the wave frequency of the reed. This in turn means a change of pitch.

This principle of the ' resonator-control ' manifests itself more or less according to the structure of the instrument. The reed of a clarinet, for example, is ' *obedient*,' whereas that of an organ is more ' *masterful*.'

Experiments have also been made whereby the same reed has been put into different instruments. The result was that the special character of the sounds produced by the instruments themselves did not change ; whence it follows that the quality of a sound depends largely on the resonating chamber.

The vocal cavities.—This brief summary of the principles of acoustics should help to give an understanding of the fundamental rules of sound production in the human voice organ, which may be compared with reed-wind instruments.

The larynx has a pair of ' free reeds ' represented by the vocal chords.[1] They distinguish themselves from mechanical reeds by the following qualities : (1) They are mobile ; (2) their tension can be varied.

The vibrations of the vocal chords are communicated to the surrounding air forcing it into waves. These air waves spread, as all waves do, in every direction. They are handed on to the air directly below and above the larynx, and thus reach on the one hand the cavities of the chest (the trachea, and the bronchi, with their ramifications in the lungs), and on the other the cavities of the pharynx, mouth, and—under favourable circumstances—the nose. As soon as they do so, resonance, reflection and resonator-control come into play. The sound waves are also handed on to the walls of the cavities. The area of propagation of the sound waves within the human body is very wide. Experiments have shown that during phonation the skull, the neck, the nose, the shoulders, and the chest are co-vibrating. The waves from the resounding walls cause changes in the physical structure of the original waves.

Thus, strictly speaking, there exists no such thing as isolated voice. For as soon as the sound waves leave the larynx they are compelled to pass through various chambers, the walls of which reflect them and bring them to resonance. How and to what extent the various chambers influence the physical and acoustic properties of sound depends on the shape and the structure of their walls. The tube through which the voice must pass, the pharynx, has apertures which lead into the nose and into the mouth respectively.

The nasal cavity can be closed off from the pharynx by the elevation of the soft palate. Not only does the soft palate approximate the posterior wall of the pharynx, but the latter moves towards the velum. The projection of the pharyngeal wall which co-operates in the closure is known as Passavant's cushion. Its nature is not yet well known, but it may tentatively be said that it consists in an elevation and concomitant folding out of the mucous membrane of the posterior pharyngeal wall through the contraction of certain muscles, especially of the palato-pharyngeal muscle.[2] Passavant's cushion, therefore, does not represent an anatomical structure, but a physiological process.

The position of the tongue may more or less obstruct the air passage into the mouth cavity. By passing through the pharynx and the mouth the primary vocal sound is endowed with various

---

[1] As to the anatomy and physiology of the vocal organ we refer to the textbooks, especially to Curry's *Mechanism of the Human Voice.*

[2] Stein, L. (1930). " Zur Frage des Passavantschen Wulstes," *Wien. med. Woch.*, No. 35.

qualities of resonance, such as intensity, volume, carrying power, 'timbre,' richness, etc. They contribute to the beauty and utility of the voice (see p. 3).

If the sound waves do not resound in the cavities of the throat and mouth, the voice makes the impression of being very poor and squeaky. This has been shown in experiments on the larynx of a corpse and observed in patients who had attempted suicide by cutting their throat just above the upper edge of the thyroid cartilage. The same sound quality can be observed in wind instruments, e.g. the clarinet, if the resonating tube is separated from the portion holding the reed.

CHAPTER XVIII

VOICE DISORDERS

Diagnostic examination.—Voice disorders must, according to our definition, be regarded as deviations from that type of voice which is commonly agreed upon. They may be based on organic defects or diseases, or they may manifest functional disintegration. In the former case, laryngological examination will show some abnormalities of the nose, pharynx, or larynx. Functional voice disturbances may exhibit organic abnormalities as well, though on close examination these generally prove to be of little import, that is to say, they are either merely co-existent or they are structural consequences of the functional disorder capable of being compensated for by functional adjustment. In addition, the constitution of the body as a whole must be examined.

Inspection of the nasal cavities (rhinoscopy) may reveal abnormalities obstructing or confining the voice passage. Such are deformities of the septum nasi, hypertrophic inflammation of the mucous membrane, growths, etc.

Démétriades [1] was able to show experimentally that the filling of the blood vessels of the nasal mucous membrane greatly influences the resonance of vocal sound. It is a well-known fact that in singing, head resonance is easier during the first stages of a cold. Démétriades believes that " . . . in case of correct conduction of sound, the normal filling of the vessels of the hard and soft parts at certain spots of the facial mask in co-operation with the correct functioning of the tongue and velum (Fröschels) plays an important part, together with the normal state of the pneumatic chambers. Probably the filling of the vessels of the pneumatic chambers of the skull, and resonance in consequence are in an unstable equilibrium ; this makes it possible to conduct the sound easily to special spots of the facial mask and to bring these spots into vibration." Experiments show that " . . . vessels filled with blood present extra good conditions for resonance. This may be due to the consistence of the blood in general (water, blood corpuscles) and to its flow in preformed channels (vessels). Thus normal filling of the vessels, i.e. physiological hyperaemia, and perhaps pathological hyperaemia akin to physiological hyperaemia, present favourable conditions for resonance." [2]

Measurements of the mouth cavity.—The cavities of the pharynx and the mouth, which offer direct entrance to the sound waves produced in the larynx, play their part in resonance and amplification of the

---

[1] Démétriades, Th. D. (1924). "Experimentelle Untersuchungen über die Bedeutung der Vasomotoren für die Schaedelresonanz und die Kopfnochenleitung," *Zeitschr. f. Hals-, Nasen-, u. Ohrenheilk*, **9**, No. 3.

[2] Démétriades, Th. D. (1925). *Zur Bedeutung des Gefässystems für die Kopfresonanz und Tonfuehrung.* I. Kongr. d. Int. Ges. f. Logopaedie u. Phoniatrie, Deuticke, Léipzig–Wien.

sound. They therefore deserve our consideration not only as to pathological processes, if such be found, but also as to their constitutional shape, which may offer more or less favourable conditions for vocal adjustment.

Erbstein's [1] method of estimating some relative measurements helps us to infer the probable vocal aptitude. In particular he correlates the form and size of the hard palate with the qualities of the sound produced.

The length (L), width (W), depth (D), and gradient (G) of the hard palate are to be put in correlation with each other. The length of the hard palate is the distance from the boundary between the hard and soft palate to the free edge of the upper middle incisors. The width of the hard palate is the distance between the opposite posterior molars of the upper jaw. The depth of the hard palate is the distance from the highest point of the hard palate to a horizontal plane cutting the neck of the upper molars. The gradient of the hard palate is the distance between its highest point and the upper middle incisors.

The results obtained by establishing a correlation between these measurements are assessed as of minimum grade (1), middle grade (2), or maximum grade (3).

The width of the hard palate equals 1, if it is smaller than half of the length, $W(1) < \dfrac{L}{2}$; likewise $W(2) = \dfrac{L}{2}$ and $W(3) > \dfrac{L}{2}$.

The depth of the hard palate is assumed to be of minimum degree if it is smaller than half of its width, $D(1) < \dfrac{W}{2}$; likewise $D(2) = \dfrac{W}{2}$; and $D(3) > \dfrac{W}{2}$.

The gradient of the hard palate depends on the location of its highest point (HP). Dividing the length of the hard palate into four quarters (I, II, III, IV), the gradient is (1) if HP lies in the third quarter or farther back; thus $G(1)$ — HP III–IV; likewise $G(2)$ — HP II; $G(3)$ — HP I.

These relative magnitudes indicate the following vocal aptitudes :—

	Bass, Contralto	Tenor, Soprano	Lyric Tenor, Color. Soprano	Baritone, Mezzo-Soprano
Width	3	1 or 2 or 3	3	2 or 3
Depth	3	3	1	2 or 3
Gradient . . .	3 or 2	3 or 2 or 1	1 or 2	2 or 3

The reader is referred to what was said on p. 182 about the interaction between the reed and the resonator.

Laryngoscopy.—The inspection of the larynx (laryngoscopy) makes sure of its anatomical condition, of the abnormalities of shape and

[1] Erbstein, M. (1929). *Vokalexpertise und objektive Bestimmung des Charakters der Singstimme.* III. Kongr. d. Int. Ges. f. Logopaedie und Phoniatrie, Deuticke, Leipzig–Wien.

magnitude of its constituent parts, of the movements of the vocal chords, structural changes of its tissues, etc.

The measurements of the vocal chords and the corresponding shape of the glottis during inspiration in persons of various vocal aptitudes appear in the following table, composed according to Erbstein's findings :—

	Bass, Contralto	Tenor, Soprano	Baritone, Mezzo-Soprano
Vocal chords .	of maximum length, thick	short, thin	approximate those of bass
Glottis . .	isosceles triangle	equilateral triangle	equilateral triangle

Functional examination.—Whatever the result of the laryngoscopic and rhinoscopic examinations may be, investigation has to be completed by systematic observations of the co-operation of the basic functions involved in phonation.

Phonation and respiration are functionally interdependent. Direct proportion exists between pitch and tension of the vocal chords, and between pitch and pressure of breath. The same proportion exists between air pressure and intensity of voice. If, therefore, the pitch of voice is to remain the same, and intensity to be increased, pressure of breath must increase while the tension of the vocal chords must decrease. Similarly, the tension of the vocal chords must increase or the vocal chords must be shortened, while the pressure of air must decrease, if the pitch is to be raised and the intensity to remain unaltered.[1] In view of D. Weiss' experiments on a model of the larynx, which indicate that from a certain maximum the pitch decreases with increasing air pressure, further investigations appear desirable.[2]

The examination of the dysphonias therefore must determine the ratio between the respiratory and phonatory activities in various registers. The duration of expiration after a deep breath must be observed during rest as well as during whispering, humming, singing, and speaking, and checked with a stop watch. It must be noted whether expiration is even or jerky ; whether inspiration is calm, moderate, quick and noiseless, or whether it is jerky or shows inspiratory stridor. Sequences of numbers, the days of the week, and meaningless syllables spoken by the patient serve as tests of economical expiration. The same properties should be examined during singing exercises. Kymograph tracings of respiration are sometimes instructive.

Testing the compass of the voice aims at finding out the pitch and the registers which present difficulties. The so-called *registers* are described by Garcia [3] as a series of consecutive, homogeneous tones progressing upwards and produced by the same mechanical principle.

[1] Müller, J. (1840). *Die Stimme des Menschen.*
[2] Weiss, D. (1936). " Physiologie der Stimme," *Monatschr. f. Ohrenheilk,* 70.
[3] Spanish singer and voice trainer, inventor of the laryngoscope (1805-1906).

The patient's ability to preserve the intensity and the pitch of a tone can either be recorded by phonography or by kymographic methods. Deviations from a given pitch can be diagnosed by listening to a tuning-fork while the patient is singing the same tone. Any deviation, be it ever so slight, is heard as a usually unpleasant ' resultant tone.' The phenomenon is based on the fact that when two different tones are sounded simultaneously, the ear perceives also two other tones which tally respectively with the difference between and with the sum of the sounded notes.

Expenditure of air must be checked together with the intensity of the voice. The ear can—according to Weber's rule—hear a deviation in the intensity of voice only if this is either increased or decreased by at least one-third. Expenditure of air is normally in proportion to intensity, e.g. forte consumes more air than piano. Abnormalities of phonation are often manifest in the reverse proportion, e.g. excessive waste of air in piano.

Fröschels has devised an apparatus which registers the surplus expenditure of air in the case of tones which may yet sound correct to the ear. A horizontal glass tube, about $2\frac{1}{2}$ ins. wide, is fixed to a tripod. An aluminium wire, about $2\frac{1}{4}$ ins. long, is fixed in the middle of this tube by means of a human hair. One end of this wire carries a little mica disc (diameter about $\frac{3}{4}$ ins.), the other end a little wax ball. The little disc is fixed at right angles to the axis of the tube, its surfaces thus facing either end of the tube. One end of the tube is closed by a thick cork plate, which has a hole through which a glass tube about $\frac{1}{2}$ in. wide protrudes into the wider tube, thus being directly opposed to the mica disc. This tube divides into two branches by means of a two-way tap. A nose-piece is attached to one of the two branches, a funnel of paper to the other. The patient sings into the funnel while holding the nose-piece in the nose. By turning the two-way tap without the patient's knowledge, either the air coming from the mouth or that coming from the nose is directed towards the mica plate. If the little disc is hit only by the quickly repeated longitudinal waves of sound vibrations, it remains in position ; but if it is hit by air which has not been transformed into sound vibrations (' wild air ') it is deviated according to the strength of this ' wild air.' This simple apparatus is of value not only for diagnosis, but also for the training of the voice.[1]

Tests of compensation (see also p. 213).—In H. Gutzmann's compensation tests the patient is asked to hold a certain note while the therapist presses his thumb gently against the thyroid cartilage. If he suddenly stops pressing, the voice under normal circumstances rises a half or a whole tone. Diseased voices generally show a much greater divergence, and will take considerable time to return to the original tone, whereas healthy voices get back quickly and, after some time, learn to show hardly any deviation at all. The thumb may press the centre of the thyroid cartilage backwards (Gutzmann), or the wings of the cartilage inwards (Fröschels).

[1] Fröschels, E. (1922). "Ein Apparat Zur Feststellung von wilder Luft." *Zeitschr. f. Hals-, Nasen- u. Ohrenheilk,* **1**, pp. 303-313.

In the Consonant-Vowel test the singer sings the syllable [va] or [za] on the same tone, and is asked to hum the [v] or [z] a little while before proceeding to [a]. If the above-mentioned compensation does not take place in time the voice rises quickly on changing to [a] owing to the sudden release of the labial or lingual resistance, Singers show lack of compensation only in case of serious vocal disorder. In the nasal sound [m] the air passage is less obstructed than in [v] or [z]. If the voice rises as described above when [ma] is pronounced, a severe degree of compensative disturbance is manifest (Gutzmann).

The initiation of a tone, i.e. its attack, may be tested by the ear or with the stethoscope. Glottal stop always indicates misuse of the voice.

Some methods of adjustment in the treatment of functional disturbances are also of diagnostic value, since they show whether and to what extent it is possible to adjust voice. Adjustment may be achieved by faradic current or by means of an intermittent current of air, pneumatically transferred to the larynx.

Vibratory massage generally has the same effect (see p. 213).

Abnormalities of articulation must also be looked for. Excessive tension of the articulating musculature, wrong positions of the articulating organs, etc., make compensation more difficult, since they have a bad effect on breathing and phonation.

CHAPTER XIX

ORGANIC VOICE DISORDERS

The vocal disorders resulting from acute or chronic inflammation of the laryngeal tissues, as well as from paresis of the laryngeal muscles are the object of *laryngological* diagnostics and treatment ; but the functional troubles which are either the natural consequence of, or have led to structural changes, can be subjected to *vocal* treatment.

NODULES OF THE VOCAL CHORDS

Causes, symptoms, and development.—' Singer's Nodules ' are the manifestation of chronic irritation of the vocal chords. This may be caused by organic factors (inflammation, etc.) or by functional disturbance, that is to say, misuse of the voice.

In any case there results excessive strain during phonation, to which the edges of the vocal chords respond in the same way as, for example, the skin responds to the constant pressure of the shoes, by producing corns, i.e. increased layers of epithelium. Fröschels, therefore, speaks of ' vocal corns.'

The free edge of the vocal chord displays these, sometimes as small triangular pointed parts, sometimes as round or oblong shapes which may reach the size of a pin-head. It would lead too far afield to discuss their greatly varied anatomical structure. Suffice it to point out that this cannot be judged by inspection ; neither can we infer from it whether or not their structure is reversible.

Nodules necessarily cause dysphony, just as a violin string sounds dull if a particle be fixed on it thus disturbing its proper vibration. We may also find sudden breaking of the voice, inability to manage certain registers, fatigue, and diplophonia.

Patients are usually not at first aware of the disease, since the initial symptom is ' mere ' fatigue. This is caused by the misuse of the vocal chords which later on leads to the formation of nodules ; fatigue may also be due to the violent efforts needed in an endeavour to make the voice sound normal, while the nodule is developing.

Nodules are not infrequently found in children who tend to shout beyond measure, as well as in some tenors and sopranos. The initial symptoms are followed by hoarseness. The manifestation of the trouble varies with the patient's natural speaking aptitude and with the singer's technique. Examination is greatly helped by stroboscopy which allows us to observe the actual mode of vibration and the way in which the nodule interferes with it.

It must not be overlooked that the quality of a given voice does not depend only upon the shape and size of the vocal chords, but also on the form of the throat, mouth, and nose as resonating chambers. A given vocal timbre is the outcome of the interaction between the vocal chords and the resonating chambers. The ear cannot always decide whether the timbre perceived is chiefly due to the mode of vibration peculiar to the vocal chords concerned or to the reinforcement of certain overtones in the resonating chambers. This is where stroboscopy comes into play. It brings before our sight the shape of the vocal chords and the form of the vibrations as they occur in the different registers. In case of vocal disorder due to nodules, it reveals which particular mode of vibration is so disturbed by the nodule as to produce hoarseness, diplophonia, breaking of the voice, and so on.

Treatment.—The method of approach can only be decided on from our conclusions as to the reversibility of the nodules. But since we have no means of ascertaining the degree of stability inherent in a given nodule, functional treatment should in most cases be tried first. Should this prove unsuccessful, surgical treatment is indicated.

Since nodules on the vocal chords are usually the result of the misuse of the vocal chords, treatment consists of resting the vocal chords, and exercises to lower the firmness of contact between, and the hypertonicity in the vocal chords. Rest is secured either by complete silence for a number of weeks or by gentle whispering. This aspirated way of speaking is recommended because in this case the opening of the glottis forms a comparatively short-based triangle through which the air passes with a mildly fricative noise. Thus irritation of the vocal chords through contact is avoided and relaxation of the vocal muscle initiated. Unfortunately, most people cannot speak in this way ; in its stead they use too much effort which produces relatively vehement friction of air against the edges of the vocal chords. Thus the noxious irritation is increased. As the patients wish the whispered sound to be very distinct they usually tend to use a forced stage whisper. They must be advised to whisper in a gentle way. Restoration of the voice can be achieved only by functional treatment demanding the greatest caution.

Respiration should be regulated if it happens to have been disordered by the vocal dysfunction (see p. 209).

Vocal treatment aims at harmonising and relaxing the laryngeal action by training the soft attack, humming, loosening the jaw, and by vibratory massage (see pp. 210 ff.). Stroboscopy often shows that tones the audible qualities of which appear correct may nevertheless be produced incorrectly. These tones should be corrected under stroboscopic control. Once their production is fairly stabilised, they should be introduced into the speaking voice.

If this briefly outlined procedure is carried out strictly for some time, the symptoms lessen distinctly. The nodule becomes smaller and voice gains in clearness. This improvement is often felt by the patient sooner than it can be assessed by the therapist.[1]

Surgical treatment is indicated if the nodule proves to be so resistant to functional influence as to render reversibility unlikely. Normal voice can be restored only if the edges of the vocal chords are made absolutely straight and do not become deformed by subsequent

[1] Stein, L. (1932). " Ueber Sängerknötchen," *Mon. f. Ohrenheilk*, **66**, pp. 1321–4.

cicatrised depression. The operation should be followed by functional treatment to abolish the abnormal way of vocalisation which originally caused the nodule, otherwise the patient is likely to relapse. In consideration of the facts mentioned above we must be guarded in making our prognostication. Professional speakers and singers must be made aware of the risk of the operation.

CHAPTER XX

PARALYSIS OF THE RECURRENT NERVE

Aetiology.—Compression of the recurrent nerve in cases of goitre, aortic aneurysm, lymphadenitis, pleuritis, and pericarditis, injury of the nerve during thyroidectomy, inflammations from chemical or toxic causes, such as alcohol, nicotine, typhoid fever, and blood poisoning, may more or less impair the innervation of the larynx muscles, thus causing paresis or paralysis of the vocal chords.

Symptoms.—The symptoms vary with the degree of the pathological process, but they sometimes do not tally with the laryngoscopic picture. If the abductor muscle of only one side is paralysed, voice is not much disturbed ; the paralysed vocal chord remains at the middle line during both respiration and phonation. Thus the glottis can be closed during the latter, and fairly adequate vibration is assured. Dysfunction of the adductor and the thyroarytenoid muscles creates dysphony varying in degree up to complete aphony in accordance with the defective closure of the glottis. The escaping air rubbing against the edges of the vocal chords produces strong fricative noises accompanied by occasional vibrations. Patients consequently tend to achieve loud speech by over-exertion, sometimes overstraining the vocal chords so much that falsetto arises. Great fatigue ensues. Patients become short of breath by reason of excessive expenditure of air.

In time the healthy vocal chord may overstep the middle line —compensatory overcrossing—but voice remains very poor. The continual over-exertion causes irritation of the laryngeal mucous membrane which, in its turn, furthers the deterioration of the voice.

Patients suffering from bilateral paralysis of the recurrent nerve are completely aphonic ; exertion may produce a poor whisper.

Treatment.—In unilateral paralysis voice may be produced by the healthy vocal chords overstepping the middle line, thus closing the glottis. This can be aided by pressure on the thyroid cartilage. The ensuing vibrations act as a sort of massage consolidating the tissues of the paralysed chord. They become harder and more resistant, thus supporting the action of the healthy vocal chord (Gutzmann). Fröschels [1] recommends breathing exercises to prevent excessive waste of breath. The complete approximation of the vocal chords is —according to him—of minor importance.

If a vocal chord is missing as a result of operation, the ventricular band tends to substitute it.

A valuable aid in treatment is faradism and vibratory massage executed during phonation.

The following example may illustrate the influence of vocal treatment in cases of paralysis of the recurrent nerve. A young man

[1] Fröschels, E. (1932). " Ueber eine neue Behandlungsmethode der Stimmstörungen bei einseitiger Recurrenslähmung," *Mon. f. Ohrenheilk,* **66,** No. 11.

received severe injury of the neck in a car accident. He was operated on at once, but it was impossible to find the recurrent nerves. After the operation the patient developed pneumonia, and was in bed for several months. He was completely aphonic. Laryngoscopy showed cadaveral position [1] of both vocal chords. Prognosis was accordingly unfavourable and the patient was greatly depressed. When he came to be treated by me a year later, laryngoscopic examination revealed the same condition. To encourage him I made him exercise a transversal pressure on the two sides of the thyroid cartilage with his thumb and forefinger to bring about a mechanical approximation of the vocal chords. The result was a harsh, croaking voice which, of course, disappeared when pressure ceased. I advised him to practise this frequently at home, pretending to him that the vocal chords would in due course get 'used' to the enforced position. To my surprise he was, after about a fortnight, able to speak with a fairly loud voice without exercising any pressure. The voice was still croaky, but the fact that his speech could be heard made him very happy, and encouraged him to greater efforts so that he was able after a short time to sing short sequences and intervals of tones. Laryngoscopy showed the vocal chords to have recovered a certain, though by no means perfect, mobility. Seen from the psychological angle, my patient, a soldier by profession, had been forced to relinquish his occupation because of the accident. The sequels of the grave injury with the unfavourable prospect of recovery had naturally given rise to feelings of frustration and inferiority. These were manifest in increased dysfunction, represented by aphonia. Vocal treatment involving encouragement restored the voice.

With regard to such cases we should beware of assuming that the degree of dysfunction manifests the actual degree of the underlying organic lesion, since the dysfunction may be increased by the psychological superstructure.[2]

[1] The term indicates that the vocal chord takes up a position approximately halfway between those of respiration and of phonation (as in a corpse). The condition is due to the flaccidity of both the abductor and adductor muscles by reason of complete paralysis of the recurrent nerve.

[2] Stein, L. (1924). "Ueber die psychologische Auffassung von organisch bedingten Funktionsstörungen," *Int. Zeitschr. f. Individualpsychol.*, 3, No. 1.

CHAPTER XXI

LARYNGECTOMY

Dissolutionary aspect.—In cases of malignant growth in the larynx the whole organ must be surgically removed, unless radium or X-ray treatment offers prospects of recovery. This matter is still controversial (see T. B. Layton, G. F. Stebbing, Lionel Colledge, Walter Howarth, Sir Alfred Webb-Johnson, C. A. Scott Ridout, Professor F. R. Nager, Professor M. Hajek, N. S. Finzi, F. Holt Diggle, Somerville Hastings, V. E. Negus).[1] In the former case the surgeon, having removed the larynx, closes the upper end of the wind pipe. Respiration can then take place only through an artificial hole in the trachea.

Phonation is consequently impossible, but the power of articulation is preserved. Every attempt to utter loud speech must obviously fail, since the vocal organ is missing and the resonating cavity disconnected from the lower respiratory tract.

It is interesting to note that this severe damage revives old evolutionary sound patterns. As the air can no longer be expelled through the mouth for the production of sounds, the patient lapses back on the earliest stage of speech evolution, viz. that of sucking; the air is drawn into the mouth, thus giving rise to clicks (see pp. 30 ff.). I have found this very often as a *spontaneous* phenomenon in cases of laryngectomy, and I am glad to find it confirmed by van Gilse,[2] especially in relation to children.

Some patients find a substitute for the normal voice now lost in a noise which is based on the activity of eructation, just as clicks are based on suction.

Since in laryngectomised patients the respiratory apparatus is disconnected from the upper respiratory and digestive organs, i.e. mouth and throat, the lower parts of the digestive apparatus (stomach and œsophagus) are utilised for voice production.

In Negus's opinion [3] the M. cricopharyngeus, the lowest part of the inferior constrictor, situated at the orifice of the œsophagus, has the function of establishing a firm closure of the œsophagus so as to prevent air from entering the œsophagus during inspiration. Air expelled from the food channel may then cause the production of sound through vibration of the contracted edges of the œsophagus.

Treatment.—Two methods of re-establishing audible speech are possible. Either the surgeon can insert an artificial larynx into the air passage, or we can make the digestive organs act as sound-producing substitutes.

---

[1] See Discussion on the Position of Radiotherapy. . . . *Proc. of the Royal Society of Medicine,* 1940, **33,** pp. 661 ff.

[2] van Gilse, P. H. G. (1939). *Niederländisch als Schnalzsprache.* 3rd Congr. of Phonetic Sciences, Laboratory of Phonetics of the University, Ghent, pp. 353 ff.

[3] Negus, l.c., p. 347.

Though the idea of applying an artificial larynx in cases of laryngectomy or atresia of the larynx might not be inapt, there are serious reasons for deciding against its application. The first reason is one of health. If an artificial larynx be inserted while the surrounding tissue is apparently freed by operation from any malignant tissue, there still exists the danger of local relapse. Secondly, the patient using the artificial larynx for phonation is highly dependent on it.

Furthermore, great tribute is due to the recent advances in laryngeal surgery. These induced Stern to reject the use of artificial larynges (though greatly appreciating the efforts by Gluck and others) and to advocate surgical methods which not only restore the bodily health of the patient, but also create new conditions helpful to the production of vibrations.[1] These efforts facilitate the work of the speech therapist, but do not render him superfluous. His work consists in substituting pseudo-voice by means of helping the patient to develop and use the pseudo-glottis. Instead of the chest, the stomach or the œsophagus now act as bellows.

The patient should first try to eructate voluntarily. If his kinesthetic sensations are not vivid enough to enable him to expel air upwards from the stomach intentionally, his attention must be drawn to this process while it is in progress as a result of taking soda water, bicarbonate of soda, or similar powders. Breathing must be eliminated during this practice. The patient is advised to inhale before each exercise, to hold the chest in the expanded position, and to give way to eructation. Repeated practice will enable him to remember the accompanying sensations and to imitate eructation at will.

The sustaining of certain positions of the head helps to give the throat more firmness. This can be increased by the use of an elastic neckband which can easily be put on and regulated by the patient himself so as to avoid pressure on the blood vessels.

The exercise should be introduced to the patient by an explicit statement that it is merely a *preliminary* exercise, and not a ' speech ' exercise. If this remark be omitted, the patient would always attempt to utilise his—now useless—breathing mechanism in an endeavour to produce normal speech.

When the patient is able to produce pseudo-voice he is shown the various vowel positions and advised to eructate at the same time, thus rendering articulation audible. We proceed to exercises of the voiced fricatives [v, w, j] and the nasals [m, n, ŋ] ; [l, r, z] and the voiced stops [b, d, g] follow.

To form voiceless sounds the patient must make economical use of the air in the mouth and throat cavities. The glottal fricative [h] can, of course, not be achieved, but must be replaced by the softly articulated velar fricative [x].

The patient can now pass on to the enunciation of syllables. To this end he is advised to eructate as long as possible, holding each vowel position. During this he must interrupt the flow of pseudo-

---

[1] Stern, H. (1929). " Der Mechanismus der Sprach- und Stimmbildung bei Laryngektomierten," *Handb. d. Hals- Nasen- Ohrenheilk*, Springer, Berlin, v, pp. 495 ff.

voice by rhythmically repeated articulatory movements (cf. Babbling, p. 33). In this manner iterated voiced syllables are achieved without difficulty. The combinations of voiceless sounds and vowels demand careful practice, since the patient must get used to substituting for pseudo-voice the expulsion of air from the mouth during the articulation of voiceless consonants.

When reiterated syllables can be pronounced successfully, the patient may proceed to modify them by altering the shapes of mouth. In this way sequences of syllables are obtained in the following order. First identical syllables, then those with different vowels, lastly those in which all syllabic elements are changed. At this stage short words may be learned. It greatly contributes to 'the patient's encouragement when his social life becomes easier by his power of uttering even simple wishes, questions, etc., such as ' bye-bye, thanks, yes, no, who, where, why, come on,' and so forth.

Gradually the number of syllables pronounced in one train is increased, thus making the formation of short sentences possible : Where are you ? [wɛʀa : ju] ; How do you do ? [xaudxudu], etc. Conversation starts with questions demanding short answers and progressing gradually to longer ones.

This treatment demands time and patience on the part of the therapist as well as of the patient. It is important to encourage the latter continuously, especially in the beginning.

Treatment is generally successful ; patients are sometimes even able to sing little songs of small compass. If, however, proper treatment brings no success, the prognosis as to the final cure of the malignant tumour is doubtful. It should, therefore, be the duty of the speech therapist to send the patient for laryngological re-examination as soon as continued fruitless endeavours arouse his suspicion. The surgeon may well at this stage discover incipient relapse and deal with it.

CHAPTER XXII

FUNCTIONAL VOICE DISORDERS

Functional voice disorder can be assumed if a thorough examination shows no mechanical impediment to the normal production of voice.

PHONASTHENIA

Aetiology.—In circumstances which do not require a great deal from the person speaking or singing, deviations from the ' normal voice ' are, as a rule, so trifling that they affect neither those producing the sound nor those listening to it ; but it is commonly known that differences of quality do exist.

As soon as the relation between the voice-producing factors and the environmental conditions, e.g. profession, is upset, vocal disturbances out of proportion arise. Here is a common example. Some one with ' normal ' voice has to give an address. During his speech he may notice a certain tiredness of the voice, soreness, dryness, even pain in his throat, which is first met by a drink of water. Later on his voice may even sound weaker, laboured, discordant, and jarring on the ear. His vocal mechanism obviously does not come up to the requirements, presented by, for instance, an unusually large room.

If such a disproportion persists, German textbooks speak of the condition as Phonasthenia [1] or Mogiphonia [2] (Fraenkel). It constitutes the mildest degree of disintegration of harmonious voice.

As all disproportion involves relativity, the reason for this can be sought in the organ itself, or in the demands made on the voice organ.

The factors impairing phonation are manifold. Local diseases of the respiratory tract, such as chronic catarrh, adenoids, chronic tonsillitis, though not affecting the vocal musculature itself, may derange muscular co-ordination, and thus cause hoarseness, fatigue, and so on. General diseases, such as exhausting illnesses (tuberculosis, etc.), constitutional diseases (Grave's disease, etc.), use of drugs (iodine), endocrine processes (puberty, pregnancy, menstruation) may have a similar effect. Over-exertion, attempts at great feats of the voice or methods of vocal training ill adapted to the pupil's vocal aptitude constitute frequent aetiological factors. Teachers of singing should keep in mind that it may prove harmful not to consider the special imagery of their pupils. They should not give, therefore, visual or motor explanations to acoustic types, and vice versa. Emotional troubles, e.g. fear of being a professional failure or of exposing oneself, or of not being able to stand the strain of singing or speaking disintegrate the basic automatism of phonation. I remember a case of phonasthenia where this trouble was caused by the patient's imagining that she would drop

---

[1] phōnē, ' sound ' ; astheneia, ' weakness.'
[2] mogis, ' by exertion.' The condition is otherwise known as ' Clergyman's Sore Throat '.

her upper dentures while singing. She did not open her mouth properly, and her muscles were so cramped that normal and correct phonation was out of the question. What made this case one of special interest was that the patient was a well-trained, talented singer.

Misuse of the vocal organ is common to all cases. For instance, a patient suffering from laryngitis tries to overcome the accompanying functional disturbance by over-compensation. This laboured phonation brings about a strain of the phonatory muscles, and often activates auxiliary muscles; this wrong innervation may then be retained although the organic disturbance may be over.

Some organ inferiorities bring about the same result, e.g. crossing of the arytenoids, wry position of the larynx, unequal heights of the vocal chords, as well as anatomical deviations in the structure of the pharynx, palate and teeth, small throat, and small ventricles (Stern). Much screaming in early childhood as well as the change of voice during puberty, especially if it lasts for a very long time, may lead to functional dysphony.

Normal change of voice does not represent an etiologic factor of great importance according to Fröschels and some voice trainers. If singing is taught during this time, it is not likely to injure the voice, provided the method is sound. This calls our attention to an important etiologic factor as an example of an unsuitable training of the voice, viz. the way children's voices (in speaking and singing) are sometimes treated at school (see p. 203).

Other patients, who do not over-compensate, try to avoid the consequences of inflammation, etc., by sparing the voice or not using it at all. The result is hypofunction and eventually habitual paresis. A parallel to this trouble in hyperrhinophonia, viz. habitual paresis of the velum after simple tonsillitis, has been described above (p. 173). The main characteristic of paretic hoarseness is a breathy voice which gives us the impression of a great waste of air. This symptom may also be produced secondarily as a manifestation of fatigue (Flatau)[1] after long and strenuous use of the voice, especially with occupations demanding much speaking; in this case organic conditions may co-exist.

The influence of disturbances of articulation must not be forgotten; especially a uvular R may make the voice sound hollow and strained. Hypertense articulation of the pharyngeal muscles and the velum also produce phonasthenic symptoms.

Cases of Phonasthenia often show a remarkable similarity to Stammering (Fröschels). Not only do these patients exhibit the same psychic symptoms (depression, anxiety, feelings of inferiority, etc.), but clearing of the throat, swallowing, and other co-movements, frequently found in Stammering, accompany phonation. Lack of space forbids us to carry the analysis so far as to draw a complete parallel between the dissolutionary patterns of Stammering and of Phonasthenia. But an attempt shall be made to reveal the gradual disintegration of the phonatory pattern in Phonasthenia, which will allow us to arrange its types in a scale indicating their severity.

[1] Flatau, T. S. (1906). *Die funktionelle Stimmschwäche (Phonasthenie) der Sänger, Sprecher und Kommandorufer*, Charlottenburg.

Primary Phonasthenia. No pathological signs can be observed laryngoscopically. Subjective symptoms in respect of voice may be absent ; but patients often complain of various sensations, such as pains in the throat or neck, sometimes radiating towards the orbit or the ear. Their stamina is failing them, and the voice loses its timbre, volume, carrying power, and precision. The compass of the voice is reduced, certain registers, the transitions, the quality of sound, and the musical intonation are impaired. I have termed this complex of symptoms ' Primary Phonasthenia,' since it forms the basis from which the other types of Phonasthenia originate and to which they are reduced in the course of readjustment before normal phonation is attained.

Hypokinetic Phonasthenia.—The vocal chords are of normal shape and colour, but the closure of the glottis is imperfect through flabbiness of the thyroarytenoid and interarytenoid muscles. The voice sounds ' veiled,' feeble, and breathy. Some female voices sound strikingly soft and weak, but clear. On first hearing the pitch appears abnormally low. Close examination reveals, however, that the average pitch of the speaking voice does not deviate from the normal pitch (b-c^1). The abnormality lies in that these patients try to speak softly in an attempt to take care of their voices. Thus they use the chest register instead of the appropriate middle register. The history of two cases described by Sokolowsky [1] showed anxiety over the possibility of tuberculosis to be the cause.

Hyperkinetic Phonasthenia.—The voice sounds muffled and may show all degrees of hoarseness down to complete aphony. The vocal chords are normal, unless there are signs of irritation, such as redness, swelling and loosening of the tissue owing to incessant exertion. Violent contractions of the musculature in the region of the sterno-cleidomastoid and the sternothyroid, of the laryngeal and pharyngeal muscles, and at times of the velum, are characteristic. These actions may be regarded as ' auxiliary forces ' mobilised by the wish to over-come the impediments in speaking sonorously. The frequent com-plaint that the throat is shut up, in conjunction with hypertense actions, indicates a regression to an early evolutionary level whereby the primary sphincteric action of the larynx, which gave birth to phonation, becomes dominant.

A severer degree of Hyperkinetic Phonasthenia is termed ' Spastic Aphonia.' It is an occupation-neurosis which occurs in neuropathic speakers, and is caused or aggravated by over-exertion, or reflexly by irritations in the larynx and in the nose. The laryngoscopic picture greatly resembles that of Hyperkinetic Phonasthenia. The vocal chords may be reddened and show distended vessels in consequence of the great exertion to which they are exposed. The voice is extremely hoarse and muffled. The patient speaks laboriously and often accom-panies his utterances by co-movements of the facial muscles. These, as well as a certain neurotic attitude, are similar in origin and

---

[1] Sokolowsky, M. (1929). " Ueber eine seltenere Form der Stimmschwäche der Sprecher," *II. Vers. d. Deutsch. Ges. f. Sprach- und Stimmheilk,*" Kabitzsch, Leipzig, pp. 154-7.

structure to those found both in Hyperkinetic Phonasthenia and in Stammering.

Ventricular band voice represents the lowest degree of vocal dissolution, and draws nearest to the primary sphincteric action of the larynx. Every phonatory attempt brings all sphincteric muscles of the larynx into action. Thus also the ventricular bands come to a firm closure and produce an unpleasant, low, squeaking, gruff and monotonous sound. The disorder is either an attempt at compensation or a purely neurotic symptom. It usually originates from dysfunction of the vocal chords, e.g. in cases of tuberculosis or syphilis of the larynx, even if cicatrised, severe submucous laryngitis, inflammation of the thyroid cartilage, and injuries, but also after exhausting influenza.[1] The tense action produces and/or furthers hypertrophic inflammation which, in turn, deteriorates the voice and leads to a vicious circle.

Often Phonasthenia combines in itself hyperkinetic and hypokinetic symptoms.[2]

Severer cases, almost without exception, show incorrect breathing as a characteristic symptom.

A concomitant sign of Phonasthenia, especially of its hyperkinetic type, is the so-called chorditis marginalis, characterised by hyperaemia of the vocal chords, especially of their free edges ; in later stages the vocal chords become livid through varicose distension of the blood vessels ; the rest of the larynx, pharynx, and nose are not affected.

It is not surprising that the glottal stop is also met with here (see p. 48).

Differential diagnosis.—Stern drew attention to Pseudo-Phonasthenia. Its symptoms may be the same as those of genuine Phonasthenia, or may greatly resemble them. It is a transitory state which usually occurs in singing pupils, singers or public speakers, who concentrate unnaturally on automatic activities of phonation.[3] It is found also in others upon whom a singing style or technique is forced irrespective of their vocal aptitudes. In consideration of the psychic elements, psychotherapy and change of the methods of voice production are very essential in these cases. The therapist must be prepared for the varying course which these disturbances often take.

Phonasthenia in connection with organic disturbances.—Functional dysphonias may coexist with diseases of organs which are not immediately concerned with phonation. Diseases of the respiratory tract and/or of the heart may affect breathing, and thus cause a phonasthenic superstructure. Erroneous diagnoses, however, are not infrequent in these cases, as phonasthenia may have developed before the organic disease, and may run parallel to it without being causally connected with it.

Vocal abnormalities result also from insufficiency of the muscles of

[1] Flatau, Th. (1928). " Zur Technik der Taschenbandstimme," *Wien. med. Woch.*, No. 29. Réthi, A. (1934). *Mon. f. Ohrenh.*, **68**, No. 5.

[2] My terms for the different types of Phonasthenia replace the misleading old terms ' spastic ' and ' paretic.' These generally indicate certain ' organic states ' which cannot be assumed to be the underlying principle of Phonasthenia.

[3] Cf. *Centipede Attitude*, p. 116.

the phonatory apparatus based on (1) acute or chronic inflammations, (2) muscular degeneration in tuberculosis, trichinosis, anemia, or infectious diseases (typhoid, diphtheria), (3) cancerous infiltration.[1]

The vocal character of Habitual and of Hysterical Aphonia is similar (Gutzmann). The voice is breathy and weak, with distinct waste of breath. Laryngoscopy usually shows bilateral paresis of the chords, sometimes paresis of the adductors, especially of the interary-tenoid muscles. The following is a characteristic case. A young girl, a medical student, had a slight irritation of the upper respiratory passages. Characteristically enough, she asked for a specially exact examination of the interarytenoid fold to be made. This question revealed to me her apprehension that a tuberculosis of the larynx was beginning, for the interarytenoid fold is known to be a spot where tuberculosis of the larynx primarily establishes itself. On my telling her that there was nothing wrong there at all, she seemed a little put out. When she came back the next day she showed aphonia with paresis of the interarytenoid muscles which disappeared promptly after psychological treatment.[2]

As the therapy of hysterical and habitual vocal disturbances is fundamentally different, correct differential diagnosis is essential. H. Stern gives the following tabulated survey of the symptoms :—

Habitual Voice Affections	*Hysterical Voice Affections*
Genesis	
Gradual development usually after catarrhs, etc.).	Sudden onset (usually after psychic trauma, more rarely reflexly in case of catarrh, etc.).
Age of Patient	
Fairly common in children.	Extremely rare with children.
Condition and Symptoms	
Condition and symptoms change little.	Objective condition and condition of voice often changes.
Vocal Disturbances	
Usually hoarseness ; habitual whispering and inspiratory stridor.	Usually aphonia, more rarely dysphonia.
Limitations of Vocal Disturbance	
Constant as to compass.	Range of tones varies with the objective condition.

---

[1] Grünwald, L. (1907). *Grundriss der Kehlkopfkrankheiten*, Lehmann, München, p. 121.
[2] Stein, L. (1927). "Ein Fall von psychogener Aphonie," *Int. Zeitschr. f. Individualpsychol.*, 5, pp. 48–50.

Clinical Examination

Sensitivity of laryngeal mucous membrane and reflexes normal or not greatly altered.	Sensitivity and reflexes generally much altered.

Atrophies

Atrophies due to inactivity occur.	No atrophies.

Hysterical Symptoms

Usually none. They may be traceable, but habitual paresis in itself is never of a hysteric nature.	Usually additional hysterical symptoms.

Other patients complain about fatigue, even exhaustion in singing or speaking, and spasmodic feelings which impede phonation. The timbre of the voice is changed and the registers of the voice are shifted upwards. In contrast with stammering, concomitant movements, and the psychological symptoms characterising the latter, are missing. Close investigation often reveals Graves' disease. Such cases are of particular interest to the consulting speech therapist, since, for lack of other signs such as goitre, he may be the only one who can make the right diagnosis through vocal examination. On the other hand, anxiety feelings and dreadful dreams may wrongly lead to the assumption of a psychogenic disorder.[1]

Prophylaxis.—School prophylaxis is essential, as is evidenced by the preponderance of hoarseness in school children. Flatau and Gutzmann mention a percentage of 41·6 hoarse children.

The following facts must be stressed : (1) Singing in choirs is noxious, as each child tries during a considerable period to shout louder than the others. (2) Songs which demand a compass greater than that of the average child are to be avoided. (3) The so-called ' school-pitch ' for speaking is harmful. According to Paulsen it is a third higher than the ordinary speaking voice of the child and much too loud. It would be interesting to know if this applies to schools of all countries.

Excessive glottal stop which Fröschels stated was found in 55 per cent. of children of eleven and in 33 per cent. after the eleventh year, is most harmful.

Consequently school and kindergarten teachers ought to have some training in speech therapy.

Treatment.—Organic factors must be taken into consideration. Abnormalities of the nasal septum, hypertrophies, growths, chronically inflamed tonsils, even if not hypertrophic, must be removed.

H. Stern [2] recommends the greatest care and caution in tonsillo-

---

[1] Segré. *Revue franc. de Phoniatrie*, No. 1.

[2] Stern, H. (1927). " Einfluss der Mandelenlfermung auf die Stimme von Sängern und Sprechern," II. Kongr. d. Int. Ges. f. Logopaedie und Phoniatrie, Deuticke, Leipzig–Wien, pp. 35–7.

tomy, especially with singers. The slightest injury to or straining of the velum or the faucial pillars must be avoided. From about the fourteenth to the eighteenth day after the operation phonetic treatment should begin in order to avoid cicatrised contractions and thickenings of the connective tissue.

In cases of definitely nervous singers, or of those with a distinctly unfavourable technique, the surgeon should refuse to carry out the operation except where health is endangered; such people will often refer defects of their technique or later deterioration of their voices to the tonsillotomy, however excellently this might have been done.

Tonsillotomy, when carried out with the necessary circumspection and caution, is never followed by any injurious consequences; on the contrary, in many cases the complaints which existed before the operation (fatigue, difficulties in singing, etc.) improve considerably or disappear completely, and the quality and compass of the voice is affected very favourably (Stern).

Local treatment of symptoms of chronic or acute irritation without any functional therapy may bring about an improvement, especially if combined with a rest cure of the voice; but it will not be completely successful unless combined with functional treatment.

Treatment of Phonasthenia and of Habitual Dysphony is initiated by a period of complete rest for about ten days.

Preliminary breathing exercises may be tried because of the disturbance of breathing so frequent in these patients (see p. 209).

When the patient has learned to inhale inaudibly and to exhale slowly, evenly, and economically, our immediate end, viz. greater conscious control over the respiratory actions, is reached.

The next step is the training of the vocal capacity. It is usually introduced by vowel-exercises with aspirated attack (see p. 210). Exercises for the soft attack (see p. 211) and humming exercises (see p. 211) follow.

In case of paresis the vocal exercises may be aided by lateral pressure against the thyroid cartilage. Hypertension is lessened by active shaking of the lower jaw; the relaxation which accompanies this shaking is transmitted to the muscles of the larynx (see p. 211). Vibratory massage is most helpful (see p. 213).

When the patient can produce vowels with the soft attack, the voiced continuant consonants are attempted in a similar way.

The treatment of ventricular band voice, in common with all hyperkinetic dysphonias, demands exercises to make the vocal mechanism relax. The rehabilitation of the voice should be based on breathing, buzzing, and humming exercises aided by vibratory massage (see pp. 209 ff.).

Treatment of hysterical aphonia. — Hysteric aphonia primarily demands psychotherapy, as the voice-disturbance is nothing but an expression of the patient's psychic maladjustment. It may happen that psychotherapy cannot be carried out owing to lack of time, etc. In these cases we must try treatments which produce closure of the glottis reflexly, in other words, which produce an emotional scream, as of pain. To this end we introduce *Muck's* probe [1] into the larynx as well as the faradic current (endo- or extralaryngeally). The reflex scream has such a suggestive influence on the patient that he begins once more to use his normal loud voice. This treatment demands great self-assurance on the part of the therapeutist if it is to be successful. It should not need to be repeated, but ought to be effective in one session. [2] Even if this method of treatment prove effective, it should nevertheless be followed by psychotherapy to prevent relapses which are otherwise not unlikely.

[1] Muck, O. (1918). *Beobachtungen und praktische Erfahrungen auf dem Gebiete der Kriegsneurosen der Stimme, der Sprache und des Gehörs*, Bergmann, Wiesbaden.
[2] The application of these methods presupposes laryngological skill.

CHAPTER XXIII

CHANGE OF VOICE AT PUBERTY

Normal change of voice.—The larynx grows during puberty. In boys it develops into that of a man in size and shape within a comparatively short time, while girls show changes in a lesser degree.

The boy's vocal chords increase by about one-third of their original length, the pitch of the voice drops an eighth approximately, and the compass is greatly extended in both directions. The new size of the larynx and of the vocal chords demands quite a different mode of innervation of the muscles; as this is only learned with time, phonation at this period of the boy's life necessarily wavers; the voice sounds hoarse and often breaks, high and low pitch following each other without transition in quick succession. There are a number of deviations from this development.

Latent change of voice.—No distinct change of voice can be detected either before, during, or after puberty, in boys or girls. Laryngoscopy may show slight signs of irritation. Very equable growth of the larynx on the one hand and good motor adaptibility on the other may account for this development.

Perverted change of voice is caused by the girl's larynx becoming as large as that of a man; the pitch of the resulting voice is accordingly low. The defect is rare.

The preservation of the infantile voice is found in cases of nanism (Biedl).

Precocious change of voice is an early symptom of pubescence which sometimes appears long before the corresponding somatic development takes place.

In *acute change of voice* the male vocal quality develops rapidly and violently; the process may be completed within three months.

Retarded change of voice is observed if the larynx starts growing two or three or more years after the somatic development has been completed. The further vocal development generally progresses on normal lines.

In *prolonged change of voice* the changing of pitch takes an excessively long time.[1]

Persisting falsetto.—The compass of the voice of boys remains between a and e[1], and may at its best reach the upper limit of the male voice (d or e). It involves a quality change towards the female voice. Gutzmann explains this disorder by the preponderance of the crico-thyroid muscle which aids the internal thyroarytenoid muscle as a tensor, this latter muscle not being up to the work in consequence of its rapid longitudinal growth. The lower horns of the thyroid cartilage are articulated against the lower lateral surfaces of the cricoid cartilage forming the crico-thyroid articulation. This is a kind

---

[1] Stern, H. (1928). " Die Notwendigkeit einer einheitlichen Nomenklatur für die Physiologie, Pathologie und Pädagogik der Stimme," *Mon. f. Ohrenh.*, **62.**

of functional hinge-joint (ginglymus) in which a rotation takes place round a transversal axis ; apart from this rotation, little sliding movements are possible. When the crico-thyroid muscle, running from the frontal surface of the thyroid cartilage to the surface of the anterior arch of the cricoid, contracts, the thyroid pivots round a transversal axis. Thus the upper rim of the arch of the cricoid and the lower rim of the thyroid cartilage are approximated. The notch of the thyroid cartilage (incisura thyroidea) describes a downward circle, thereby increasing its distance from the arytenoid cartilages, the posterior attachment of the vocal chords. As a result the vocal chords are stretched and so tensed.

X-ray pictures taken by Jörgen Möller and Fischer while a singer was holding a note first in the chest register and then in falsetto showed the triangle between the lower rim of the thyroid cartilage and the upper rim of the cricoid cartilage to be much narrower in falsetto, and thus proved the considerable influence of the crico-thyroid muscle in the production of falsetto.

Persisting falsetto generally exposes the patients to the derision of those around them, which often causes open or hidden depression ; but there are usually no symptoms of compulsion. The prognosis under treatment is usually good even later in life.

Differential diagnosis.—Exact examination, especially with regard to constitutional and neurological signs and symptoms is necessary. This will prevent the confusion of persisting falsetto with the falsetto occurring in cases of endocrine disturbance or castration before puberty, or the breaking of the voice which sometimes is a symptom of Syringomyelia [1] (Stern).

Treatment.—Mechanical aid in the form of appropriate pressure on the thyroid cartilage neutralises the hypertension of the crico-thyroid muscle (Bresgen, Kayser, Gutzmann) by approximating the two ends of the vocal chords, thereby producing a somewhat deep, sometimes coarse voice. The production of this sound must be supervised with much caution for some days. The patient soon becomes familiar with the new innervation. The pressure can then be lessened gradually until he can produce the proper tone without external aid.

When the patient can produce one tone without failure the formation of a somewhat higher tone may cautiously be attempted (an interval of one or two semitones). The two tones should be formed in one breath and by continuous vocalisation. The therapist demonstrates the second tone accompanying it by a moderate lifting of his arm. The lifting movements of the arm by becoming signs associated with the patient's muscular activities, facilitate the finding of the right innervation in further practice.

The compass is gradually extended by practising intervals (third, fourth, fifth). When the patient has mastered these, he may attempt to speak words and short sentences. The correct intonation should first be made conscious to the patient, detached from articulation, for

---

[1] Cavity formation in the spinal cord and in the midbrain, manifest in anaesthesia, trophic changes (painless swellings, spontaneous fractures), and wasting of the muscles.

the very conception of a word or sentence inevitably evokes the habitual falsetto.

Humming exercises (see p. 211) and, later on, voice strengthening exercises (see p. 212) are used to improve the quality and carrying power of the voice. Vibratory massage during phonation aids the relaxation of the vocal muscles.

It is important to note that the low pitch characteristic of the male voice can never be achieved by developing the tones in the downward direction, but only by starting at the lowest possible tone and working up to the appropriate range of tones.

When the male voice has been produced, the patients are often discontented because of the ' booming ' resonance of the new voice in their ears. Although this sensation generally loses its unpleasant effect after a while, the therapist must not neglect this fact, as it prevents some patients from carrying on earnestly enough with the vocal exercises.

Psychological help, i.e. encouragement, is essential. The patients have been continually discouraged, as the trouble is mostly believed to be constitutional and, therefore, incurable. I can remember a patient who, having been assured of the incurability of his voice by many doctors in his country, tried a pilgrimage to the Holy Land as the last resort. As chance would have it, he met a man there who gave him my name. I was able to cure him, and he firmly believed me to be a ' messenger of God ' !

The chances for curing *Perverted Change of Voice* are not very great, as there are no means of achieving a passive shortening of the vocal chords or of stimulating them into the necessary activity. One can speak and sing to the patient and try to induce him to imitate. Faradism helps, as it stimulates the vocal chords into greater tension.

CHAPTER XXIV

VOCAL TREATMENT

On the following pages a selection of useful exercises is given to which reference has been made in the respective chapters.[1]

Breathing exercises.—In some cases breathing exercises provide a useful basis for further treatment. " An increased supply of breath is required for every form of physical exercise : movement, singing, speaking. . . . For singing and speaking, an increased volume of air is required to make sound, a more sustained flow being needed for singing than for speaking. The mechanism of increased respiration is the same in every case, and there is no difference in the method of air *supply* for whatever purpose it may be required, but different activities demand special methods of breath *control.* . . . The aim, therefore, is to develop normal breathing for action, eliminating effort as far as possible."[2]

I. Stand upright with legs comfortably apart, feet parallel, hands hanging by the sides, shoulders straight and flat. Lift arms quickly sidewards on inspiration, clapping the backs of the hands against each other above the head.

Always inhale inaudibly through mouth and nose, unless told to do it differently for a special reason. Keep the mouth comfortably open with the upper lip slightly lifted, the lower jaw hanging loosely and the tongue lying flat in the mouth. Exhale aspiratedly and evenly while the arms return slowly to their original position.

II. Position as for I. Arms bent, hands on the hips. Move elbows and shoulders quickly backwards on inhalation, and return slowly to the original position on exhalation.

III. Position as for I. Hands clasped at the nape of the neck. Throw arms back on inhalation and return slowly to the original position on exhalation.

IV. Clasp the hands behind the back above the waist level. Stretch the arms downwards quickly on inhalation. Return slowly to the original position on exhalation, the hands gliding upwards along the back.

V. Inhale and exhale in the way practised in exercises I-IV, and register the movements of the chest and of the abdomen with the hands.

VI. Inhale and exhale as in V, but stop exhalation several times.

VII. Inhale and exhale as in V and VI, with arms hanging loosely at the sides.[3]

---

[1] It should be noted that such exercises can be applied only if the psychological attitude of the patient is one which makes him strive after such aids. Wherever possible the exercises should be the speech part of behavioural patterns.

[2] Thurburn, G. L. (1939). *Voice and Speech*, p. 51. See also Fogerty, E. (1937). *Speech Craft*, pp. 26 ff.

[3] Cf. Gutzmann (1912), *Sprachheilkunde*, pp. 147 ff.

Blowing exercises.—The aim is to relieve the respiratory musculature and to help even and economical exhalation.

I. Blow softly and as long as possible through the rounded lips.

II. Blow while articulating [f].

III. Blow while articulating [s].

IV. Repeat these three exercises with rhythmic interruptions instead of in a continuous flow.

Training of voice attack.—Vocal training should be based on the mastery of the attacks (see pp. 26 ff.). Exercises should be introduced by a demonstration of the activities of the vocal chords. Illustrating their approximation with the corresponding movements of the second and third fingers, we can point out that they would certainly press against one another if we approximated them too rapidly. If approximated slowly, they will not overstep the mark, and will lie close without pressure.

Aspirated attack.—In phonation we want to prevent the vocal chords from pressing against each other, that is to say, we want a gradual approximation. This task can only be accomplished step by step. The first step is made by aspirated exhalation. Here the glottis is narrowed, the vocal chords being arrested half-way. The escaping air produces a friction between the chords, which serves as an indicator for their action. Thus if we hear aspiration, we may be sure that the glottis can by no means be constricted. As we have no sensation of what is going on in the larynx, this audible effect serves as an indicator of our action.

To familiarise oneself with the right pattern of the required aspiration, one may recall that this is perhaps one of the most primitive of noises ever made by man. It is the common interjectional expression of relief. The patient should first be made to picture this behavioural attitude (see p. 212). Once this action is fairly canalised, it may be followed by phonation. As the vocal chords are arrested during aspiration, they do not gain an excessive speed ; the glottal stop is therefore unlikely to follow.

The patient should next glide into voice by way of aspiration. His action can now be divided into two bars. During the first one aspiration is produced, during the second voice appears—aspirated attack.

The patient must be reminded that no further activity of the articulatory organs is required.

Strictly speaking ' voice ' cannot be obtained of itself, as it necessarily undergoes modification in the cavities in and above the larynx. What should be aimed at is therefore a vocal sound with the least possible articulatory action. Thus the organs of speech should take up the position which they hold when they are at rest, the mouth and pharynx cavities opening slightly by relaxation of the muscles concerned. Thereby a so-called indefinite vowel such as [ə] in English [əlait] (alight), [bʌtə] (butter), [ðə haus] (the house), [fər evə] (for ever) is enunciated.

The *vowel*-character should not, however, be mentioned to the patient at this stage ; for any reference to actual speech-patterns belonging to higher levels of language differentiation would rouse pathological attitudes connected with the patient's misconceptions as to the speech-sounds.

I. Practise the aspirated attack as in laughter : [hə hə hə : hə : : hə : : : . . .].

II. The same, introducing intervals of two, three, four, or five notes.

Soft attack.—The technique now begins to take on the character of experiment. The patient is instructed to produce the sound sequence just practised (see exercises above), but to use only the minimum of breath during the first bar. He should imagine that he wishes to take the therapist by surprise as to the moment in which voice is initiated. This modification of the former exercise brings about a smooth approximation of the vocal chords without there being any noticeable friction. Voice is produced when the vocal chords are closely approximated. The listener gets the impression and the speaker senses that phonation is easy. The result obtained is the soft attack.

Humming exercises help to establish the pattern of the soft attack and of relaxed vocalisation. I. Vocalise while keeping the [v] position. II. The same with [z]. III. The same with [w]. IV. Staccato exercises on vowels. V. Spiess' exercise is the most valuable help for achieving breath control and relaxation of the vocal musculature. V*a*. Hum through a glass tube 4 inches long and about ⅔ of an inch wide. The sound of the voice during this exercise ought to be of a metallic, trumpet-like character, and should be prolonged as much as possible. V*b*. Hum as in V*a*, and close the nose while humming. V*c*. Hum as in V*a*, and close the tube. V*d*. Hum as in V*a*, and close the nose and the tube alternately. It is essential that the sound should progress without any interruption or alteration. In order to observe whether superfluous air escapes through Spiess' glass tube, we use a thin strip of paper held before the opening of the tube during humming. If the exercise is executed correctly the paper does not move even if the nose is closed.

Exercises to loosen the jaw.—I. Shaking of jaw. II. Rattling of jaws. In both exercises the tongue must lie flat. The mouth should be comfortably open. The lower jaw hanging loosely in its joint is rhythmically moved from one side to the other, or up and down, while the speed is gradually increased. The patient must feel no tension in the masticatory muscles.

Tongue exercises.—I. Roll up the tongue. Bend the tip backward towards the uvula. II. Roll out the tongue with the tip touching the frenulum and the body of the tongue pressing forward against the edges of the upper teeth. III. Practise I and II alternately, first slowly, then more quickly. IV. Roll the tongue into a tube and protrude it between the lips ; pull it back until the tip is behind the incisors, then repeat the exercise. V. Utter [da da da . . .] before a mirror and keep the tongue against the front teeth ; the tongue must be flat and quite relaxed. Begin the exercise with the tongue slightly between the teeth to prevent its tendency to glide back. You may let it glide back only when you can hold it without difficulty in the proper position for any length of time.

'*Breath eating.*'—Fröschels recommends his method of 'breath eating' in the treatment of Stammering and hyperkinetic dysphonias. According to him speech 'is' chiefly breathing ; the speaking movements 'are' but those of eating. Since eating movements are naturally relaxed, the patient is enabled to attain the relaxed pattern of action by actually 'eating breath' while he is speaking or singing.

The initiator of this method overlooked, however, that his explanation does not account for *articulate* speech. The activities involved in the latter 'are' neither breathing nor eating. It can only be said that these two actions have evolved into speaking. The highly integrated function thus achieved naturally retains certain properties inherent in eating or breathing, such as 'relaxedness.' Fröschels' method is therefore of some help in vocal exercises in so far as articulateness plays a minor part. In stammerers it can lead to relaxation only if its bio-psychological value is clearly understood by the patient. He must be carefully guided along the track which leads to the aforementioned integration (see pp. 49 ff.). Fröschels [1] seems to have realised the difficulties which this aim presents. He therefore bases his method upon philosophical grounds which cannot here be described at length. Suffice it to say that he discriminates between a punctiform time ('being') and a flowing time ('becoming'). The union of the two times in man he calls a miracle and yet regards it as a reality. The efficiency of his 'lightning treatment' consists—we are told—in that the patient can on the basis of the above conception be freed from the misbelief that he is identical with the individual of yesterday. He can see that, though he yielded to his disorder yesterday, he need not do so to-day.

From practical experience we doubt that stammerers, unless exceptionally suggestible, would respond to this purely verbal elucidation. They verbally agree, but their behaviour contradicts this.

Yawning exercises.—These exercises come into play if patients are unable to achieve the soft attack and relaxed vocalisation.

The vowels should be started by actual yawning, since this conveys the pattern of relaxation.

Sighing promotes correct and easy exhalation and prevents laboured articulation by gliding the voice over a sequence of tones. At a later stage the *image* of sighing promotes the desired function.

Voice strengthening exercises.—I. Hold a low-pitched note in the chest register. II. Sing low-pitched intervals (second, third, fourth) in the chest register. III. Sing low-pitched sequences of two or three tones up and down. Syllables like [nia-i, nio-i, niu-i] should be used for these exercises ; first repeat the same syllable several times, then change ; [n, a, o, u] should be clearly articulated and enunciated loudly and prolongedly, but without any strain. If the [i] is incorrect it must not be practised at the end of a syllable but only in the middle : [nia, nio, . . .]. The [i] in the foregoing syllables should first be short, and lengthened only when articulation and resonance become correct. There may be countless variations of such exercises. [2]

[1] Fröschels, E. (1934). "Eine psychotherapeutische Methode," *Med. Klin.*, No. 11.
[2] Cf. Thurburn, l.c.

Gradually the auxiliary sounds are omitted ; the final vowel is first short, then by degrees held longer and longer : [nia, nia :, nia : : ; ja, ja :, ja : : ; ana, ana :, ana : : ; anda, anda : ; ada, ada : , . . .]. Change the initial vowel : [ana, ena, ina, ona, una], and so forth. Change the end vowel : [ana, ane, ani, ano, anu], etc.

Syllables containing back vowels and diphthongs, such as [nui, noi, mui, mau, tau, ty-toe-toi . . .] promote chest resonance.

There follow words and short sentences containing such sounds, e.g. joy—hoist ; hoist the oyster ; Hugh threw a blue shoe ; sails remained safe in hail and rain ; the cat sat on the mat ; he eats a piece of cheese on the heath for tea ; etc.

First of all texts [1] with the vowels most favourable for the patient ought to be chosen, i.e. those vowels with which a higher point on the melodic scale can be reached with the least difficulty (Fröschels) ; later on the semi-vowels [j], [w], as well as the voiced continuant consonants [l, m, n, r] ; later still texts with mostly voiced consonants ; at last sentences with breathed consonants and combinations of consonants.

Whether the practice of high-pitched vowels should precede that of the low-pitched ones or follow these, must be decided individually. The slightest improvement in the quality of the voice must decide in favour of the exercise which reproduced it. The most generally approved exercises must give way to rare ones, or even to new experiments if they show no satisfactory result.

In cases of Phonasthenia in concurrence with lack of self-control and concentration, a combination of rhythmic movements with the vocal exercises may prove helpful, e.g. the throwing and catching of a ball or a ring, and so on ; children should march to certain rhythms, knock or tap rhythmically, etc.

Methods of compensation, such as vibratory massage, rearward pressure on the thyroid cartilage, and faradism aid the treatment.

In vibratory massage the vibrating part of the apparatus is put against the region of the larynx ; the patient should execute vocal exercises during the massage. Vibratory massage may also be done by movements of the therapist's (later on the patient's) fingers. This needs great flexibility and gentleness, which can only be achieved through long and careful training.

In faradism the two electrodes are gently pressed against the sides of the thyroid cartilage, and a weak current is sent through the larynx, while the patient is performing the humming or voice strengthening exercises. When the patient can hold tones tolerably well during faradism, the intensity of the current is gradually reduced to vanishing-point. The patient should try to go on singing or humming, and should not be influenced by the feeling of impotence which is bound to occur on reduction of the current.

[1] See Fogerty, l.c. ; Thurburn, l.c.

CHAPTER XXV

SPEECH AND VOICE DISORDERS IN WAR

The present war calls for a few remarks on how war casualties may advance our knowledge, and on what methods of treatment may be of help.

Minute examination of the mental and linguistic behaviours of *aphasiacs* in conjunction with the neurological signs will further our knowledge of linguistic disintegration (see pp. 77 ff.). Neurological examination should be particularly helpful in the sometimes difficult discrimination between *organic Aphasia* resulting from lesions due to blast, and *hysterical Aphasia*. The latter is often accompanied by functional deafness, thus reflecting infantile Hearing-Mutism (see pp. 95 ff.).

In this case psychological treatment should be directed towards the abolishment of the patient's withdrawal from the external world and re-establishment of the ' listening ' function.[1] " The rough-and-ready application of a second shock (or excitement) to cure a previous ' shock,' " is to be condemned, since it is " apt to convert mutism into stuttering." [2]

Similar considerations apply to *Dyslalia* which may occur in cases of hysteria after blast concussion. Exact and complete descriptions of the linguistic state with due regard to rendering both the articulatory shapes and the sounds in phonetic notation (see pp. 57 f.) are desirable. Such efforts will also help to discriminate dyslalic disorders from dysarthric ones (see pp. 168 ff.). Trifling disturbances of gait, of breathing, and of sensibility, symptoms of exhaustion after much speaking, twitching of the facial muscles will confirm the latter opinion, and so help to avoid unnecessary psychotherapeutic attempts. Dyslalia engendered by concussion or by psychic trauma symbolises a distinctly infantile attitude. Psychotherapy should therefore endeavour to re-establish that social attitude which involves the cortical control necessary for checking excessive sound changes (see pp. 164 f.). Normal speech will then soon reappear, since former normal speech-patterns are not destroyed, but distorted through lack of inhibition.

Blast concussion often causes clonic *Stammering* or revives a stammer which was overcome or concealed in childhood. In the course of recovery aphasiacs often develop clonic stammering.

The differential diagnosis between these genuine stammerers and malingerers will be easy by way of the methods described on p. 126.

In treatment due regard should be paid to the dissolutionary state of the patient ; the principles laid down on pp. 112 ff. apply equally to ' war stammerers.' The first requirement is to remove these patients to a base hospital as soon as the physical condition permits this. There psychological treatment should be carried out by a qualified

[1] See Hurst, A., and Miller, E. (1940). *Proc. of the Roy. Soc. of Med.*, March.
[2] Myers, C. S. (1940). *Shell Shock in France*, Cambridge University Press.

speech therapist along the lines shown on pp. 128 ff. He will have to pay due regard to the discrimination between underlying, co-existing, and superimposed psychic factors. Any attempt to counteract the clonic stammer by way of simple suggestion, minimising, or strong faradism [1] leads to hypertonicity, concealment of the symptoms, distrust, aggression, and so forth, which will greatly hamper the efforts of the speech therapist. Many reported cases of 'recovery' have on close examination proved to be concealed stammers.

Injuries of the pharynx may cause Hyperrhinophonia (see pp. 172 ff.). Injection of paraffin wax into the musculature of the posterior pharyngeal wall (see p. 178) has proved most helpful where plastic surgery was hampered through insufficiency of the remaining tissue.

Extirpation of the larynx or cicatrisation of the glottis after injury require the establishing of the *pseudo-voice* (see pp. 195 ff.).

Phonasthenia, impairing the ability to give vigorous commands, responds well to rest cure, but should in the forces at home be given treatment along the lines indicated on pp. 203 ff. to prevent relapse.

Hysterical aphonia, sometimes with consequent inflammatory signs due to overstraining, and contraction of the ventricular bands, occurs frequently. It can in the great majority of cases be made to disappear by ether administered [2] rapidly to the stage of intoxication, with vigorous suggestion, electricity, or Muck's probe (see pp. 204 ff.). This symptomatic treatment should be completed by the analysis of the neurotic background.

[1] Fröschels, E. (1917). " Die Entstehung des tonischen Sotterns," *Med. Klin.* Myers, l.c., pp. 43–4.
[2] Hurst, A. (1940). *Medical Diseases of War*, Arnold, London, p. 66.

BIBLIOGRAPHY

This list contains only a small and arbitrary selection of books which the reader might profitably use for further study. Books to which reference has been made in the text are not included.

CHAPTER I

Russell, B. (1940). *Inquiry into Meaning and Truth.* Allen & Unwin, London.
Ayer, A. C. (1936). *Language, Truth and Logic.* Gollancz, London.
Ayer, A. C. (1940). *The Foundation of Empirical Knowledge.* Macmillan, London.
Benjamin, A. C. (1937). *Introduction to the Philosophy of Science.* Macmillan, London.

CHAPTER II

Bergson, H. (1928). *Creative Evolution.* Macmillan, London.
Hocart, A. M. (1933). *The Progress of Man.* Methuen, London.
Jennings, H. S. (1930). *The Biological Basis of Human Nature.* Faber & Faber, London.
Kidd, B. (1921). *A Philosopher with Nature.* Methuen, London.
Langdon-Brown, W. (1938). *Thus We Are Men.* Kegan Paul, London.
Lloyd-Morgan, C. (1922). *Emergent Evolution.* Williams & Norgate, London.
Meek, A. (1930). *The Progress of Life.* Arnold, London.
Nouy, L. du (1936). *Biological Time.* Methuen, London.
Sherrington, C. (1940). *Man on His Nature.* Cambridge University Press.
Starling's *Principles of Human Physiology* (1941). Churchill, London.
Bechterew, V. M. (1933). *General Principles of Human Reflexology.* Jarrolds, London.
Langdon-Brown, W. (1923). *The Sympathetic Nervous System in Disease.* Milford, London.
Berman, L. (1935). *The Glands Regulating Personality.* Macmillan, London.
Wittkower, E. (1936). *Der Einfluss der Gemütsbewegungen.* Vienna–Leipzig.
Berry, R. J. A. (1939). *Your Brain and Its Story.* Oxford University Press.
Watson, J. B. (1925). *Behaviourism.* Kegan Paul, London.
Woodworth, R. S. (1931). *Contemporary Schools of Psychology.* Methuen, London.
MacMurray, J. (1939). *The Boundaries of Science. A Study in the Philosophy of Psychology.* Faber & Faber, London.
Driesch, H. (1927). *Mind and Body.* Methuen, London.
Gardner, M. (1933). *General Psychology.* Harper & Brothers, New York–London.
MacDougall, W. (1923). *An Outline of Psychology.* Methuen, London.
MacDougall, W. (1936). *Psycho-Analysis and Social Psychology.* Methuen, London.
Pratt, C. C. (1939). *The Logic of Modern Psychology.* Macmillan, New York.
Miller, E. (1926). *Types of Mind and Body.* Kegan Paul.
Stout, G. F. (1928). *Analytic Psychology.* Allen & Unwin, London.
Hazlitt, V. (1933). *The Psychology of Infancy.* Methuen, London.
Koffka, K. (1924). *The Growth of Mind.* Kegan Paul, London.
Piaget, J. (1929). *The Child's Concept of the World.* Kegan Paul, London.
Campion, G. G. (1923). *Elements in Thought and Emotion.* University of London Press.
MacCurdy, J. (1925). *The Psychology of Emotion.* Kegan Paul, London.
Smith, W. W. (1922). *The Measurement of Emotion.* Kegan Paul, London.
Campion, G. G. and Smith, G. E. (1934). *The Neural Basis of Thought.* Kegan Paul, London.

Titchener, R. (1909). *Lectures on the Experimental Psychology of the Thought Processes.* Macmillan, New York.
Cattell, R. B. (1936). *A Guide to Mental Testing.* University of London Press.
Knight, R. (1933). *Intelligence and Intelligence Tests.* Methuen, London.
Spearman, C. (1925). *Measure of Intelligence for Use in Schools.* Methuen, London.
Terman, L. M. (1919). *The Measurement of Intelligence.* Harrap, London.
Thorndike, E. L. et al. (1926). *The Measurement of Intelligence.* Bur. Publ. Teach. Coll., Columbia University.
Pavlov, I. P. (1927). *Conditioned Reflexes.* Oxford University Press.
Bradby, M. K. (1920). *The Logic of the Unconscious Mind.* Frowde, and Hodder & Stoughton, London.
Price, M. (1914). *The Unconscious.* Macmillan, New York.

CHAPTERS III–IV

Frazer, J. G. (1907). *Questions on the Customs, Beliefs and Languages of Savages.* Cambridge University Press.
Lewis, M. M. (1936). *Infant Speech.* Kegan Paul, London.
Low, A. A. (1936). *Studies in Infant Thought and Speech.* University of Illinois.
MacCarthy, D. (1930). *The Language Development of the Pre-School Child.* University Minneapolis Press.
Markey, J. F. (1928). *The Symbolic Process and Its Integration in Children.* Kegan Paul, London.
Piaget, J. (1932). *The Language and Thought of the Child.* Kegan Paul, London.
Carnap, R. (1937). *Logical Syntax of Language.* Kegan Paul, London.
Critchley, M. (1938). *The Language of Gesture.* Arnold, London.
Eisenson, J. (1938). *The Psychology of Speech.* Harrap, London.
Partridge, E. (1938). *The World of Words.* Kegan Paul, London.
Sapir, E. (1921). *Language.* Harcourt, Brace.
Zipf, G. K. (1936). *The Psycho-Biology of Language.* Routledge, London.
Jespersen, O. (1918). *Chapters on English.* Allen & Unwin, London.
Bell, A. G. (1907). *The Mechanism of Speech.* Funk & Wagnalls, New York.
Jespersen, O. and Pedersen, H. (1926). *Phonetic Transcription and Transliteration.* Oxford University Press.

CHAPTER V

Crookshank, F. G. (1927). *Diagnosis.* Kegan Paul, London.
Hawlett, R. T. (1923). *Pathology.* Churchill, London.
Newsholme, H. P. (1929). *Health, Disease, and Integration.* Allen & Unwin, London.
Talbot, E. S. (1898). *Degeneracy.* Scott.
White, W. A. (1926). *The Meaning of Disease.* Williams & Wilkins, Baltimore.
Adler, A. (1924). *The Practice and Theory of Individual Psychology.* Kegan Paul, London.
Dicks, H. V. (1939). *Clinical Studies in Psychopathology.* Arnold, London.
Gillespie, R. D. (1933). *Mind in Daily Life.* Methuen, London.
Gordon, R. G. (1934). *The Neurotic and his Friends.* Methuen, London.
Hollingworth, H. L. (1931). *Abnormal Psychology.* Methuen, London.
MacDougall, W. (1926). *An Outline of Abnormal Psychology.* Methuen, London.
Mitchell, T. W. (1922). *Medical Psychology.* Methuen, London.
Alexander, F. M. (1924). *Constructive Conscious Control of the Individual.* Methuen, London.
Glover, E. (1939). *Psycho-Analysis.* Bale & Curnow, London.
Woodworth, R. (1931). *Contemporary Schools of Psychotherapy.* Methuen, London.
Ross, T. A. (1936). *An Enquiry into Prognosis in the Neuroses.* Cambridge University Press.
Gordon, R. G., Harris, N. G. and Rees, J. R. (1936). *An Introduction to Psychological Medicine.* Oxford University Press.

CHAPTER VI

MacAllister, A. H. (1937). *Clinical Studies in Speech Therapy*. University of London Press.
Travis, L. E. (1931). *Speech Pathology*. Appleton, London.
Wyllie, J. (1894). *The Disorders of Speech*. Oliver & Boyd, Edinburgh.

CHAPTERS VII–IX

Kinnier Wilson, S. A. (1928). *Aphasia*. Kegan Paul, London.
Stinchfield, S. M. and Young, E. M. (1938). *Children with Delayed or Defective Speech*. Oxford University Press.
Ewing, A. W. G. and Ewing, I. R. (1938). *The Handicap of Deafness*. Longmans, Green & Co., London.
Goldstein, M. A. (1933). *Problems of the Deaf*. St. Louis.
Kerridge, P. M. T. (1937). *Hearing and Speech in Deaf Children*. His Majesty's Stationery Office, London.
Kerridge, P. M. T. and Fry, D. B. (1939). *Tests for the Hearing of Speech by the Deaf*. H. K. Lewis, London.

CHAPTERS X–XII

Appelt, A. (1938). *The Real Cause of Stammering*. Methuen, London.
Bluemel, C. S. (1930). *The Mental Aspects of Stammering*. Williams & Wilkins, Baltimore.
Coriat, J. H. (1928). *Stammering. A Psychoanalytic Interpretation*. Nerv. and Ment. Dis. Publ. Co., New York–Washington.
Fletcher, J. M. (1928). *The Problem of Stuttering*. Longmans, Green & Co., New York.
Fogerty, E. (1930). *Stammering*. Allen & Unwin, London.
Ladell, R. M. (1940). *The Stammerer Unmasked*. Pitman, London.
Kingdon-Ward, W. (1941). *Stammering*. Hamish Hamilton, London.

CHAPTERS XIII–XVI

Berry, J. and Legge, T. P. (1912). *Hare Lip and Cleft Palate*. London.
Brown, G. V. I. (1936). *Surgery of Oral Diseases and Malformations*. Lea & Fabiger, Philadelphia.
Shaw, D. M. (1927). *Dental Prosthetic Mechanics*. Arnold, London.

CHAPTER XVII

Aïkin, W. A. (1932). *The Voice*. Longmans, London.
Behnke, E. and Browne, L. (1885). *The Child's Voice*. S. Low, London.
Paget, R. (1930). *Human Speech*. Kegan Paul, London.
Pear, T. H. (1931). *Voice and Personality*. Chapman & Hall, London.
White, E. G. (1938). *Science and Singing*. Dent, London.
MacLachlan, N. W. (1936). *New Acoustics*. Oxford University Press.
Stevens, S. S. and Davis, A. H. (1938). *Hearing*. Chapman & Hall, London.
Ballenger, H. C. (1940). *A Manual of Otology, Rhinology and Laryngology*. Kimpton, London.
Thomson, S. and Negus, V. E. (1937). *Diseases of the Nose and Throat*. Cassell, London.
Tarneaud, J. (1937). *Sémeiologie Stroboscopique des Maladies du Larynx*. Maloine, Paris.

CHAPTERS XVIII–XXV

Evetts, E. T. (1933). *Vocal Disorders*. Dent, London.
Tarneaud, J. (1935). *La Nodule de la Corde Vocale*. Maloine, Paris.

CHAPTER XXVI

Good, M. E. (1930). *Hear with Your Eyes.* Methuen, London.
Hast, H. G. (1925). *The Singer's Art.* Methuen, London.
Mellor, E. (1934). *How is Your Breathing?* Methuen, London.
Reaney, P. H. (1923). *The Elements of Speech Training.* Methuen, London.
Rich, K. (1932). *The Art of Speech.* Methuen, London.
Barrows, S. T. and Hall, K. H. (1936). *Games and Jingles for Speech Development.* Expression Company, Boston.
Wood, A. L. (1934). *Jingle Book for Speech Correction.* E. P. Dutton & Co., New York.

GLOSSARY

Amyotrophic lateral sclerosis. Degeneration of the cells of the anterior horn of the spinal cord, the nuclei of the medulla, and the pyramidal tracts. Symptoms : weakness and wasting of the muscles.

Angular gyrus. Convolution of the brain adjacent to the lower part of the parietal lobe.

Anterior horn. On a cross-section of the spinal cord the grey matter is arranged in a shape resembling the letter H. Each half of this figure has a posterior and an anterior horn. Sensory fibres terminate in the former, motor ones spring from the latter.

Anterior poliomyelitis. Inflammatory process in the anterior part of the grey matter of the spinal cord, leading to motor paralysis with muscular wasting and tremor. No sensory or trophic disturbances.

Aortic aneurysm. Dilatation of the aorta (the large vessel springing from the left ventricle of the heart). Breathlessness accompanies it, if it compresses the left recurrent nerve which hooks round the arch of the aorta.

Archicapillaries. Primordial form of the capillaries.

Arytenoids. (Arytenoid cartilages.) Twin four-sided cartilages articulated on the superior posterior face of the cricoid cartilage. Posterior attachment of the vocal chords.

Assimilation. In philology a process by which two neighbouring or not too distant sounds in a sequence are made alike.

Atresia. Narrowing or closing of a natural aperture by cicatrisation or by a membrane.

Biogenetic law. The development of the individual is a recapitulation of the evolution of the race.

Botulism. Food-poisoning caused by the bacillus botulinus which occurs in ill-preserved meat or fish.

Bradylalia. Slowness of enunciation.

Bulbar paralysis. (Glosso-labial-laryngeal paralysis.) Degenerative waste of the nuclei in the medulla oblongata and in the pons. Symptoms : atrophy of the motor fibres. Hence disability to actuate the muscles of the face, the tongue, the palate and the throat.

Cerebellum. Part of the brain which controls the equilibrium of the body, the maintenance of the reflex tonus of the musculature, and the co-ordination and regulation of muscular activity.

Chorditis marginalis. Inflammation affecting solely the edges of the vocal chords.

Chromosomes. Bodies in the germ cells regarded as the vehicles of heredity.

Cochlear. Pertaining to the cochlea, i.e. the snail-shaped part of the inner ear which contains the sensory cells of the auditory nerve.

Congenital spastic paraparesis. (Little's disease.) Rigidity and spasticity of the musculature due to cerebral haemorrhagic processes before or at birth.

Construction. Arrangement of words expressing relations (syntactic c.). Arrangements of parts of words, resulting in differences of form or structure (morphological c.).

Copula. Word connecting subject and predicate.

Corpus mamillare. White protuberance on the base of the brain.

Cyclothymia. Milder form of manic-depressive psychosis.

Cytoplasm. The protoplasm of the cells.

Dementia paralytica. (General paralysis of the insane.) Chronic inflammation of the brain and its surrounding membranes (meninges). Late effect of syphilitic infection. Characterised chiefly by irritability, weakness of memory, progressive mental enfeeblement, and disturbances of co-ordination.

Dementia praecox. Endogenous mental enfeeblement beginning insidiously in adolescence.

Diplegia. Paralysis of both sides of the body.

Dysphagia. Disability to swallow.

Dyspnoea. Difficulty in breathing.

Encephalitis. Inflammation of the brain.

Epithelium. A layer of cells forming the top layer of the skin, and lining ducts and hollow organs.

Faradism. Application of induced electric currents for the stimulation of muscles more or less deprived of their nervous control.

Faucial pillars. Two (anterior and posterior) folds of mucous membrane sheathing the tonsils, extending from the soft palate to the root of the tongue and the lateral wall of the pharynx respectively.

Fistulous ulcer. A narrow channel connecting two cavities or connecting a cavity and the surface of the body, due to ulcerative disintegration.

Flexion. Inflexion, i.e. the modification of words by means of suffixes, infixes, prefixes, change of the vowel of the base, etc., thereby indicating number, case, tense, etc.

Flexionless. Incapable of flexion.

Formants. Overtones, independent of the fundamental tone, which are characteristic of the diverse speech sounds.

Friedreich's disease. (Hereditary ataxia.) Sclerosis (hardening), hypoplasia (diminished development) or degeneration of the spinal cord (pyramidal tracts, Goll's column). Symptoms : unsteady gait, tremor, ataxy, retarded development.

Genes. Particles of the chromatin (substance of the chromosomes), being the representatives of the various hereditary features.

Gradation. Vowel changes occurring in words sprung from a common base ; e.g. Engl., sing, sang, sung, song.

Grave's disease. (Exophthalmic goitre.) Enlargement of the thyroid gland. Main symptoms : nervousness, heart palpitation, tremors, metabolic disturbances, protrusion of the eyeballs.

Hebephrenia. Type of dementia praecox, characterised by decay of the personality, mental enfeeblement, delusions, apathy and depression.

Hemiplegia. Paralysis of one side of the body.

Hepato-lenticular degeneration. (Wilson's disease.) Progressive degeneration of the corpus striatum, concurring with cirrhosis of the liver. Main symptom : muscular rigidity.

Hereditary ataxia. See Friedreich's disease.

Hyperkinetic. Term applied to movements of a quasi-spastic character.

Hypokinetic. Term applied to movements of a quasi-paretic character.

Hysteria. Neurosis tending to liberate the patient from a disagreeable situation (flight into disease). Symptoms : loss of memory, multiple personality, convulsions, paralysis, muscular contractions.

Idiopathic. Term applied to diseases developing independently, not constituting a symptom of another disease.

Indication. Sign pointing to the cause or particularly to the treatment of a disease.

Infantile paralysis. Inflammation of the anterior portion of the grey matter of the spinal cord, affecting mainly children. Manifest in paralysis of diverse muscle groups.

Inferior constrictor. One of the constrictors of the pharynx ; covers the region of the larynx and part of the œsophagus.

Inner capsula. A vital bundle of nerve fibres in the cerebrum, connecting the white matter of the hemispheres with the pyramidal tracts.

Insula (the " island " of Reil). Lobe of the brain lying at the bottom of the Sylvian fissure, separating the frontal lobe from the temporal lobe.

Labialisation. Modification of a speech-sound by action of the lips.

Lalling. Baby talk.

Lambdoid. Resembling the sound [l] or the letter L.

Laryngectomy. Extirpation of the larynx in cases of malignant growth.

Libidinal. Pertaining to libido.

Libido. Psycho-analytic term embracing all forces emanating from the primary sex instinct.

Lipoid. Fat-like chemical substance.

Lymphadenitis. Inflammation of the lymphatic glands.

Mediastinum. The space between the two lungs.

Metazoa. Collective term denoting multicellular organisms as opposed to protozoa, i.e. organisms consisting of a single cell.

Mongolism. Mental defect associated with a peculiar physiognomy recalling that of the Mongols. Causation obscure. Physical characteristics : small round skull, flattened face, slit-like eyes. Mental symptoms : good-natured, imitative, impulsive, unbalanced, reasoning poor.

Morphology. The science of external forms and structures of animals, plants, and languages.

Multiple sclerosis. (Disseminated sclerosis.) Relapsing disease with scattered greyish patches due to the destruction of the sheaths of the nerve fibres. Symptoms : motor weakness, inco-ordination, dysarthria, paraesthesiae (disturbances of sensation), retro-bulbar neuritis (inflammatory or degenerative affections of the optic nerve behind the retina), vertigo, diminished emotional control.

Myasthenia gravis. Weakness and wasting of the muscles, and severe fatigue after even slight efforts. Owing to "lymphorrhages" (i.e. collections of small round cells resembling lymphocytes) lying between or within the muscle fibres.

Myotonia congenita. (Thomsen's disease.) Hereditary disease characterised by prolonged tonic contraction and retarded relaxation of the musculature. Nature obscure.

Nanism. Dwarfishness.

Nares. Nostrils.

Nucleus. Aggregate of nerve cells.

Ontogenetic. Pertaining to ontogeny, i.e. the development of an individual.

Oral-erotic attitude. Psycho-analytic term applied to an early stage (first nine months) when the child's libido is directed on to the activities of the mouth (sucking, seeking the mother's breast).

Paranoia. Type of insanity characterised mainly by delusions and ideas of persecution, leading to ultimate decay of the personality.

Paresis. Slight paralysis.

Parkinsonism. Syndrome consisting of slow and feeble voluntary movements, muscular rigidity, and tremors, owing to degeneration mainly of the ganglion cells of the corpus striatum.

Parotitis. Mumps. Inflammation of the parotid gland.

Pericarditis. Inflammation of the pericardium, the membrane surrounding the heart.

Phylogenetic. Pertaining to phylogeny, i.e. the evolution of the species (race).

Pleuritis. Inflammation of the pleura, the membrane surrounding the lungs and lining the inner surface of the chest wall.

Pragmatist. One who adheres to the doctrine of pragmatism which puts philosophy and all knowledge into relation with life and action. According to it the truth of a judgment or opinion depends on whether it furthers life.

Prefrontal gyrus. Convolution of the frontal lobe.

Progressive muscular atrophy. Wasting and weakness of the musculature owing to disease of the spinal neuron.

Proprioceptive stumuli arise in the organs themselves and help in regulating their movements.

Pseudo-bulbar palsy. Term applied to a state of impairment of voluntary control over emotional expression. Resembles bulbar palsy, but is caused by lesions above the medulla.

Psychosis. Mental disease.

Schizophrenia. Type of dementia praecox. Main symptom : split of the personality in adolescence, associated with deterioration of the entire personality, disorders of feeling, conduct and thought, and withdrawal of interest from the environment.

Semantics. (Semasiology.) Study of the development of meaning.

Semasiological. Pertaining to semantics.

Septum nasi. Partly bony, partly cartilaginous wall dividing the interior of the nose into two cavities.

Sequelae. Symptoms or effects liable to follow a disease.

Softening of the brain. Occurs when an area of the brain is deprived of its normal blood supply through inflammation, or blood clots.

Staccato. A passage in which each note is sung or played in a sharply detached, abrupt manner. In singing, the staccato effect should not be produced by the glottal stop.

Sternocleido-mastoid muscle. Runs from the sternum and the clavicle to the mastoid process of the temporal bone.

Sternothyroid muscle. Runs from the sternum and the cartilages of the first and second ribs to the thyroid cartilage.

Stroboscopy. Examination of fast regular vibrations by means of intermittent light. Thereby only a short phase of each vibration is perceived at a time and so the whole vibration seems to be slowed down.

Subcortical. Term applied to structures situated below the cortex of the brain.

Submucous laryngitis. Inflammation affecting mainly the tissues underneath the mucous membrane of the larynx.

Supramarginal gyrus. Convolution of the brain adjacent to the parietal lobe.

Sylvian fissure. A deep impression dividing the frontal and temporal lobes of the brain.

Synergic. Term applied to the co-operation of two or more antagonistic muscles in performing an action.

Syringomyelia. Cavity formation in the grey matter of the spinal cord and the bulb. Main symptom : progressive muscular atrophy.

Tachylalia. Excessively rapid speech.

Tonus. State of tension in a muscle.

Transitions. Stages in the musical scale at which the singer is compelled to modify his activities in order to proceed smoothly from one register to the next higher.

Trophic. Term applied to the influence which nerves exert with regard to the health and nourishment of the parts which they supply.

Turbinal. Bony projection springing from the lateral wall of the nasal cavity, lined by a thick vascular mucous membrane.

Vegetative. Pertaining to or connected with the growth of a living being as opposed to its psychological activities.

Velarisation. Anticipatory elevation of the back of the tongue in the vicinity of the velum during the articulation of consonants followed by a velar vowel [u, o].

Ventricle. Deep depression between the vocal chord and the ventricular band.

Vestibular organ. Hinder part of the inner ear concerned with the balancing sense.

Visceral. Pertaining to the viscera, the bowels.

INDEX

15

For Product Safety Concerns and Information please contact our EU
representative GPSR@taylorandfrancis.com
Taylor & Francis Verlag GmbH, Kaufingerstraße 24, 80331 München, Germany

* 9 7 8 1 1 3 8 3 5 8 8 9 8 *